Mental Health Disorders

SOURCEBOOK

Fifth Edition

Health Reference Series

Fifth Edition

Mental Health Disorders
SOURCEBOOK

*Basic Consumer Health Information about
Healthy Brain Functioning and Mental Illnesses,
Including Depression, Bipolar Disorder, Anxiety
Disorders, Posttraumatic Stress Disorder, Obsessive-
Compulsive Disorder, Psychotic and Personality
Disorders, Eating Disorders, Impulse Control
Disorders, and More*

*Along with Information about Medications and
Treatments, Mental Health Concerns in Specific Groups,
Such as Children, Adolescents, Older Adults, Minority
Populations, and People in Poverty, a Glossary of
Related Terms, and Directories of Resources for
Additional Help and Information*

Edited by
Karen Bellenir

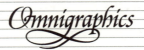

Omnigraphics

155 W. Congress, Suite 200, Detroit, MI 48226

Bibliographic Note
Because this page cannot legibly accommodate all the copyright notices, the Bibliographic Note portion of the Preface constitutes an extension of the copyright notice.

Edited by Karen Bellenir

Health Reference Series

Karen Bellenir, *Managing Editor*
David A. Cooke, MD, FACP, *Medical Consultant*
Elizabeth Collins, *Research and Permissions Coordinator*
Cherry Edwards, *Permissions Assistant*
EdIndex, Services for Publishers, *Indexers*

* * *

Omnigraphics, Inc.
Matthew P. Barbour, *Senior Vice President*
Kevin M. Hayes, *Operations Manager*

* * *

Peter E. Ruffner, *Publisher*

Copyright © 2012 Omnigraphics, Inc.
ISBN 978-0-7808-1275-8
E-ISBN 978-0-7808-1276-5

Library of Congress Cataloging-in-Publication Data

Mental health disorders sourcebook : basic consumer health information about healthy brain functioning and mental illnesses, including depression, bipolar disorder, anxiety disorders, posttraumatic stress disorder, obsessive-compulsive disorder, psychotic and personality disorders, eating disorders, impulse control disorders ... / edited by Karen Bellenir. -- 5th ed.
     p. cm. -- (Health reference series)
  Summary:"Provides basic consumer health information about the signs, symptoms, and treatment of various mental illnesses, and the special mental health concerns of children and adolescents, older adults, and other groups, along with tips for maintaining mental wellness. Includes index, glossary of related terms, and other resources"-- Provided by publisher.
  Includes bibliographical references and index.
  ISBN 978-0-7808-1275-8 (hardcover : alk. paper) 1. Mental illness. 2. Psychiatry. I. Bellenir, Karen.
  RC454.4.M458 2012
  616.89--dc23
                                                                2012026342

∞

Table of Contents

Visit www.healthreferenceseries.com to view *A Contents Guide to the Health Reference Series*, a listing of more than 16,000 topics and the volumes in which they are covered.

Part Three: Mental Health Treatments

Part Four: Pediatric Mental Health Concerns

Part Five: Other Populations with Distinctive Mental Health Concerns

Part Six: Mental Illness Co-Occurring with Other Disorders

Part Seven: Additional Help and Information

Preface

About This Book

Mental health encompasses thoughts, actions, and feelings. Mentally healthy individuals are able to cope with life's challenges, handle stressful situations, deal with anger, maintain meaningful relationships with others, and enjoy life. Despite the benefits, maintaining a healthy mind is not always possible, and mental disorders are common. According to statistics compiled by the Substance Abuse and Mental Health Services Administration, approximately 5% of the U.S. adult population was diagnosed with, or had experienced within the past year, a mental illness sufficiently serious to cause functional impairment.

Mental Health Sourcebook, Fifth Edition discusses how the brain works, the components of mental wellness, and the processes that lead to illness. It offers information about the major types of mental illness and their treatments, including affective disorders, anxiety disorders, psychotic disorders, personality disorders, and disorders that impact behavior, including impulse control disorders, addictions, and eating disorders. A special section looks at pediatric issues in mental health and another examines the distinctive concerns of other specific populations. Information is also included about the relationship between mental health and chronic illnesses, such as cancer, epilepsy, heart disease, pain, and sleep disorders. The book concludes with a glossary of mental health terms, a list of crisis hotlines, and a directory of mental health organizations.

How to Use This Book

This book is divided into parts and chapters. Parts focus on broad areas of interest. Chapters are devoted to single topics within a part.

Part One: The Brain and Mental Health explains the components of healthy brain functioning and the processes that can go awry leading to mental illness. It also discusses lifestyle and other factors that can help reinforce mental wellness.

Part Two: Mental Illnesses begins with information about the link between suicide and mental illness and facts about suicide prevention. It goes on to describe the various classifications of mental health disorders, including depressive and other affective disorders, anxiety disorders, psychotic disorders, personality disorders, and other disorders that impact behavior.

Part Three: Mental Health Treatments addresses the different ways mental health disorders are diagnosed and treated. It offers guidelines for identifying mental health emergencies, explains the services available from different types of mental health professionals, and discusses medications used to help control symptoms of mental illness. The part concludes with a chapter about complementary and alternative medicine for mental health care, which includes facts about dietary, physical, and spiritual therapies.

Part Four: Pediatric Mental Health Concerns describes the special issues that arise when children and teens have psychiatric needs. It offers specific details about some of the most commonly occurring mental health issues among young people, including attention deficit hyperactivity disorder, autism spectrum disorder, bipolar disorder, depression, and learning disabilities.

Part Five: Other Populations with Distinctive Mental Health Concerns addresses concerns among men, women, older adults, and other groups for whom special considerations may impact mental wellness. These include people dealing with the psychological impact of prejudice and discrimination, trauma or disaster, cultural isolation, and poverty.

Part Six: Mental Illness Co-Occurring with Other Disorders explains the ways physical conditions can sometimes affect psychological well-being. It discusses some specific disorders commonly associated with changes in mental health status, including cancer, diabetes, epilepsy, heart disease, and stroke. It also addresses issues related to sleep disorders and mental functioning, and it examines the complex relationship between mental health and the experience of pain.

Part Seven: Additional Help and Information provides a glossary of mental health terms, a list of toll-free helplines and hotlines for people in crisis, and a directory of mental health organizations.

Bibliographic Note

This volume contains documents and excerpts from publications issued by the following U.S. government agencies: Centers for Disease Control and Prevention; National Cancer Institute; National Institute of Child Health and Human Development; National Institute of Diabetes and Digestive and Kidney Diseases; National Institute of Mental Health; National Institute of Neurological Disorders and Stroke; National Institute on Aging ; National Institute on Drug Abuse; National Institutes of Health; Office on Women's Health; Substance Abuse and Mental Health Services Administration; U.S. Department of Veterans Affairs; U.S. Navy; and the Weight-Control Information Network.

In addition, this volume contains copyrighted documents from the following organizations and individuals: A.D.A.M., Inc.; American Academy of Family Physicians; American Diabetes Association; American Psychological Association; Anxiety and Depression Association of America; Assertive Community Treatment Association; Victoria Balenger, PhD; Beyond Blue Ltd. (Australia); BSCS; Cleveland Clinic Foundation; Cleveland Sleep Research Center; Family Caregiver Alliance; Geriatric Mental Health Foundation; Hartford Hospital; HeartHealthyWomen.org; Helpguide.org; March of Dimes Birth Defects Foundation; Mautner Project: The National Lesbian Health Organization; Mental Health Association of Westchester; Merck & Co., Inc.; Mind (UK); NAMI, the National Alliance on Mental Illness; National Council on Problem Gambling; National Sleep Foundation; National Stroke Association; Nemours Foundation; PsychCentral; Regents of the University of California (University of California, San Francisco, Center for HIV Information); Regents of the University of Michigan (University of Michigan Depression Center); Royal College of Psychiatrists (UK); SAVE: Suicide Awareness Voices of Education; Schizophrenic.com; Washington State Department of Enterprise Services (Employee Assistance Program); and the World Health Organization.

Full citation information is provided on the first page of each chapter or section. Every effort has been made to secure all necessary rights to reprint the copyrighted material. If any omissions have been made, please contact Omnigraphics to make corrections for future editions.

Acknowledgements

In addition to the organizations listed above, special thanks are due to research and permissions coordinator, Liz Collins, and prepress services provider, WhimsyInk.

About the Health Reference Series

The *Health Reference Series* is designed to provide basic medical information for patients, families, caregivers, and the general public. Each volume takes a particular topic and provides comprehensive coverage. This is especially important for people who may be dealing with a newly diagnosed disease or a chronic disorder in themselves or in a family member. People looking for preventive guidance, information about disease warning signs, medical statistics, and risk factors for health problems will also find answers to their questions in the *Health Reference Series*. The *Series*, however, is not intended to serve as a tool for diagnosing illness, in prescribing treatments, or as a substitute for the physician/patient relationship. All people concerned about medical symptoms or the possibility of disease are encouraged to seek professional care from an appropriate health care provider.

A Note about Spelling and Style

Health Reference Series editors use *Stedman's Medical Dictionary* as an authority for questions related to the spelling of medical terms and the *Chicago Manual of Style* for questions related to grammatical structures, punctuation, and other editorial concerns. Consistent adherence is not always possible, however, because the individual volumes within the *Series* include many documents from a wide variety of different producers and copyright holders, and the editor's primary goal is to present material from each source as accurately as is possible following the terms specified by each document's producer. This sometimes means that information in different chapters or sections may follow other guidelines and alternate spelling authorities. For example, occasionally a copyright holder may require that eponymous terms be shown in possessive forms (Crohn's disease *vs.* Crohn disease) or that British spelling norms be retained (leukaemia *vs.* leukemia).

Locating Information within the Health Reference Series

The *Health Reference Series* contains a wealth of information about a wide variety of medical topics. Ensuring easy access to all the fact sheets, research reports, in-depth discussions, and other material contained within the individual books of the *Series* remains one of our highest priorities. As the *Series* continues to grow in size and scope, however, locating the precise information needed by a reader may become more challenging.

A Contents Guide to the Health Reference Series was developed to direct readers to the specific volumes that address their concerns. It presents an extensive list of diseases, treatments, and other topics of general interest compiled from the Tables of Contents and major index headings. To access *A Contents Guide to the Health Reference Series*, visit www.healthreferenceseries.com.

Medical Consultant

Medical consultation services are provided to the *Health Reference Series* editors by David A. Cooke, MD, FACP. Dr. Cooke is a graduate of Brandeis University, and he received his M.D. degree from the University of Michigan. He completed residency training at the University of Wisconsin Hospital and Clinics. He is board-certified in Internal Medicine. Dr. Cooke currently works as part of the University of Michigan Health System and practices in Ann Arbor, MI. In his free time, he enjoys writing, science fiction, and spending time with his family.

Our Advisory Board

We would like to thank the following board members for providing guidance to the development of this *Series*:

- Dr. Lynda Baker, Associate Professor of Library and Information Science, Wayne State University, Detroit, MI

- Nancy Bulgarelli, William Beaumont Hospital Library, Royal Oak, MI

- Karen Imarisio, Bloomfield Township Public Library, Bloomfield Township, MI

- Karen Morgan, Mardigian Library, University of Michigan-Dearborn, Dearborn, MI

- Rosemary Orlando, St. Clair Shores Public Library, St. Clair Shores, MI

Health Reference Series *Update Policy*

The inaugural book in the *Health Reference Series* was the first edition *of Cancer Sourcebook* published in 1989. Since then, the *Series* has been enthusiastically received by librarians and in the medical community. In order to maintain the standard of providing high-quality health information for the layperson the editorial staff at Omnigraphics felt it was necessary to implement a policy of updating volumes when warranted.

Medical researchers have been making tremendous strides, and it is the purpose of the *Health Reference Series* to stay current with the most recent advances. Each decision to update a volume is made on an individual basis. Some of the considerations include how much new information is available and the feedback we receive from people who use the books. If there is a topic you would like to see added to the update list, or an area of medical concern you feel has not been adequately addressed, please write to:

Editor
Health Reference Series
Omnigraphics, Inc.
155 W. Congress, Suite 200
Detroit, MI 48226
E-mail: editorial@omnigraphics.com

Part One

The Brain and Mental Health

Chapter 1

Mental Health Begins with Healthy Brain Functions

Chapter Contents

Section 1.1

Brain Basics

Excerpted from "Brain Basics," National Institute of Mental
Health (www.nimh.nih.gov), November 2, 2011.

The Brain and Mental Health

Mental disorders are common. You may have a friend, colleague,
or relative with a mental disorder, or perhaps you have experienced
one yourself at some point. Such disorders include depression, anxiety
disorders, bipolar disorder, attention deficit hyperactivity disorder
(ADHD), and many others.

Some people who develop a mental illness may recover completely;
others may have repeated episodes of illness with relatively stable periods in between. Still others live with symptoms of mental illness every
day. They can be moderate or serious and cause severe disability.

Through research, we know that mental disorders are brain disorders. Evidence shows that they can be related to changes in the
anatomy, physiology, and chemistry of the nervous system. When the
brain cannot effectively coordinate the billions of cells in the body, the
results can affect many aspects of life.

Scientists are continually learning more about how the brain grows
and works in healthy people, and how normal brain development and
function can go awry, leading to mental illnesses.

The Growing Brain

Neurons are the basic working unit of the brain and nervous system. These cells are highly specialized for the function of conducting
messages. A neuron has three basic parts:

- **Cell body** which includes the nucleus, cytoplasm, and cell organelles. The nucleus contains DNA and information that the
cell needs for growth, metabolism, and repair. Cytoplasm is the
substance that fills a cell, including all the chemicals and parts
needed for the cell to work properly including small structures
called cell organelles.

- **Dendrites** branch off from the cell body and act as a neuron's point of contact for receiving chemical and electrical signals called impulses from neighboring neurons.

- **Axon** which sends impulses and extends from cell bodies to meet and deliver impulses to another nerve cell. Axons can range in length from a fraction of an inch to several feet.

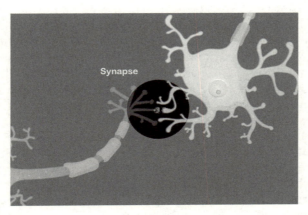

Figure 1.1. *Illustration of axon terminal and neuron with highlight of synapse.*

Each neuron is enclosed by a cell membrane, which separates the inside contents of the cell from its surrounding environment and controls what enters and leaves the cell, and responds to signals from the environment; this all helps the cell maintain its balance with the environment.

Synapses are tiny gaps between neurons, where messages move from one neuron to another as chemical or electrical signals.

The brain begins as a small group of cells in the outer layer of a developing embryo. As the cells grow and differentiate, neurons travel from a central "birthplace" to their final destination. Chemical signals from other cells guide neurons in forming various brain structures. Neighboring neurons make connections with each other and with distant nerve cells (via axons) to form brain circuits. These circuits control specific body functions such as sleep and speech.

The brain continues maturing well into a person's early 20s. Knowing how the brain is wired and how the normal brain's structure develops and matures helps scientists understand what goes wrong in mental illnesses.

Scientists have already begun to chart how the brain develops over time in healthy people and are working to compare that with brain development in people mental disorders. Genes and environmental cues both help to direct this growth.

Every cell in our bodies contains a complete set of DNA (deoxyribonucleic acid). DNA, the "recipe of life," contains all the information inherited from our parents that helps to define who we are, such as our looks and certain abilities, such as a good singing voice. A gene is a segment of DNA that contains codes to make proteins and other important body chemicals. DNA also includes information to control which genes are expressed and when, in all the cells of the body.

As we grow, we create new cells, each with a copy of our original set of DNA. Sometimes this copying process is imperfect, leading to a gene mutation that causes the gene to code for a slightly different protein. Some mutations are harmless, some can be helpful, and others give rise to disabilities or diseases.

Genes aren't the only determinants of how our bodies function. Throughout our lives, our genes can be affected by the environment. In medicine, the term environment includes not only our physical surroundings but also factors that can affect our bodies, such as sleep, diet, or stress. These factors may act alone or together in complex ways, to change the way a gene is expressed or the way messages are conducted in the body.

Epigenetics is the study of how environmental factors can affect how a given gene operates. But unlike gene mutations, epigenetic changes do not change the code for a gene. Rather, they effect when a gene turns on or off to produce a specific protein. Scientists believe epigenetics play a major role in mental disorders and the effects of medications. Some, but not all mutations and epigenetic changes can be passed on to future generations.

Further understanding of genes and epigenetics may one day lead to genetic testing for people at risk for mental disorders. This could greatly help in early detection, more tailored treatments, and possibly prevention of such illnesses.

The Working Brain

Neurotransmitters

Neurotransmitters send chemical messages between neurons. Mental illnesses, such as depression, can occur when this process does not work correctly. Communication between neurons can also be electrical, such as in areas of the brain that control movement. When electrical signals are abnormal, they can cause tremors or symptoms found in Parkinson disease.

Serotonin: Serotonin helps control many functions, such as mood, appetite, and sleep. Research shows that people with depression often have lower than normal levels of serotonin. The types of medications most commonly prescribed to treat depression act by blocking the recycling, or reuptake, of serotonin. As a result, more serotonin stays in the synapse for the receiving neuron to bind onto, leading to more normal mood functioning.

Dopamine: Dopamine is mainly involved in controlling movement and aiding the flow of information to the front of the brain, which is linked to thought and emotion. It is also linked to reward systems in the brain. Problems in producing dopamine can result in Parkinson disease, a disorder that affects a person's ability to move as they want to, resulting in stiffness, tremors or shaking, and other symptoms. Some studies suggest that having too little dopamine or problems using dopamine in the thinking and feeling regions of the brain may play a role in disorders like schizophrenia or attention deficit hyperactivity disorder (ADHD).

Glutamate: The most common neurotransmitter, glutamate, has many roles throughout the brain and nervous system. Glutamate is an excitatory transmitter: when it is released it increases the chance that the neuron will fire. This enhances the electrical flow among brain cells required for normal function and plays an important role during early brain development. It may also assist in learning and memory. Problems in making or using glutamate have been linked to many mental disorders, including autism, obsessive compulsive disorder (OCD), schizophrenia, and depression.

Brain Regions

We have many specialized brain systems that work across specific brain regions to help us talk, help us make sense of what we see, and help us to solve a problem. Some of the regions most commonly studied in mental health research are listed below.

Amygdala: The brain's "fear hub," which activates our natural "fight-or-flight" response to confront or escape from a dangerous situation is called the amygdala. The amygdala also appears to be involved in learning to fear an event, such as touching a hot stove, and learning not to fear, such as overcoming a fear of spiders. Studying how the amygdala helps create memories of fear and safety may help improve treatments for anxiety disorders like phobias or post-traumatic stress disorder (PTSD).

Prefrontal cortex (PFC): The PFC is the seat of the brain's executive functions, such as judgment, decision making, and problem solving. Different parts of the PFC are involved in using short-term or "working" memory and in retrieving long-term memories. This area of the brain also helps to control the amygdala during stressful events. Some research shows that people who have PTSD or ADHD have reduced activity in their PFCs.

Anterior cingulate cortex (ACC): The ACC has many different roles, from controlling blood pressure and heart rate to responding when we sense a mistake, helping us feel motivated and stay focused on a task, and managing proper emotional reactions. Reduced ACC activity or damage to this brain area has been linked to disorders such as ADHD, schizophrenia, and depression.

Hippocampus: The hippocampus helps create and file new memories. When the hippocampus is damaged, a person can't create new memories, but can still remember past events and learned skills, and carry on a conversation, all which rely on different parts of the brain. The hippocampus may be involved in mood disorders through its control of a major mood circuit called the hypothalamic-pituitary-adrenal (HPA) axis.

Section 1.2

Brain Function and Mental Illness

Excerpted from *The Science of Mental Illness*. Copyright © 2005 by BSCS. All rights reserved. Reprinted with permission. Reviewed by David A. Cooke, MD, FACP, 2011–2012.

Defining Mental Illness

We can all be "sad" or "blue" at times in our lives. We have all seen movies about the madman and his crime spree, with the underlying cause of mental illness. We sometimes even make jokes about people being crazy or nuts, even though we know that we shouldn't. We have all had some exposure to mental illness, but do we really understand it or know what it is? Many of our preconceptions are incorrect. A mental illness can be defined as a health condition that changes a person's thinking, feelings, or behavior (or all three) and that causes the person distress and difficulty in functioning. As with many diseases, mental illness is severe in some cases and mild in others. Individuals who have a mental illness don't necessarily look like they are sick, especially if their illness is mild. Other individuals may show more explicit symptoms such as confusion, agitation, or withdrawal. There are many different mental illnesses, including depression, schizophrenia, attention deficit hyperactivity disorder (ADHD), autism, and obsessive-compulsive disorder. Each illness alters a person's thoughts, feelings, and/or behaviors in distinct ways.

Not all brain diseases are categorized as mental illnesses. Disorders such as epilepsy, Parkinson disease, and multiple sclerosis are brain disorders, but they are considered neurological diseases rather than mental illnesses. Interestingly, the lines between mental illnesses and these other brain or neurological disorders is blurring somewhat. As scientists continue to investigate the brains of people who have mental illnesses, they are learning that mental illness is associated with changes in the brain's structure, chemistry, and function and that mental illness does indeed have a biological basis. This ongoing research is, in some ways, causing scientists to minimize the distinctions between mental illnesses and these other brain disorders. In this

9

text, we will restrict our discussion of mental illness to those illnesses that are traditionally classified as mental illnesses, as listed in the previous paragraph.

Mental Illness and the Brain

The term mental illness clearly indicates that there is a problem with the mind. But is it just the mind in an abstract sense, or is there a physical basis to mental illness? As scientists continue to investigate mental illnesses and their causes, they learn more and more about how the biological processes that make the brain work are changed when a person has a mental illness.

The Basics of Brain Function

Before thinking about the problems that occur in the brain when someone has a mental illness, it is helpful to think about how the brain functions normally.

The brain is an incredibly complex organ. It makes up only two percent of our body weight, but it consumes 20 percent of the oxygen we breathe and 20 percent of the energy we take in. It controls virtually everything we as humans experience, including movement, sensing our environment, regulating our involuntary body processes such as breathing, and controlling our emotions. Hundreds of thousands of chemical reactions occur every second in the brain; those reactions underlie the thoughts, actions, and behaviors with which we respond to environmental stimuli. In short, the brain dictates the internal processes and behaviors that allow us to survive.

How does the brain take in all this information, process it, and cause a response? The basic functional unit of the brain is the neuron. A neuron is a specialized cell that can produce different actions because of its precise connections with other neurons, sensory receptors, and muscle cells. A typical neuron has four structurally and functionally defined regions: The cell body, dendrites, axons, and the axon terminals.

Near its end, the axon divides into many fine branches that have specialized swellings called axon terminals or presynaptic terminals. The axon terminals end near the dendrites of another neuron. The dendrites of one neuron receive the message sent from the axon terminals of another neuron.

The site where an axon terminal ends near a receiving dendrite is called the synapse. The cell that sends out information is called the presynaptic neuron, and the cell that receives the information is called the postsynaptic neuron. It is important to note that the synapse is not a physical connection between the two neurons; there is no cytoplasmic connection between the two neurons. The intercellular space between the presynaptic and postsynaptic neurons is called the synaptic space or synaptic cleft. An average neuron forms approximately 1,000 synapses with other neurons. It has been estimated that there are more synapses in the human brain than there are stars in our galaxy. Furthermore, synaptic connections are not static. Neurons form new synapses or strengthen synaptic connections in response to life experiences. This dynamic change in neuronal connections is the basis of learning.

Neurons communicate using both electrical signals and chemical messages. Information in the form of an electrical impulse is carried away from the neuron's cell body along the axon of the presynaptic neuron toward the axon terminals. When the electrical signal reaches the presynaptic axon terminal, it cannot cross the synaptic space, or synaptic cleft. Instead, the electrical signal triggers chemical changes that can cross the synapse to affect the postsynaptic cell. When the electrical impulse reaches the presynaptic axon terminal, membranous sacs called vesicles move toward the membrane of the axon terminal. When the vesicles reach the membrane, they fuse with the membrane and release their contents into the synaptic space. The molecules contained in the vesicles are chemical compounds called neurotransmitters. Each vesicle contains many molecules of a neurotransmitter. The released neurotransmitter molecules drift across the synaptic cleft and then bind to special proteins, called receptors, on the postsynaptic neuron. A neurotransmitter molecule will bind only to a specific kind of receptor.

The binding of neurotransmitters to their receptors causes that neuron to generate an electrical impulse. The electrical impulse then moves away from the dendrite ending toward the cell body. After the neurotransmitter stimulates an electrical impulse in the postsynaptic neuron, it releases from the receptor back into the synaptic space. Specific proteins called transporters or reuptake pumps carry the neurotransmitter back into the presynaptic neuron. When the neurotransmitter molecules are back in the presynaptic axon terminal, they can be repackaged into vesicles for release the next time an electrical impulse reaches the axon terminal. Enzymes present in the synaptic space degrade neurotransmitter molecules that are not taken back up into the presynaptic neuron.

The nervous system uses a variety of neurotransmitter molecules, but each neuron specializes in the synthesis and secretion of a single type of neurotransmitter. Some of the predominant neurotransmitters in the brain include glutamate, GABA [gamma-aminobutyric acid], serotonin, dopamine, and norepinephrine.

11

Investigating Brain Function

Mental health professionals base their diagnosis and treatment of mental illness on the symptoms that a person exhibits. The goal for these professionals in treating a patient is to relieve the symptoms that are interfering with the person's life so that the person can function well. Research scientists, on the other hand, have a different goal. They want to learn about the chemical or structural changes that occur in the brain when someone has a mental illness. If scientists can determine what happens in the brain, they can use that knowledge to develop better treatments or find a cure.

The techniques that scientists use to investigate the brain depend on the questions they are asking. For some questions, scientists use molecular or biochemical methods to investigate specific genes or proteins in the neurons. For other questions, scientists want to visualize changes in the brain so that they can learn more about how the activity or structure of the brain changes. Historically, scientists could examine brains only after death, but new imaging procedures enable scientists to study the brain in living animals, including humans. It is important to realize that these brain imaging techniques are not used for diagnosing mental illness. Mental illnesses are diagnosed by the set of symptoms that an individual exhibits. The imaging techniques described in the following paragraphs would not enable the mental health professional to diagnose or treat the patient more effectively. Some of the techniques are also invasive and expose patients to small amounts of radiation. Research studies using these tests are generally not conducted with children or adolescents.

One extensively used technique to study brain activity and how mental illness changes the brain is positron emission tomography (PET). PET measures the spatial distribution and movement of a radioactive chemical injected into the tissues of living subjects. Because the patient is awake, the technique can be used to investigate the relationship between behavioral and physiological effects and changes in brain activity. PET scans can detect very small (nanomolar) concentrations of tracer molecules and achieve spatial resolution of about 4 mm. In addition, computers can reconstruct images obtained from a PET scan in two or three dimensions.

PET requires the use of compounds that are labeled with positron-emitting isotopes. A positron has the same mass and spin as an electron but the opposite charge; an electron has a negative charge and a positron has a positive charge. A cyclotron accelerates protons into the nucleus of nitrogen, carbon, oxygen, or fluorine to generate these isotopes. The additional proton makes the isotope unstable. To become stable again, the proton must break down into a neutron and a positron. The unstable positron travels away from the site of generation and dissipates energy along the way. Eventually, the positron collides with an electron, leading to the emission of two gamma rays at 180 degrees from one another. The gamma rays reach a pair of detectors that record the event. Because the detectors respond only to simultaneous emissions, scientists can precisely map the location where the gamma rays were generated. The radioactive chemicals used for PET are very short lived. The half-life (the time for half of the radioactive label to disintegrate) of the commonly used radioisotopes ranges from approximately 2 minutes to less than 2 hours, depending on the specific compound. Because a PET scan requires only small amounts (a few mcg) of short-lived radioisotopes, this technique can be used safely in humans.

PET scans can answer a variety of questions about brain function, including where the neurons are most active. Scientists use different radiolabeled compounds to investigate different biological questions. For example, radiolabeled glucose can identify parts of the brain that become more active in response to a specific stimulus. Active neurons metabolize more glucose than inactive neurons. Active neurons emit more positrons, and this shows as red or yellow on PET scans compared with blue or purple in areas where the neurons are not highly active. (Different computer enhancement techniques may use a different color scheme, but the use of a spectrum with red indicating high activity and blue indicating low activity is common.) Scientists can use PET to measure changes in the activity of specific brain areas in a person who has a mental illness. Scientists can also investigate how the mentally ill brain changes after a person receives treatment.

PET imaging is not the only technique that researchers use to investigate how mental illness changes the brain. Different techniques provide different information to scientists. Another important technique is magnetic resonance imaging (MRI). Unlike PET, which reveals changes in activity level, MRI is used to look at structural changes in the brain. For example, MRI studies reveal that the ventricles, or spaces within the brain, are larger in individuals who have schizophrenia compared with those of healthy individuals.

Other techniques that scientists use to investigate function in the living brain include single photon emission computed tomography (SPECT), functional magnetic resonance imaging (fMRI), and electroencephalography (EEG). Each technique has its own advantages, and each provides different information about brain structure and function. Scientists often use more than one technique when conducting their research.

13

The Causes of Mental Illnesses

At this time, scientists do not have a complete understanding of what causes mental illnesses. If you think about the structural and organizational complexity of the brain together with the complexity of effects that mental illnesses have on thoughts, feelings, and behaviors, it is hardly surprising that figuring out the causes of mental illnesses is a daunting task. The fields of neuroscience, psychiatry, and psychology address different aspects of the relationship between the biology of the brain and individuals' behaviors, thoughts, and feelings, and how their actions sometimes get out of control. Through this multidisciplinary research, scientists are trying to find the causes of mental illnesses. Once scientists can determine the causes of a mental illness, they can use that knowledge to develop new treatments or to find a cure.

The Biology of Mental Illnesses

Most scientists believe that mental illnesses result from problems with the communication between neurons in the brain (neurotransmission). For example, the level of the neurotransmitter serotonin is lower in individuals who have depression. This finding led to the development of certain medications for the illness. Selective serotonin reuptake inhibitors (SSRIs) work by reducing the amount of serotonin that is taken back into the presynaptic neuron. This leads to an increase in the amount of serotonin available in the synaptic space for binding to the receptor on the postsynaptic neuron. Changes in other neurotransmitters (in addition to serotonin) may occur in depression, thus adding to the complexity of the cause underlying the disease.

Scientists believe that there may be disruptions in the neurotransmitters dopamine, glutamate, and norepinephrine in individuals who have schizophrenia. One indication that dopamine might be an important neurotransmitter in schizophrenia comes from the observation that cocaine addicts sometimes show symptoms similar to schizophrenia. Cocaine acts on dopamine-containing neurons in the brain to increase the amount of dopamine in the synapse.

Risk Factors for Mental Illnesses

Although scientists at this time do not know the causes of mental illnesses, they have identified factors that put individuals at risk. Some of these factors are environmental, some are genetic, and some are social. In fact, all these factors most likely combine to influence whether someone becomes mentally ill.

Environmental factors such as head injury, poor nutrition, and exposure to toxins (including lead and tobacco smoke) can increase the likelihood of developing a mental illness.

Genes also play a role in determining whether someone develops a mental illness. The illnesses that are most likely to have a genetic component include autism, bipolar disorder, schizophrenia, and ADHD. For example, the observation that children with ADHD are much more likely to have a sibling or parent with ADHD supports a role for genetics in determining whether someone is at risk for ADHD. In studies of twins, ADHD is significantly more likely to be present in an identical twin than a fraternal twin. The same can be said for schizophrenia and depression. Mental illnesses are not triggered by a change in a single gene; scientists believe that the interaction of several genes may trigger mental illness. Furthermore, the combination of genetic, environmental, and social factors might determine whether a case of mental illness is mild or severe.

Social factors also present risks and can harm an individual's, especially a child's, mental health. Social factors include severe parental discord, death of a family member or close friend, parent's mental illness, parent's criminality, overcrowding, economic hardship, abuse, neglect, and exposure to violence.

Treating Mental Illnesses

At this time, most mental illnesses cannot be cured, but they can usually be treated effectively to minimize the symptoms and allow the individual to function in work, school, or social environments. To begin treatment, an individual needs to see a qualified mental health professional. The first thing that the doctor or other mental health professional will do is speak with the individual to find out more about his or her symptoms, how long the symptoms have lasted, and how the person's life is being affected. The physician will also do a physical examination to determine whether there are other health problems. For example, some symptoms (such as emotional swings) can be caused by neurological or hormonal problems associated with chronic illnesses such as heart disease, or they can be a side effect of certain medications. After the individual's overall health is evaluated and the condition diagnosed, the doctor will develop a treatment plan. Treatment can involve both medications and psychotherapy, depending on the disease and its severity.

Chapter 2

The Components of Mental Health

Chapter Contents

Section 2.1

Myths about Mental Health

From "Myths and Facts about Mental Health," Substance Abuse and Mental Health Services Administration (SAMHSA), October 30, 2009.

Myths and Facts about Mental Health

Often people are afraid to talk about mental health because there are many misconceptions about mental illnesses. It's important to learn the facts to stop discrimination and to begin treating people with mental illnesses with respect and dignity. Here are some common myths and facts about mental health.

Myth: There's no hope for people with mental illnesses.

Fact: There are more treatments, strategies, and community supports than ever before, and even more are on the horizon. People with mental illnesses lead active, productive lives.

Myth: I can't do anything for someone with mental health needs.

Fact: You can do a lot, starting with the way you act and how you speak. You can nurture an environment that builds on people's strengths and promotes good mental health. For example:

- Avoid labeling people with words like "crazy," "wacko," "loony," or by their diagnosis. Instead of saying someone is a "schizophrenic" say "a person with schizophrenia."

- Learn the facts about mental health and share them with others, especially if you hear something that is untrue.

- Treat people with mental illnesses with respect and dignity, as you would anybody else.

- Respect the rights of people with mental illnesses and don't discriminate against them when it comes to housing, employment, or education. Like other people with disabilities, people with mental health needs are protected under Federal and State laws.

Myth: People with mental illnesses are violent and unpredictable.

Fact: In reality, the vast majority of people who have mental health needs are no more violent than anyone else. You probably know someone with a mental illness and don't even realize it.

Myth: Mental illnesses cannot affect me.

Fact: Mental illnesses are surprisingly common; they affect almost every family in America. Mental illnesses do not discriminate—they can affect anyone.

Myth: Mental illness is the same as mental retardation.

Fact: The two are distinct disorders. A mental retardation diagnosis is characterized by limitations in intellectual functioning and difficulties with certain daily living skills. In contrast, people with mental illnesses—health conditions that cause changes in a person's thinking, mood, and behavior—have varied intellectual functioning, just like the general population.

Myth: Mental illnesses are brought on by a weakness of character.

Fact: Mental illnesses are a product of the interaction of biological, psychological, and social factors. Research has shown genetic and biological factors are associated with schizophrenia, depression, and alcoholism. Social influences, such as loss of a loved one or a job, can also contribute to the development of various disorders.

Myth: People with mental illnesses cannot tolerate the stress of holding down a job.

Fact: In essence, all jobs are stressful to some extent. Productivity is maximized when there is a good match between the employee's needs and working conditions, whether or not the individual has mental health needs.

Myth: People with mental health needs, even those who have received effective treatment and have recovered, tend to be second-rate workers on the job.

Fact: Employers who have hired people with mental illnesses report good attendance and punctuality, as well as motivation, quality of work, and job tenure on par with or greater than other employees. Studies by the National Institute of Mental Health (NIMH) and the National Alliance for the Mentally Ill (NAMI) show that there are no differences in productivity when people with mental illnesses are compared to other employees.

Myth: Once people develop mental illnesses, they will never recover.

Fact: Studies show that most people with mental illnesses get better, and many recover completely. Recovery refers to the process in which people are able to live, work, learn, and participate fully in their communities. For some individuals, recovery is the ability to live a fulfilling and productive life. For others, recovery implies the reduction or complete remission of symptoms. Science has shown that having hope plays an integral role in an individual's recovery.

Myth: Therapy and self-help are wastes of time. Why bother when you can just take one of those pills you hear about on TV?

Fact: Treatment varies depending on the individual. A lot of people work with therapists, counselors, their peers, psychologists, psychiatrists, nurses, and social workers in their recovery process. They also use self-help strategies and community supports. Often these methods are combined with some of the most advanced medications available.

Myth: Children do not experience mental illnesses. Their actions are just products of bad parenting.

Fact: A report from the President's New Freedom Commission on Mental Health showed that in any given year 5–9 percent of children experience serious emotional disturbances. Just like adult mental illnesses, these are clinically diagnosable health conditions that are a product of the interaction of biological, psychological, social, and sometimes even genetic factors.

Myth: Children misbehave or fail in school just to get attention.

Fact: Behavior problems can be symptoms of emotional, behavioral, or mental disorders, rather than merely attention-seeking devices. These children can succeed in school with appropriate understanding, attention, and mental health services.

Section 2.2

Good Mental Health

"Mental Health: Good Mental Health," Office on Women's Health
(www.womenshealth.gov), March 29, 2010.

Your mental health is very important. You will not have a healthy body if you don't also take care of your mind. People depend on you. It's important for you to take care of yourself so that you can do the important things in life—whether it's working, learning, taking care of your family, volunteering, enjoying the outdoors, or whatever is important to you.

Good mental health helps you enjoy life and cope with problems. It offers a feeling of well-being and inner strength. Just as you take care of your body by eating right and exercising, you can do things to protect your mental health. In fact, eating right and exercising can help maintain good mental health. You don't automatically have good mental health just because you don't have mental health illness. You have to work to keep your mind healthy.

Nutrition and Mental Health

The food you eat can have a direct effect on your energy level, physical health, and mood. A "healthy diet" is one that has enough of each essential nutrient, contains many foods from all of the basic food groups, provides the right amount of calories to maintain a healthy weight, and does not have too much fat, sugar, salt, or alcohol.

By choosing foods that can give you steady energy, you can help your body stay healthy. This may also help your mind feel good. The same diet doesn't work for every person. In order to find the best foods that are right for you, talk to your health care professional.

Some vitamins and minerals may help with the symptoms of depression. Experts are looking into how a lack of some nutrients—including folate, vitamin B12, calcium, iron, selenium, zinc, and omega-3—may contribute to depression in new mothers. Ask your doctor or another health care professional for more information.

Exercise and Mental Health

Regular physical activity is important to the physical and mental health of almost everyone, including older adults. Being physically active can help you continue to do the things you enjoy and stay independent as you age. Regular physical activity over long periods of time can produce long-term health benefits. That's why health experts say that everyone should be active every day to maintain their health.

If you are diagnosed with depression or anxiety, your doctor may tell you to exercise in addition to taking any medications or receiving counseling. This is because exercise has been shown to help with the symptoms of depression and anxiety. Your body makes certain chemicals, called endorphins, before and after you work out. They relieve stress and improve your mood. Exercise can also slow or stop weight gain, which is a common side effect of some medications used to treat mental health disorders.

Sleep and Mental Health

Your mind and body will feel better if you sleep well. Your body needs time every day to rest and heal. If you often have trouble sleeping—either falling asleep, or waking during the night and being unable to get back to sleep—one or several of the following ideas might be helpful to you:

- Go to bed at the same time every night and get up at the same time every morning. Avoid "sleeping in" (sleeping much later than your usual time for getting up). It will make you feel worse.

- Establish a bedtime "ritual" by doing the same things every night for an hour or two before bedtime so your body knows when it is time to go to sleep.

- Avoid caffeine, nicotine, and alcohol.

- Eat on a regular schedule and avoid a heavy meal prior to going to bed. Don't skip any meals.

- Eat plenty of dairy foods and dark green leafy vegetables.

- Exercise daily, but avoid strenuous or invigorating activity before going to bed.

- Play soothing music on a tape or CD that shuts off automatically after you are in bed.

- Try a turkey sandwich and a glass of milk before bedtime to make you feel drowsy.

- Try having a small snack before you go to bed, something like a piece of fruit and a piece of cheese, so you don't wake up hungry in the middle of the night. Have a similar small snack if you awaken in the middle of the night.

- Take a warm bath or shower before going to bed.

- Place a drop of lavender oil on your pillow.

- Drink a cup of herbal chamomile tea before going to bed.

You need to see your doctor if:

- You often have difficulty sleeping and the solutions listed above are not working for you

- You awaken during the night gasping for breath

- Your partner says that your breathing stops when you are sleeping

- You snore loudly

- You wake up feeling like you haven't been asleep

- You fall asleep often during the day

Stress and Mental Health

Stress can happen for many reasons. Stress can be brought about by a traumatic accident, death, or emergency situation. Stress can also be a side effect of a serious illness or disease.

There is also stress associated with daily life, the workplace, and family responsibilities. It's hard to stay calm and relaxed in our hectic lives. With all we have going on in our lives, it seems almost impossible to find ways to de-stress. But it's important to find those ways. Your health depends on it.

Common symptoms include:

- Headache

- Sleep disorders

- Difficulty concentrating

- Short-temper

- Upset stomach

- Job dissatisfaction

- Low morale
- Depression
- Anxiety

Remember to always make time for you. It's important to care for yourself. Think of this as an order from your doctor, so you don't feel guilty. No matter how busy you are, you can try to set aside at least 15 minutes each day in your schedule to do something for yourself, like taking a bubble bath, going for a walk, or calling a friend.

Section 2.3

Good Emotional Health

What is good emotional health?

People who have good emotional health are aware of their thoughts, feelings and behaviors. They have learned healthy ways to cope with the stress and problems that are a normal part of life. They feel good about themselves and have healthy relationships.

However, many things that happen in your life can disrupt your emotional health and lead to strong feelings of sadness, stress or anxiety. These things include:

- Being laid off from your job
- Having a child leave or return home
- Dealing with the death of a loved one
- Getting divorced or married
- Suffering an illness or an injury
- Getting a job promotion
- Experiencing money problems

- Moving to a new home
- Having a baby

"Good" changes can be just as stressful as "bad" changes.

How can my emotions affect my health?

Your body responds to the way you think, feel and act. This is often called the "mind/body connection." When you are stressed, anxious or upset, your body tries to tell you that something isn't right. For example, high blood pressure or a stomach ulcer might develop after a particularly stressful event, such as the death of a loved one. The following can be physical signs that your emotional health is out of balance:

- Back pain
- Change in appetite
- Chest pain
- Constipation or diarrhea
- Dry mouth
- Extreme tiredness
- General aches and pains
- Headaches
- High blood pressure
- Insomnia (trouble sleeping)
- Lightheadedness
- Palpitations (the feeling that your heart is racing)
- Sexual problems
- Shortness of breath
- Stiff neck
- Sweating
- Upset stomach
- Weight gain or loss

Poor emotional health can weaken your body's immune system, making you more likely to get colds and other infections during emotionally difficult times. Also, when you are feeling stressed, anxious or upset, you may not take care of your health as well as you should. You may not feel like exercising, eating nutritious foods or taking medicine that your doctor prescribes. Abuse of alcohol, tobacco or other drugs may also be a sign of poor emotional health.

Why does my doctor need to know about my emotions?

You may not be used to talking to your doctor about your feelings or problems in your personal life. But remember, he or she can't always tell that you're feeling stressed, anxious or upset just by looking at you. It's important to be honest with your doctor if you are having these feelings.

First, he or she will need to make sure that other health problems aren't causing your physical symptoms. If your symptoms aren't caused by other health problems, you and your doctor can address the emotional causes of your symptoms. Your doctor may suggest ways to treat your physical symptoms while you work together to improve your emotional health.

If your negative feelings don't go away and are so strong that they keep you from enjoying life, it's especially important for you to talk to your doctor. You may have what doctors call "major depression." Depression is a medical illness that can be treated with individualized counseling, medicine or with both.

How can I improve my emotional health?

First, try to recognize your emotions and understand why you are having them. Sorting out the causes of sadness, stress and anxiety in your life can help you manage your emotional health. The following are some other helpful tips.

Express your feelings in appropriate ways: If feelings of stress, sadness or anxiety are causing physical problems, keeping these feelings inside can make you feel worse. It's OK to let your loved ones know when something is bothering you. However, keep in mind that your family and friends may not be able to help you deal with your feelings appropriately. At these times, ask someone outside the situation—such as your family doctor, a counselor or a religious advisor—for advice and support to help you improve your emotional health.

Live a balanced life: Try not to obsess about the problems at work, school or home that lead to negative feelings. This doesn't mean you have to pretend to be happy when you feel stressed, anxious or upset. It's important to deal with these negative feelings, but try to focus on the positive things in your life too. You may want to use a journal to keep track of things that make you feel happy or peaceful. Some research has shown that having a positive outlook can improve your quality of life and give your health a boost. You may also need to find ways to let go of some things in your life that make you feel stressed and overwhelmed. Make time for things you enjoy.

Develop resilience: People with resilience are able to cope with stress in a healthy way. Resilience can be learned and strengthened with different strategies. These include having social support, keeping a positive view of yourself, accepting change, and keeping things in perspective.

Calm your mind and body: Relaxation methods, such as meditation, are useful ways to bring your emotions into balance. Meditation is a form of guided thought. It can take many forms. For example, you may do it by exercising, stretching or breathing deeply. Ask your family doctor for advice about relaxation methods.

Take care of yourself: To have good emotional health, it's important to take care of your body by having a regular routine for eating healthy meals, getting enough sleep and exercising to relieve pent-up tension. Avoid overeating and don't abuse drugs or alcohol. Using drugs or alcohol just causes other problems, such as family and health problems.

Chapter 3

Lifestyles and Mental Health

Chapter Contents

Section 3.1

Eating Well and Mental Health

Eating Well

This information is for everyone who wants to eat healthily. It is particularly for people who feel that their mental health problem or its treatment has affected them in the way they eat.

Eating well—what does it mean?

This can actually mean a lot of different things to different people. Broadly speaking it means eating in a way so that:

- our weight remains normal—not too low and not to high;
- our weight remains stable—not going up and down all the time;
- all necessary food groups and vitamins are available;
- eating becomes and remains an enjoyable experience.

Why is eating well important?

Eating well helps us to prevent many diseases which are linked with being overweight. Diseases include high blood sugar, high blood pressure, heart problems, stroke, cancer, joint problems, and sleeping difficulties just to name a few. Eating well also makes us feel emotionally well.

Why is eating well important for people with mental health problems?

People with mental health problems are more likely to have a weight problem. The reasons for this are not fully clear. For instance, some people always feel tired and just not up to any activity. Others always feel hungry.

Some of this may be related to the mental health problem itself; however, it has increasingly become clear that weight problems may also be a side-effect of some treatments. This does not mean one should stop treatment because one might become mentally unwell again. Sometimes it is possible to swap to another medication. Alternatively, one can try to become more physically active or switch to better eating habits.

This text looks at eating habits. Let's start with finding out what foods there are.

Foods can essentially be divided into three groups:

- Carbohydrates or sugar based foods
- Fats
- Proteins

A word of advice: The Royal College of Psychiatrists can only give general information but not consider individual cases. If in doubt, you should discuss your diet with your nurse, a doctor, or a dietitian. Also, the guidance given here applies to adults only and not to children who have different dietary needs. If you are pregnant or suffer from certain physical health problems your dietary requirements may also be different.

Carbohydrates

What are they?

Carbohydrates are essentially made up of sugar. There are simple carbohydrates made up of just one or several sugar units (glucose or fructose) and there are complex carbohydrates made up of long chains of sugars. These long sugar chains are called starch. Complex carbohydrates often contain a lot of fiber. Simple carbohydrates are broken down easily in the body and may give an instant but short-term effect. Complex carbohydrates take longer to break down but have a longer effect. Each gram of carbohydrate provides approximately four calories of energy.

What are they used for?

Carbohydrates are the main fuel of the body. For instance, muscles work most effectively on glucose although they can also burn fat. The brain can only operate on glucose and does not use fat or proteins as fuel.

31

Examples: Simple carbohydrates are found in foods like glucose, sugar, jam, honey, sweets, etc. They are also found in many fizzy drinks and sports drinks. Complex carbohydrates are found in foods like vegetables, fruits, grains such as wheat and rice, or from products such as pasta, cereals, beans and potatoes.

What is the glycemic index?

This is a measure of how fast a food is broken down into single sugar units, i.e. glucose. The longer it takes, the lower the glycemic index (GI). The glycemic index does not only depend on the length of the sugar chain, but also on the fiber content. That is why white rice and white bread, where the outer layer is removed from the grain, have a much higher glycemic index than brown rice and brown bread. Foods with a low glycemic index are often called "good carbs" and foods with a high glycemic index are called "bad carbs".

What happens if I eat too many carbohydrates?

If you eat more carbohydrates than your body needs to burn as fuel then the excess will be converted into fat and stored.

Which carbohydrates should I eat?

Try to eat "good carbs" with a low glycemic index. Goods carbs include fruits, vegetables, and legumes such as beans, pasta, brown rice, basmati rice, whole meal bread, and potatoes.

Fats

What are they?

Fats are made up of chains of fatty acids. There are three different types of fatty acids which are defined by their chemical structure and by their ability to take up additional hydrogen atoms. This sounds very theoretical but has very important health applications as they differ in their ability to promote bad (LDL) or good (HDL) cholesterol. One gram of fat yields approximately eight calories.

Unsaturated fats are made up of fatty acids that can store additional hydrogen atoms. If only one hydrogen atom can be taken up they are monounsaturated, and if several can be taken up they are called polyunsaturated. Unsaturated fats are usually liquid, this means they are oils. They can lower blood cholesterol levels.

Saturated fats cannot store an additional hydrogen atom. They are already fully loaded, in other words saturated. They are solid and they raise cholesterol.

Trans-fats are unsaturated. They can be produced from oils by introducing some hydrogen atoms into oils so that they become solid. Trans-fats are mainly used for industrial food production.

What are they used for?

Fats serve many different purposes. They are an important energy store which can be activated when the body has run of glucose. Fat deposits insulate the body against the cold. Fatty acids are also important components for cell membranes and hormones and may even have a role in keeping us mentally stable. Fats are needed to make use of some vitamins such as vitamin A, D, E and K.

Examples: Unsaturated fats are found in foods like vegetable oils, for instance sunflower- and olive oil, olives, nuts, seeds, and avocados.

Saturated fats are mainly found in animal products such as milk, butter, cheese, cream, and meats and dairy products such yogurts, puddings or ice cream. Note that coconut products including coconut paste or milk are also high in saturated fats.

Trans-fats are found in hardened vegetable oils such as margarine and spreads. Mass-produced foods like cakes, biscuits and chips may contain large amounts of trans-fats.

What happens if I eat too many fats?

The fat deposits of the body will be extended.

Which fats should I eat?

Try to eat unsaturated fats such as vegetable oils, seeds, and nuts. Remember that even "good fats" have a lot of calories and thus need to be eaten in moderation. Try to use skimmed and semi-skimmed milk instead of whole milk and whole-milk products.

What about omega-3 fatty acids?

Omega-3 fatty acids are unsaturated fatty acids which cannot be produced by the body itself. This means that they are so-called "essential" fatty acids. Omega-3 fatty acids are supposed to have a range of health benefits such as lowering cholesterol, preventing heart and joint disease, and improving learning.

Omega-3 fatty acids may also keep us mentally more stable and may be tried as supplements in people who suffer from mood problems and schizophrenia. They may help prevent relapse in bipolar disorder. There is not enough evidence to recommend them as an alternative to antidepressants.

Note: Omega-3 fatty acids taken as supplements may interact with blood thinning drugs.

Which foods contain omega-3 fatty acids?

Omega-3 fatty acids can be found in oily fish such as cod, salmon, and mackerel. They can also be founds in plant sources such as flax-seed and walnuts.

How safe is omega-3 from fish sources?

For most people the benefits will outweigh any concern about possible contamination. However, if you are pregnant make sure to check with a health professional about how many portions of fish you can eat in a week.

Proteins

What are they?

Proteins are made of amino acids. They can be divided in essential amino acids which the body cannot produce itself and non-essential amino acids which the body can manufacture itself. Complete proteins contain essential amino-acids whereas incomplete proteins do not contain essential amino acids. One gram of protein yields approximately four calories.

What are they used for?

Proteins are the main building blocks of the body and make up our muscles. They form enzymes and hormones which are the key to virtually all body functions. Last but not least amino acids are the basis of our genes and the underlying script of our individual genetic information. Proteins can also be used as an energy source but this is not very effective and may lead to muscle wasting. This is usually the body's last resource.

Examples: Complete proteins are derived from animal products such as meat, fish and milk. Incomplete proteins can be derived from vegetable sources such as grains, pulses and nuts.

What happens if I eat too many proteins?

Problems usually only occur if you eat excessive amounts or if the main organs which process proteins, i.e. the liver and the kidney, do not work properly. Then the body may get overloaded. Many protein products also contain saturated fat and may lead to weight gain and high cholesterol.

Which proteins should I eat?

Try to eat a varied diet of proteins which provide you with a source of essential amino acids. Even most vegetarian diets are suitable, but people eating a strict vegan diet may not get all amino acids they need. Try to stick to lean protein options such as fish, lean meat, skimmed or semi-skimmed milk or dairy products, and whole grains and pulses. Note that refined wheat and white rice are low in protein because the outer layer of the grain which contains the proteins is removed.

Eating a balanced diet: The British Food Standards Agency defines a balanced diet as a diet of varied foods. You find examples of recommend foods in the previous respective sections under the question which carbohydrates, fats and proteins should I eat.

The agency recommends (http://www.food.gov.uk/healthiereating/healthycatering/healthycatering02):

- basing the diet on starchy foods
- five portions of fruit and vegetables
- moderate amount of meats
- at least two portions of fish a week
- moderate amounts of dairy products
- replacing fats such as butter and margarine with vegetable oils whenever possible
- avoiding sugar
- limiting the daily intake of salt to no more than 6 grams

Watching your weight: Some of the recommended foods are not always good options if you want to slim down. For instance avocados and nuts have a low glycemic index and contain unsaturated fatty acids. Nevertheless, they are high in calories. For instance, one medium sized avocado has about 230 calories. That is as much as eating twelve tomatoes.

Avoid processed foods whenever you can but stick to the original food source. For instance, one serving of chips (French fries) (100g) has about 360 calories. This is as much as eating ten medium-sized boiled potatoes (500g).

Drinking well: Many patients with mental health problems always feel thirsty. Part of the problems may be medications leading to a dry mouth. However, drinks can have a lot of calories too.

Low calorie choices include:

- Water
- Tea and coffee (without sugar)
- Skimmed milk (in moderation)
- "Lite" diet soft drinks

Avoid:

- Alcohol
- Regular fizzy drinks
- Whole milk
- Smoothies

What about fruit juice?

It is usually better to eat the whole fruit rather than fruit juice. You may also feel less hungry if you eat the fruits rather than drinking the juice. One large glass of apple juice (300 ml) contains as many calories as three apples.

What about vitamins, trace elements and supplements?

Many people like to use supplements but very few people need them to correct a clear-cut deficiency having resulted in poor health. Most people who take supplements do so in the hope that these carry substantial health benefits, e.g. protecting against cancer, improving the immune system, and supporting mental health. However, scientific evidence about the benefits of supplements remains mostly ambiguous with a few exceptions. Note that supplements are not a substitute for a healthy balanced diet. If you decide to take a supplement do not exceed the recommended daily intake regarded as safe. If you are smoking do not take beta-carotene since the combination may increase your risk of cancer.

What are antioxidants?

Most processes in the body require oxygen. But oxygen can do good as well as harm such as damaging body cells. Antioxidants are substances which neutralize such harmful substances. They are contained in many vitamins such as vitamin A, C, and E and some trace elements such as selenium. They are contained in many fruits and vegetables such as oranges, strawberries, spinach, tomatoes, carrots, and broccoli just to name a few. Green tea is another good source of antioxidants. Selenium can be found in pasta, bread, eggs, poultry, beef, and some fish such as cod.

What about calcium?

Calcium is important to keep bones and teeth healthy. This is particularly important in people with mental health problems because some medications increase the risk of osteoporosis. Calcium may also be helpful to prevent or alleviate premenstrual stress. Good sources of calcium include milk, dairy products and fish such as sardines where the bones are eaten. Broccoli and kale also contains calcium. However, calcium can only work if it is combined with vitamin D. Good sources of vitamin D include oily fish, some cereals and eggs. Getting out and about and being exposed to sunlight is another good way to get vitamin D (as long as you take care not to burn).

The Royal College of Psychiatrists has produced a leaflet on supplements commonly suggested for mental health problems (http://mentalhealthuk.org/mentalhealthinfoforall/treatments/complementary therapy.aspx). You will find further about vitamin E, omega-3 fatty acids, selenium, folic acid and S-adenosylmethionine (SAME).

Diets for Mental Health Problems

What is the best diet for schizophrenia?

There is no specific schizophrenia diet but you should eat a balanced varied diet according to the above recommendations. Ensuring that you eat enough foods rich in omega-3 fatty acids seems a good idea. If you tend to gain weight or have experienced weight gain as a side effect of your medication you should try to eat "good carbs," i.e. carbohydrates with a low glycemic index, which are not easily broken down into glucose. Make sure that you also get calcium in your diet by including dairy products ideally based on skimmed milk to keep the fat intake down.

What is the best diet for mood disorders?

The same principles as above apply. Ensuring enough omega-3 fatty acids may help to keep your mood stable. If you take lithium you should not drink too many caffeine containing drinks such as tea and coffee since this may reduce your lithium levels. Some vegetables such as artichokes and celery may do the same if eaten in large amounts.

Selenium, folic acid (folate), and tryptophan are substances which have all been implicated in keeping one's mood stable.

Tryptophan is needed to make serotonin. However, it is not clear how good they are when taken as supplements and you should seek medical advice if you want to use such supplements. Particularly avoid taking too much selenium as this can lead to poisoning. Instead of using a supplement right away, you may try to eat a balanced diet which contains these substances in sufficient amounts.

Selenium is found in cereals, meats, fish and egg. Selenium is also found in Brazil nuts. These can be extremely rich in selenium so that one should only eat them occasionally. Folic acid can be found in cereals and breads which have been enriched with folic acid. This is also called fortified. Folic acid is also found in brown rice, leafy green vegetables, peas, and broccoli as well as orange juice and bananas. Finally tryptophan can be found in poultry, meats, some fish such as salmon and halibut and also bananas.

What about chocolate?

Chocolate contains tryptophan but dark chocolate is better than milk chocolate and is even thought to lower cholesterol. However, chocolate of whatever sort is high in calories and should only be eaten in small amounts.

What is the best diet for epilepsy?

A so-called ketogenic diet maybe of help in children with epilepsy which cannot be controlled. A ketogenic diets is a diet high in fat and low in carbohydrates. The most widely diet used of this type is the Atkins diet. Such a diet can be quite hard to sustain long term though. The idea of the ketogenic diet is to switch the main fuel of the brain from glucose (sugar) to ketones, which are produced when fat is broken down. Some adults who suffer from uncontrollable epilepsy may also benefit but research findings are much less clear. Seek specialist advice before going on such a diet.

What is the best diet for ADHD?

Again, there are no clear recommendations as research is only just developing in this area. Some research has shown that people with ADHD have lower levels of omega-3 fatty acids or may not be able to tolerate gluten. Gluten is a protein found in wheat, rye, and barley. Even the ketogenic diet has been suggested but findings are only based on animal experiments.

What about grapefruits and grapefruit juice?

Grapefruits are powerful stuff and they can change the way our body metabolizes medication. Particularly, grapefruits or grapefruit juice can significantly increase the concentration of many medications including some types of antidepressants, antipsychotics, and sedatives. Changes are more likely if grapefruits and grapefruit juice are consumed in large amounts but one cannot even exclude such changes on occasional use.

What about orthomolecular medicine?

Orthomolecular medicine aims at treating or preventing health problems, including mental health problems, through supplements and vitamins. Vitamins are often recommended in large doses, so-called megavitamins. Orthomolecular medicine remains controversial and very few studies have been conducted in this area. These largely suggest that orthomolecular medicine may not be helpful. Large doses of vitamins and supplements may be harmful or even toxic. That is why the Food Standard Agency has set recommended levels of daily intake for most vitamins and supplements.

Ten Tips to Eat Well on a Budget

Many people think that eating well costs a lot of money. However, eating well can be surprisingly cheap. Here are ten tips which may help you to eat well but cheaply.

1. Avoid ready meals and take-outs. They are often rich in fat and sugars and may not provide good value for money.

2. Avoid buying snacks such as crisps, ice creams, and sweets apart from the occasional treat.

3. Shop seasonal fruits and vegetables. For instance, oranges and bananas are winter fruits whereas strawberries and peaches

are summer fruits. Broccoli and parsnips are winter vegetables whereas and zucchinis (courgettes) and peppers are summer vegetables. Buying fruits and vegetables out of season can be expensive.

4. Buy fresh foods such as fruit, vegetables, and meats in small amounts and more often since they go bad easily.

5. Avoid canned foods if possible. For instance dried beans and pasta are less expensive than canned beans and processed pasta. Also canned fruits can be more expensive than seasonal fresh fruit but have fewer vitamins.

6. Avoid fizzy drinks and fruit juices. They are often quite expensive. Use water and fruit instead.

7. Compare prices in local shops and supermarkets and take advantage of special offers.

8. Use generic supermarket brands instead of classic brands. They often contain the same ingredients but are cheaper.

9. Cook and eat together with others and share the costs.

10. Make a shopping list and plan your food budget every week. If you feel you cannot do this on your own, ask for help. For instance a key worker may be able to help.

Section 3.2

Sleep and Mental Health

"A good day starts with a good night sleep."—Mansoor Ahmed, M.D., F.A.A.S.M.

We may not have a clear understanding of the functions of sleep, but its importance and its impact on our daytime mood and mental functionality becomes apparent when we actually don't sleep. Or have a disturbed sleep. More than any other specialty, there is a profound link between sleep, cognition, and psychiatry. This may be due to the fact that cognition, mood, and sleep-wake share many structural mechanistic pathways. Sleep disturbances are in fact so common in psychiatric illnesses that they are considered to be an integral component of diagnostic criteria for many these conditions. Furthermore, as compared to general population, co-morbid sleep disorders, such obstructive sleep apnea (OSA), restless legs syndrome (RLS), and circadian rhythm disorders appear to be more common in patients with psychiatric conditions. These sleep disorders have serious multisystem consequences, including mental health and cognitive symptoms. If they remain unrecognized and untreated, these disorders may result in further worsening of sleep and psychiatric conditions. Recognizing the fact that sleep is important for mental health and that sleep disturbances are fairly common in patients with psychiatric disorders, a close collaboration between sleep and psychiatric healthcare providers is critical for optimum management of these conditions.

Interest in behavior, sleep, and dreaming has existed since the dawn of the history. From Hippocrates and Aristotle to Freud, including other great thinkers, many have attempted to unravel the mechanism of sleep and psychological basis of dreaming. The most important of all discoveries related to sleep was the recognition that sleep is not simply a uniform state of unresponsiveness as it was thought for centuries.

In 1953–55, Dr. Nathaniel Klietman and his fellow, Dr. Charles De-
ment, demonstrated sleep as a cyclic phenomenon alternating between
non-rapid eye movement (NREM) and rapid eye movement (REM) sleep.
REM sleep, also known as paradoxical or active sleep, occurs when the
EEG pattern shows an active mind while body muscles are temporarily paralyzed. Much earlier Freud also noted muscle paralysis during
sleep that hindered dreamers from acting out their dreams. REM sleep
appears to play an important role in memory consolidation and affects
regulation, including the emotional tone related to past events. NREM
sleep is divided into light sleep and slow wave sleep, also known as delta
sleep. Slow wave sleep appears to play a role in recuperation of central
nervous system (CNS) and certain memory domains.

The discovery of REM and NREM sleep in 1953 was the beginning
of the modern era of sleep research and sleep medicine as a discipline.
It is becoming clear that sleep medicine is truly a multidisciplinary science. There is hardly any medical, mental, or psychiatric condition that
doesn't affect sleep, and there is hardly any system physiology that is
not affected by sleep and sleep disorders. For example, in obstructive
sleep apnea (OSA) repeated disturbances in gas exchange, autonomic
system changes, and the sleep fragmentation that accompany apnea
affect multiple physiological systems leading to metabolic and cardiovascular abnormalities and neuropsychiatric symptoms. A significant
majority of patients evaluated at the sleep clinic exhibit frequent symptoms of psychopathology, which may or may not be due to psychiatric
illness. Research and clinical evidence concerning the association of
sleep disorders with psychiatric problems is growing quickly. Sleep is
now recognized by psychiatrists and psychologists as the neurobiological
substrate for many emotional and behavioral disorders. Even a simple
loss of sleep (i.e., sleep restriction) can trigger maniac episodes in vulnerable patients with underlying bipolar mood disorders. Conversely,
sleep restriction under proper circumstances, has been shown to improve
mood in patients with depression. Data from a large number of studies
examining neurobiological mechanisms provide strong evidence that
sleep, circadian rhythm control, and mood share many common neuro-
circuitries and neurotransmitters. This may explain the fact that several
psychiatric disorders have prominent sleep symptoms.

Not only are sleep disturbances such as insomnia and non-
restorative sleep quite common in many psychiatric disorders, but they
may actually precede the development and diagnosis of a psychiatric
disorder. Furthermore, studies have shown the presence of persistent
sleep disturbances, such as insomnia, despite apparent improvement
in underlying primary psychiatric condition. The presence of persistent

insomnia in patients with major depression receiving treatment, suggests a poor prognostic value including an increased risk of suicide.

Despite the fact that sleep disorders are common, with profound negative implications on psychiatric illnesses, sleep disorders may remain undiagnosed, despite the relative ease of diagnosis in many cases.

On many occasions, physicians who have exhausted all routine laboratory tests and medical interventions in an effort to diagnose and treat a patient with undiscovered sleep problems refer the patient to a psychiatrist. In a study by S. Mosko and colleagues, 66.5% of 206 patients evaluated at sleep center reported one episode of major depression in the previous five years and 25.7% described themselves as depressed on presentation. Additional studies have established substantial risk of developing major depression and generalized anxiety in patients with sleep disorders.

Despite strong mechanistic and clinical links between sleep and psychopathology, current clinical practices of both sleep medicine and psychiatry lack optimal collaboration. Also it is only since 1996 that the American Medical Association has recognized sleep medicine as a specialty. Perhaps this may also explain a lack of or delay in clinical integration between sleep, psychiatry, and other medical disciplines. A close integration is, therefore, very much needed to optimize the clinical care of patients who have either underlying primary sleep or psychiatric disorders.

The following material briefly summarizes the clinical data on the nature of sleep disturbances in psychiatric disorders. This review also provides some practical basic guidelines on how to recognize presence of common sleep disorders and the beneficial role of appropriate sleep therapies on mood and psychiatric symptoms. (The effects of psychotherapeutic agents on sleep are beyond the scope of this review.)

Primary Psychiatric and Behavioral Disorders and Effects on Sleep and Daytime Wakefulness

Sleep in Anxiety Disorders

Anxiety disorders are among the most common of mental disorders. Many patients with general anxiety disorder (GAD) (44%), posttraumatic stress disorder (PTSD), and panic disorder (61%) suffer from insomnia. Difficulty falling or maintaining sleep or non-restorative sleep is one of the six features used to establish the diagnosis of GAD. Furthermore, daytime irritability and fatigue can be considered a consequence of sleep disturbances.

Patients with panic disorders have poor sleep efficiency and reduced total sleep time. Panic attacks emerging from sleep (during NREM) are reported in 50% of patents.

PTSD patients suffer from a myriad of severe sleep problems characterized by insomnia and nightmares. Polysomnography (PSG) evaluation usually reveals fragmented sleep, frequent arousals, and reduced slow wave sleep. REM sleep abnormalities may include increased REM sleep latency, disrupted REM sleep continuity, and higher REM density including increased eye movement frequency. Abnormal behavior during sleep such as shouting, yelling, and dream enactment is commonly observed. Nightmares, predominantly emerging from REM sleep, occur in up to 90% of PTSD patients. These nocturnal sleep disturbances may also contribute to daytime somatic symptoms

Besides the underlying psychiatric conditions and associated changes in sleep-arousal mechanisms, other unrelated, sleep disorders including restless legs syndrome (RLS) and periodic leg movements during sleep (PLMS) and circadian misalignment can further contribute and aggravate pre-existing sleep disturbances in these individuals.

It is important to note that certain selective serotonin receptor inhibitors (SSRI) and serotonin norepinephrine receptor inhibitors (SNRI) commonly used to treat anxiety disorders, can also contribute to the pathogenesis of RLS/PLMS conditions. Similarly, underlying OSA can result in sleep maintenance insomnia. Some studies have shown an increased incidence of OSA in patients with PTSD. Ironically under these circumstances, utilization of hypnotics, a common clinical practice, may not have any effect on insomnia and may even aggravate it.

On many occasions, maladaptive cognitive behavior, such as fear of insomnia, provokes bedroom anxiety may further exacerbate insomnia. Many of these patients also develop the habit of looking at the clock repeatedly which further aggravates underlying anxiety and frustration as well as insomnia.

Mood Disorders

Major depression and bipolar disorders are prevalent, and associated disability is one of the highest reported for any disease, second only to ischemic cardiac disease. These disorders are commonly associated with sleep disturbances, and these disturbances are part of the diagnostic criteria.

In a majority of the patients with mood disorders, insomnia and sleep disturbance may exist for years before the diagnosis of depression is established. Furthermore, subjective and objective sleep disturbance such as the REM parameters may persist even during a period of clinical remission and herald poor prognosis.

Although insomnia is the most common symptom, hypersomnolence sometimes manifests itself as a symptom of depression. Cyclic insomnia and hypersomnolence can be a clue to an underlying bipolar mood disorder. Objective sleep evaluation by PSG has been studied more extensively than any other psychiatric disorder, and most patients have shown non-specific objective changes.

The sleep parameter changes include: 1) Disturbed sleep continuity including delayed sleep onset, frequent awakening, and early morning awakening; 2) reduced slow wave sleep; and 3) REM sleep abnormalities, particularly reduced REM latency and increased REM density (i.e., increased rate of rapid eye movement during REM sleep). There may be evidence that duration of the depressive episode may correlate with the degree of observed sleep abnormalities.

Schizophrenia

Schizophrenia is a disorder of thought and cognitive impairment and considered as the most devastating neuropsychiatric illness. Underlying sleep disturbances can be severe and include profound insomnia and reversal of the sleep-wake cycle. A clinically stable patient on treatment may continue to have early and middle of the night insomnia. Sleep architecture in those patients is characterized by poor sleep efficiency and difficulty in achieving persistent sleep. Unlike depression, no specific abnormalities in REM sleep have been found in schizophrenia these patients.

Attention Deficit Hyperactivity Disorder (ADHD)

Insomnia is frequently reported in ADHD. Besides sleep disturbances related to ADHD, other comorbid conditions can result in insufficient and poor quality sleep, such as OSA, RLS, and delayed sleep phase syndrome (DSPS), potentially aggravating the ADHD symptoms.

It is of utmost importance to carefully tease out the potential problems affecting sleep before confirming or rejecting the diagnosis of ADHD. Sleep disturbances disrupt the attention and arousal mechanisms, presumably by perturbations in neurotransmitter pathways, notably noradrenergic and dopaminergic pathways. Successful implementation of strategies to address the underlying issues causing sleep disturbances help with improvement in sleep and potentially helps with daytime neurobehavioral symptoms.

Primary Sleep Disorders and Relationship to Mood-Psychiatric Illness

There are more than 80 recognized sleep disorders. Many of these sleep disorders are associated with a higher incidence of anxiety and depression. Some common sleep disorders such as OSA, RLS, and circadian disorders appear to be more prevalent in patients with psychiatric conditions. These sleep disorders have serious multisystem consequences including mental health and cognitive symptoms. If they remain unrecognized and untreated, these disorders may result in further worsening of sleep and psychiatric conditions.

Obstructive Sleep Apnea (OSA)

Sleep apnea is a serious and most common sleep disorder affecting 12 million Americans. A majority of the OSA sufferers remains undiagnosed. This condition is far more common in obese individuals with hypertension—particularly resistant hypertension—diabetes, and congestive heart failure. In general, OSA is characterized by loud snoring and repeated episodes of breathing cessation during sleep resulting in sleep fragmentation and non-restorative sleep. The resulting daytime consequences include: a) sleepiness, fatigue, other neuro-cognitive abnormalities; b) increased risk of hypertension and stroke; and c) metabolic abnormalities.

Patients with depression as well as OSA appear worse off than those with OSA only. Depressive symptoms persist in at least some patients in short-term studies of treatment for OSA. Direct treatment of depression in OSA might improve acceptance of therapy, reduce sleepiness and fatigue, and improve quality of life

OSA: Important Facts

- An estimated 12 million Americans suffer from sleep-disordered breathing.

- Sleep apnea causes daytime sleepiness in an estimated 1 out of 25 (4 percent) middle aged men and 1 out of 50 (2 percent) middle aged women.

- Up to 93 percent of women and 82 percent of men with signs and symptoms of moderate-to-severe sleep-disordered breathing remain undiagnosed.

- The symptoms of sleep-disordered breathing (such as snoring) are more likely to be reported by men than women.

- Women are much more likely to develop sleep apnea after menopause.

- African Americans, Hispanics, and Pacific Islanders are more likely to develop sleep apnea than Caucasians.

- The risk of sleep apnea increases with age. At least 1 out of 10 people over the age of 65 suffers from sleep apnea.

- More than half of people with sleep apnea are overweight.

Restless Legs Syndrome (RLS) and Periodic Leg Movements during Sleep (PLMS)

Sleep disturbance due to RLS and PLMS can lead to daytime sleepiness, anxiety or depression, and confusion or slowed thought processes. PLMS always coexists with RLS, but may occur independent of RLS. Most often RLS occurs in middle-aged and older adults. Idiopathic RLS can occur at a young age as well. RLS is always more severe during the evening hours and at night; in more severe cases, it can also occur during daytime. Other common symptoms include creepy crawly sensations in legs (arms and whole body can be involved) with an urge to move, usually when sitting or lying down. Moving legs or walking relieves the symptoms at least temporarily.

Once diagnosed, treatment for the condition is available and can be very effective.

Circadian Rhythm Disorders

These disorders are commonly termed as disruptions in the internal biological clock. Such disruptions can either be advanced or delayed phase. In delayed sleep phase disorder (DPSD), where the sufferers are also called "night owls," people are unable to sleep until very late in the night or early morning hours. DPSD is more common in children and adolescents. Whereas, those with advanced sleep phase disorder (ASPD) fall asleep in the early evening hours, resulting in early morning awakening—as early as midnight to 2:00 a.m. ASPD is more commonly seen in the elderly.

In both situations, the circadian mismatch can have a negative impact on school and work performance, as well as having social consequences.

Narcolepsy and Other Sleep Disorders of Hypersomnolence

Although narcolepsy is not a common sleep disorder, it can be extremely debilitating for sufferers. The same can be said about hypersomnia, whether it is the result of narcolepsy or due to other sleep disorders or underlying psychiatric disorders.

Section 3.3

Physical Activity and Mental Health

Introduction

Exercise keeps our hearts and bodies healthy. But how?

We often talk about the mind and body as though they are completely separate—but they aren't. The mind can't function unless your body is working properly—but it also works the other way. The state of your mind affects your body.

So—if you feel low or anxious, you may do less and become less active—which can make you feel worse. You can get caught in a harmful cycle.

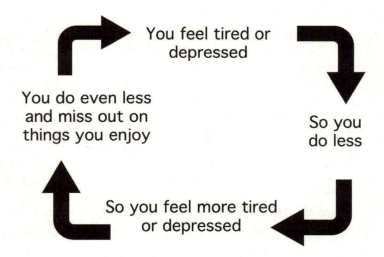

Figure 3.1. *A Harmful Cycle.*

Why bother with exercise?

To work properly, your body needs regular exercise—and most of us feel good when we are active.

Until the last 100 years or so, you had to be quite active to just live your everyday life. Now, in modern Western societies, so much of what we used to do is done by machines. We drive cars, so we walk less, vacuum cleaners make cleaning easy, and washing is done by a machine. At work we may not even have to move around in the office—it's enough to sit at the computer. It doesn't help that modern high-energy foods make us put on too much weight—or that, (in the West at least) food has never been cheaper or easier to buy.

So how can you start to get more active, day to day? You may be turned off by the word *exercise* because:

- I've never done it.
- I wasn't good at sports at school.
- I would feel silly.
- Other people would make fun of me.
- It won't help unless it hurts: "No pain, no gain."
- It's sweaty and uncomfortable.
- I'm too tired.
- I would rather do something else.
- It's expensive.
- I think it will make me feel worse.
- I don't have anyone to do it with.
- I don't know where, when, or how to start.

But—it doesn't have to be about running around a track or working out in a gym. It can just be about being more active each day—perhaps just walking more, or taking the stairs rather than the lift. If medical problems stop you from doing one thing, there may be others that you can do.

What happens if you don't do very much?

Some people can get away with doing very little and live to a ripe old age—but most of us can't. Broadly speaking, the less you do, the more likely you are to end up with:

- low mood/depression;
- tension and worry.

If you keep active, you are:
- less likely to be depressed, anxious or tense;
- more likely to feel good about yourself;
- more likely to concentrate and focus better;
- more likely to sleep better;
- more likely to cope with cravings and withdrawal symptoms if you try to give up a habit such as smoking or alcohol;
- more likely to be able to keep mobile and independent as you get older;
- possibly less likely to have problems with memory and dementia.

So—don't worry about not doing enough—get started by building a bit more physical activity into your daily life now. Even a small change can boost your morale, give you a sense of achievement, and help you to feel better in yourself.

What might work for me?

Activity should:
- Be enjoyable—if you don't know what you might enjoy, try a few different things.
- Help you to feel more competent, or capable. Gardening or DIY projects can do this, as well getting you more active.
- Give you a sense of control over your life—that you have choices you can make (so it isn't helpful if you start to feel that you have to exercise). The sense that you are looking after yourself can also feel good.
- Help you to escape for a while from the pressures of life.
- Be shared. The companionship involved can be just as important as the physical activity.

Why does exercise work?

We are not yet exactly sure. There are several possibilities:
- Most people in the world have always had to keep active to get food, water, and shelter. This involves a moderate level of

activity and seems to make us feel good. We may be built—or "hard wired"—to enjoy a certain amount of exercise. Harder exercise (perhaps needed to fight or flight from danger) seems to be linked to feelings of stress, perhaps because it is needed for escaping from danger.

- Exercise seems to have an effect on certain chemicals in the brain, like dopamine and serotonin. Brain cells use these chemicals to communicate with each other, so they affect your mood and thinking.

- Exercise can stimulate other chemicals in the brain called *brain derived neurotrophic factors*. These help new brain cells to grow and develop. Moderate exercise seems to work better than vigorous exercise.

- Exercise seems to reduce harmful changes in the brain caused by stress.

How much exercise is enough for me?

- Firstly—any exercise is better than none.

- BUT a moderate level of exercise seems to work best.

- This is roughly equivalent to walking fast, but being able to talk to someone at the same time.

- You need to do about 30 minutes of moderate physical exercise on at least five days of every week. This can be done in one 30-minute session or broken up into shorter 10- or 15-minute sessions.

- This can not only lower the risk of heart disease, diabetes, and cancer, but also seems to help depression—so you get a double benefit.

- Don't start suddenly—build more physical activity into your life gradually, in small steps.

When should I exercise?

As regularly as you can. There will be days when you just don't feel like exercise—you may feel tired or be too busy or anxious about something. If you keep to your routine and exercise at times like this, you will almost certainly feel better. Why?

If you are tired, exercise tends to give you energy. If you are worried, it can take your mind off your concerns for a while. Even if you can't "exercise," a 15-minute walk can help you to clear your mind and relax. You may find it helpful to listen to music at the same time.

It's best not to do too much in the evening. Being active will generally help you to sleep but, if you exercise late in the evening, you may find it difficult to settle.

Eating and energy levels: Caffeine and high energy snacks will boost your energy quickly—but after an hour or so you will probably feel more tired than you did before. A short walk will boost your energy level for much longer.

Exercise and coping: If you are active you will probably find it easier to deal with life's problems and challenges. So, if those problems stop you from regularly exercising, it's worth remembering that finding time for exercise may well help you to deal with such problems.

Exercise can also help you to cope better by improving how you feel about yourself and getting you together with other people.

How well does exercise work for depression?

For mild depression, physical activity can be as good as antidepressants or psychological treatments like cognitive behavioral therapy (CBT).

It can certainly be harder to get active when you are depressed. But being active lifts your mood and gives you a sense of being in control and in touch with other people.

In some areas in the UK, GPs (family doctors) can prescribe exercise.

What's the downside?

Not much. If you are normally very active, you may get depressed if, for any length of time, you can't exercise because of an injury. If this does happen, you can carry on with exercises using those parts of your body that are not injured. This will help you to keep fit, feel more in control, and keep in touch with other people. It can help to set yourself targets—both for the next few days and longer, for the next weeks or months.

Some people with eating disorders use exercise to lose too much weight.

Some athletes (such as those in weight-related sports like horse racing, boxing, and gymnastics) are more likely to develop eating disorders.

Physical exercise can cause injuries and some health problems—but you are much more likely to get ill if you don't keep active. If in doubt, ask your doctor.

Getting Down to It

Any physical activity needs to be something that you can do regularly. But lots of things can stop you, especially if you feel depressed. You may feel that you:

- don't have the energy;
- don't feel confident enough;
- don't know anybody to exercise with;
- don't have the right clothes;
- can't afford it;
- just aren't the "exercise or sporty type";
- won't feel any different for doing it.

Exercise can be about playing sport or doing hard-core exercise—if you want that. For other people, it is just about being more physically active and sitting around less. It doesn't have to be hard—but try to do something every day.

Some things aren't expensive—walking is free and jogging just needs a pair of trainers (cheap ones are fine). If you have a bike already, try cycling to work (or for any regular journey)—you may even save some money.

But Don't Overdo It!

If you haven't been active for a while, doing too much when you start can make you more tired—particularly if you also have a health problem (including depression) that makes you tired. One day you may have the energy to be really active but feel completely exhausted the next.

Whatever you choose to do, start with something easy—like walking round the block. Build your level up gradually, perhaps by just doing a minute or two more—or a few meters more—each day. Try to do something most days, even if you feel tired.

Start by working out how much you do already—you can use a pedometer to show you how many steps you take every day. Or you could keep a diary for a few days of how long you spend doing active things. Then set yourself some goals. Make sure they are:

- **S:** Specific (clear)
- **M:** Measurable—you will know when you've achieved them

53

- **A:** Achievable—you can achieve them
- **R:** Relevant—they mean something to you
- **T:** Time-based—you set yourself a time limit to achieve your goals.

They need to be things you can see yourself doing—and take pride in, so you feel good about yourself. You may be able to do it on your own or with some help from others.

Nobody's perfect. You will have setbacks when you can't meet a short term goal, or just feel too tired to do anything. Recognize it when it happens, but don't worry about it. Tomorrow is another day and short term setbacks don't matter in the bigger picture of your longer-term goals. And, if you need to, do ask someone else to give you a hand.

References

Management of depression in primary and secondary care. National Institute for Clinical Excellence (NICE), 2004.

Taylor AH & Faulkner, G (2008). Inaugural Editorial. *Mental Health and Physical Activity*, vol 1, issue 1, pages 1–8. A new academic journal with a specific focus on the relationship between physical activity and mental health. www.elsevier.com/wps/find/journaldescription .cws_home/714078/description#description

Thayer RE. *Calm Energy: How people regulate mood with food and exercise*. Oxford University Press, New York 2001.

Section 3.4

Keeping Mentally Fit As You Age

Today, thoughts of aging gracefully have been replaced by efforts to age successfully. As we age and look forward to longer life expectancies than past generations, we strive to age with good health. How do we do this? By eating nutritiously. Limiting alcohol. Keeping physically active. Staying connected with our friends and family. Seeking medical treatment when necessary. These are the right steps toward healthy aging. And with good health, we can enjoy life and pursue new dreams and endeavors as we age.

Good health includes both physical and mental well-being. And the two go hand in hand. A healthy mind contributes to a healthy body. The mind, like the body, benefits from low blood pressure, low cholesterol, nourishing food, a healthy weight, and physical activity.

There are many healthy lifestyle choices we can make to keep our bodies healthy and avoid illness and disability. There are additional steps we can take to help preserve healthy minds.

What changes in mental abilities can we expect as we age? What's normal?

As we age, we can expect certain changes in our bodies and minds. We may not see and hear as well as we did in our 20s. We may not be able to remember recent events or details as well or as quickly as we did in our 30s. Beginning in our 30s, our brain's weight, the network of nerves, and its blood flow begin to decrease. Our brains adapt, however, and grow new patterns of nerve endings.

While certain changes in our mental abilities are inevitable as we age, much remains the same. We retain our intellect. Our ability to change and be flexible remains. Old dogs can learn new tricks. We just might need a little more time. We keep our ability to grow intellectually and emotionally.

55

What can I do to keep my mind healthy?

For the last several years, new research has emerged that shows there are many things we can do to keep our minds healthy. Many of the same things we do to keep our bodies healthy contribute to healthy minds. Physical activity and a diet that helps lower cholesterol levels and blood pressure also helps to keep our minds healthy by allowing our bodies to deliver oxygen-rich blood to our brains. In addition, activities that stimulate our minds, like crossword puzzles, reading, writing, and learning new things, help to keep our brains healthy. Staying engaged with the people around us and our communities plays an equally big part in staying mentally fit.

Following are some specific recommendations to keep a healthy mind and ward off mental health problems.

Be physically active. The benefits are numerous. Being physically active helps prevent bone density loss, maintain balance, and ward off illnesses (like heart disease, stroke, and some cancers). For some, illness and disability can bring on or contribute to mental illness. For example, those who live with diabetes, cancer, and heart disease can also suffer from depression.

Regular physical activity helps to:

- Maintain and improve memory
- Maintain and improve mental ability
- Prevent dementia (impaired intellectual functioning) including Alzheimer's disease
- Make us happy and prevent and alleviate depression
- Improve energy levels

How does exercise do all that? Physical activity—whether it's walking, running, swimming, dancing (we have a lot of choices)—helps to:

- Decrease heart rate
- Decrease blood pressure
- Decrease blood cholesterol
- Strengthen the heart and increase the flow of oxygen to the brain
- Improve reaction time
- Improve mobility

If you are thinking about starting an exercise program, talk first with your doctor. Start slowly, take proper precautions (for example, walk in well-lit areas in sturdy shoes), and have fun. Remember, you don't have to be athletic to benefit from regular physical activity.

Keep blood pressure down. Blood pressure below 120/80 mmHg is considered healthy and helps reduce the risk of stroke, which is tied to dementia including Alzheimer's disease. High blood pressure damages blood vessels, which increases one's risk of stroke, kidney failure, heart disease, and heart attack. Nearly two-thirds of adults over age 65 have high blood pressure, 140/90 mmHg or higher. Those with blood pressure between 120/80 mmHg and 139/89 mmHg are considered to have prehypertension, which means that while the blood pressure is not too high, they are likely to develop it in the future. To reduce or keep blood pressure at a healthy level, keep your weight down, don't smoke, exercise regularly, eat a healthy diet, and limit salt, alcohol, and caffeine.

Keep your cholesterol levels low. High blood cholesterol is a risk factor for heart disease as well as dementia. The higher your blood cholesterol level, the greater your chance of disease and illness. An excess of cholesterol (a fat-like substance) in your blood can build up on the walls of your arteries. This causes them to harden and narrow, which slows down and can block blood flow. A blood cholesterol level of less than 200 mg/dL is considered healthy, 200–239 mg/dL is borderline high, and 240 mg/dL and above is high. Heredity, age, and gender can affect cholesterol levels. Cholesterol rises with age and women's levels tend to rise beginning after menopause. Healthy changes to diet, weight, and physical activity can help improve blood cholesterol levels.

Eat your vegetables... and more. We've heard it all our lives, the good advice to eat our vegetables. The same diet that can help us stay strong and healthy provides the nutrition necessary for a healthy brain. It starts with a diet rich in fruits and vegetables, whole grains, and nonfat dairy products. Experiment and find out how you best like to eat the good things that your entire body needs. There's an endless variety to suit every taste.

Some specific dietary recommendations for a healthy brain

Folate is a B vitamin found in foods such as spinach and asparagus. Folic acid is the synthetic form used in supplements and fortified foods. Folate is necessary for the health of our cells, and helps to prevent anemia and changes to DNA (the building blocks of cells) that could lead to cancer. Folate is also necessary to maintain normal levels of homocysteine, an amino acid in the blood. Good sources of folate and folic acid include fortified breakfast cereals, dark-green leafy vegetables, asparagus, strawberries, beans, and beef liver.

The vitamins E and C are important antioxidants found in foods that help guard against cell damage and may reduce the risk of cancer and heart disease. While there's no conclusive evidence, vitamins E and C may help boost mental ability and prevent dementia.

For adults, the recommended dietary allowance (RDA) of vitamin E is 15 milligrams per day from foods. Foods naturally rich in vitamin E include nuts, such as almonds, vegetable oils, seeds, wheat germ, spinach, and other dark-green leafy vegetables.

The RDA of vitamin C for adults is 75 milligrams per day for women and 90 milligrams per day for men. Vitamin C is found in oranges, grapefruits, asparagus, Brussels sprouts, broccoli, bell peppers, collard greens, cabbage, cauliflower, kale, potatoes, spinach, and turnip greens.

Monitor your medication use. Be sure to read labels and carefully follow your physician's instructions. Some medications come with certain precautions such as avoiding alcohol or not combining with other medications, even over-the-counter drugs and herbal remedies. Some memory loss, some forms of dementia, and other problems of the brain can be traced back to harmful drug combinations or inappropriate drug use.

Drink moderately. If you don't drink, don't start. If you do drink, limit yourself to no more than one drink a day if you are over the age of 65 and do not have a drinking problem. One drink is 12 ounces of beer, 1.5 ounces of distilled spirits, or 5 ounces of wine.

Give up smoking. If you are a smoker, don't wait until you are debilitated by a serious disease before considering quitting. Smoking significantly increases one's chance of having a stroke and developing lung and other cancers, emphysema, chronic bronchitis, chronic obstructive pulmonary disease (COPD), heart attacks, and peripheral vascular disease.

According to the American Lung Association, when an older person quits smoking, circulation improves immediately and lungs begin to heal. After one year, the additional risk of heart disease caused by smoking is cut almost in half, and the risk of stroke, lung disease, and cancer decreases.

Maintain a healthy weight. People who are obese or overweight are at increased risk for heart disease, high blood pressure, diabetes, arthritis-related disabilities, and some cancers. The health risks of being overweight include high blood pressure, high cholesterol, heart disease, and stroke. Being underweight also carries risks including poor memory and decreased immunity. Ask your health care provider how much you should weigh and for suggestions on reaching that weight. Whatever your weight, a healthy diet and regular exercise will only improve your overall health.

Take care of your teeth by brushing and flossing and seeing your dentist regularly. Recent studies have linked chronic inflammation caused by gum disease to a number of health problems, including Alzheimer's disease and heart disease. So, take care of your teeth not only to maintain a dazzling smile and the ability to chew your favorite foods but also to ward off disease.

Keep mentally fit. Just as we exercise our bodies to keep them in working order, so must we exercise our brains to stay mentally agile and adept. It's the use-it-or-lose-it theory. By engaging in mentally stimulating activities, we can maintain our brain functions as we age. We can continue to grow new connections among the billions of brain cells we possess by learning new things. This activity may help to ward off dementia like Alzheimer's disease. So, work out your brain daily. Stimulate new areas of your brain and grow more connections among brain cells by intellectually challenging yourself. Solve a puzzle, learn a new musical instrument, read a challenging book, play a board or card game, attend a lecture or play, or write a short story.

Reduce stress. Just as stress can wear our bodies down and increase blood pressure and the risk of heart disease, it can also affect the way we think, our moods, and ability to remember. In fact, the hormones our bodies release when we are under stress may shrink the brain, affecting memory and learning. Stress can also cause or contribute to depression and anxiety.

- To deal with stress, first identify its causes and determine what changes you can make to avoid it. For example, if rush-hour traffic is causing you stress, time your driving or change your route to avoid heavy traffic. If party planning and gift buying during the holidays overwhelm you, simplify and concentrate on those aspects you really look forward to, like getting together with friends and family.

- Talk it out. Sometimes talking through your stress with a friend or therapist, or even writing in a journal, helps to put things in perspective.

- Relax. Whether it's by taking walks, playing golf, hitting a tennis ball, or meditating, find ways to release your stress and take a break.

- Get moving. Physical activity on most days of the week helps our bodies keep mental stress in check.

- Give yourself a break. If you must live with a stressful situation, take mini-vacations. Whether it's 20 minutes or several days, take time to relax and enjoy the things and people you find pleasurable.

Protect your brain. A history of head injury or loss of consciousness can affect the health of your brain. Falls are the leading cause of brain injury in the elderly, according to the Brain Injury Association of America. Takes steps to protect your head and the precious matter inside.

- To avoid falls, exercise regularly to improve your balance.

- Clear your home of hazards like clutter on the floor. Make sure you have proper lighting.

- In the car, wear your seatbelt. Ask someone else to drive in situations where you are not as comfortable as you once were, such as nighttime driving or driving in bad weather.

- On your bike, wear a helmet.

- When walking or running, wear proper shoes with good support and stay in well-lit areas.

- If your balance seems a bit unsteady, talk to your doctor about any medications you may be taking.

Stay socially connected. The support we receive from our friends, family, and colleagues helps maintain our mental health. Studies have shown that those who are engaged with family and community groups take longer to show the symptoms of Alzheimer's disease than those who are socially isolated. So stay or become connected. Join a book club or a volunteer group and interact with the world around you.

Look on the bright side. A positive outlook and emotions contribute to a healthy mind and body. Focus on the good in the world and the activities and people that make you happy.

Stay connected spiritually. If nurturing your spiritual side has had meaning for you, keep up that aspect of your life. Those with a strong faith often find support and comfort from their beliefs and their community. So whatever your religious or spiritual beliefs, stay connected. This connection can help prevent and relieve depression and may guard against dementia.

How can I help my memory?

- Don't expect to remember everything. In today's busy world, we're all overloaded with information. When necessary, use lists, calendars, reminders, and other memory aides. For example, write down appointments on your calendar and keep a list of chores in your pocket.

- Develop routines to help you remember. Take medicines the same time every day. Leave your keys in the same place.

- Visual memory tends to be better than auditory memory. That is, it's easier to remember what we see than what we hear. Using both at the same time will enhance memory. For example, if you need to pick up fruit at the grocery store, picture blueberries in the produce isle.

- Associating stories with new things or ideas is also helpful.

- Increasing attention improves learning and memory. When learning something new, limit the distractions (turn off the TV and choose a quiet room), and focus your attention.

- More time helps learning and recall. Allow yourself additional time and have patience.

What's not normal as we get older? What might indicate an illness?

While some forgetfulness is normal in older age, persistent memory loss is not. And because we experience more loss as we age (family members who move away, the death of loved ones), we are bound to experience more sadness. However, prolonged periods of sadness or depression are not normal as we age.

If you experience any of the following warning signs listed below, or notice that an older relative or friend is experiencing any of these, seek help. Older adults can first start by talking to friends or loved ones, and find help from their family physician, internist, psychiatrist, or geriatric psychiatrist, to name just a few professionals who can provide assistance.

Warning Signs

The following are not normal characteristics of aging and can indicate an illness. Discuss these symptoms with your physician.

- Depressed mood or sadness lasting longer than two weeks

- Unexplained crying spells

- Loss of interest or pleasure in the things and people that were previously enjoyable

- Jumpiness or tiredness, lethargy, fatigue, or loss of energy

- Irritability, quarrelsomeness

- Loss or increase in appetite or weight change

- Sleep change such as insomnia (not being able to sleep) or sleeping more than usual

- Feelings of worthlessness, inappropriate guilt, hopelessness, helplessness

- Decreased ability to think, concentrate, or make decisions

- Repeated thoughts of death or suicide, suicide attempts—Seek help from a medical professional immediately.

- Aches and pains, constipation, or other physical problems that cannot otherwise be explained

- Confusion and disorientation

- Memory loss, loss of recent, short-term memory

- Social withdrawal

- Trouble handling finances, working with numbers, paying the bills

- Change in appearance, standard of dress

- Problems maintaining the home, the yard

What might trigger or contribute to mental illness?

- Physical disability

- Physical illness

  - With diseases of the heart and lungs, the brain may not get enough oxygen, which affects mental ability and behavior.

- Diseases of the adrenal, thyroid, pituitary, or other glands can affect emotions, perceptions, memory, and thought processes
- A change in environment such as moving into a new home
- Loss or illness of a loved one
- A combination of medications
    - On average, older adults take more medications than others. Because our metabolism slows down as we age, drugs can remain longer in an older person and reach toxic levels more quickly
- Drug-alcohol interactions can cause confusion, mood changes, symptoms of dementia
- Alcohol or drug abuse and misuse
- Poor diet
    - Dental problems can contribute to a poor diet. Some older adults may avoid foods that are difficult to chew.

If I suspect a problem, what should I do?

- Talk with your physician. Explain how you feel and describe what is not normal for you. Have a list of all medications, and vitamin, mineral, and herbal supplements.
- Talk to a trusted friend, family member, or spiritual advisor.

Talking with Your Doctor, Pharmacist, or Other Health Care Providers

- Have a list of all medications, herbal remedies, and vitamin, mineral, and herbal supplements.
- Don't be shy or embarrassed. Explain how you feel.
- Ask questions. Take a list and pencil if necessary.
- Remind your doctors and pharmacist about your medical history.
- Ask for advice and instructions in clear writing, free of medical jargon.
- Ask for a follow-up visit if all your questions cannot be answered during your appointment.
- If you have questions once at home, don't hesitate to phone your doctor.

Chapter 4

Developing and Reinforcing Mental Wellness

Chapter Contents

Section 4.1

Becoming More Resilient

Resilience means being able to adapt to adversity, to bounce back, having the ability to roll with the punches. When we are resilient, we use inner strengths to rebound quicker from misfortune and setbacks—whether it's job loss, illness, natural disaster, or the loss of a loved one.

In contrast, when lacking in resilience, we tend to dwell on the problem, feel victimized, become overwhelmed, and turn to unhealthy coping mechanisms like substance abuse. We may even develop mental illness problems such as depression and anxiety.

Resilience is not about toughing it out or living by old clichés such as "grin and bear it." Resilience doesn't make our problems go away, but it can give us the ability to see past them, get on with daily tasks, remain generally optimistic, and find enjoyment in life. Being resilient does not mean being stoic or going it alone. In fact, being able to reach out to others for support is a key component of resilience.

If we are not as resilient as we would like to be, we can learn how to become more resilient. Learning resilience involves behaviors, thoughts, and actions that almost anyone can learn:

- **Get connected:** Build strong, positive relationships with family and friends who listen and offer support. Get involved in your faith community, civic groups, or volunteer opportunities.

- **Use humor and laughter:** Humor is a helpful coping mechanism. If need be, turn to movies, funny books, and comedians for a laugh.

- **Learn from your experiences:** Recall how you coped in the past, and build on what helped you through those rough times.

- **Remain hopeful and optimistic:** Look forward to the future, even if it's just a glimmer of how things might improve. Expect good results, and, every day, look for something—anything—that signals change for the better.

- **Take care of yourself:** Tend to your own needs and feelings. Play, exercise, get plenty of sleep, and eat well. As on the airplane, put your own oxygen mask on first so you'll be able to help the others.

- **Accept and anticipate change:** Change and uncertainty are a natural part of life. Be flexible.

- **Work towards goals:** Do something, no matter how small, that gives you a sense of accomplishment. It may be finishing a project or making that difficult phone call.

- **Take action:** Most likely, your problems will not disappear on their own. Figure out what needs to be done, make a plan to do it, and then do it.

- **Learn new things about yourself:** Look back on experiences and think about how you changed as a result. You may be stronger than you thought.

- **Think better of yourself:** Congratulate yourself for enduring. Be justifiably proud of yourself, and nurture that self-confidence and self-esteem so that you know you are a strong, capable and self-reliant person.

- **Maintain perspective:** Look at your situation within the larger context of your life, and that of the world. Keep a long-term perspective and know that your situation can improve

Section 4.2

Stress and How to Handle It

From "Stress and Your Health Fact Sheet," Office on Women's
Health (www.womenshealth.gov), March 17, 2010.

What is stress?

Stress is a feeling you get when faced with a challenge. In small
doses, stress can be good for you because it makes you more alert and
gives you a burst of energy. For instance, if you start to cross the street
and see a car about to run you over, that jolt you feel helps you to jump
out of the way before you get hit. But feeling stressed for a long time
can take a toll on your mental and physical health. Even though it may
seem hard to find ways to de-stress with all the things you have to do,
it's important to find those ways. Your health depends on it.

What are the most common causes of stress?

Stress happens when people feel like they don't have the tools to
manage all of the demands in their lives. Stress can be short-term or
long-term. Missing the bus or arguing with your spouse or partner
can cause short-term stress. Money problems or trouble at work can
cause long-term stress. Even happy events, like having a baby or getting married can cause stress. Some of the most common stressful life
events include the following:

- Death of a spouse
- Death of a close family member
- Divorce
- Losing your job
- Major personal illness or injury
- Marital separation
- Marriage
- Pregnancy

- Retirement
- Spending time in jail

What are some common signs of stress?

Everyone responds to stress a little differently. Your symptoms may be different from someone else's. Here are some of the signs to look for:

- Not eating or eating too much
- Feeling like you have no control
- Needing to have too much control
- Forgetfulness
- Headaches
- Lack of energy
- Lack of focus
- Trouble getting things done
- Poor self-esteem
- Short temper
- Trouble sleeping
- Upset stomach
- Back pain
- General aches and pains

These symptoms may also be signs of depression or anxiety, which can be caused by long-term stress.

Do women react to stress differently than men?

One recent survey found that women were more likely to experience physical symptoms of stress than men. But we don't have enough proof to say that this applies to all women. We do know that women often cope with stress in different ways than men. Women "tend and befriend," taking care of those closest to them, but also drawing support from friends and family. Men are more likely to have the "fight or flight" response. They cope by "escaping" into a relaxing activity or other distraction.

Can stress affect my health?

The body responds to stress by releasing stress hormones. These hormones make blood pressure, heart rate, and blood sugar levels go up. Long-term stress can help cause a variety of health problems, including these:

- Mental health disorders, like depression and anxiety
- Obesity
- Heart disease
- High blood pressure
- Abnormal heart beats
- Menstrual problems
- Acne and other skin problems

Does stress cause ulcers?

No, stress doesn't cause ulcers, but it can make them worse. Most ulcers are caused by a germ called *Helicobacter pylori*. Researchers think people might get it through food or water. Most ulcers can be cured by taking a combination of antibiotics and other drugs.

What is post-traumatic stress disorder?

Post-traumatic stress disorder (PTSD) is a type of anxiety disorder that can occur after living through or seeing a dangerous event. It can also occur after a sudden traumatic event. This can include situations like the following:

- Being a victim of or seeing violence
- Being a victim of sexual or physical abuse or assault
- The death or serious illness of a loved one
- Fighting in a war
- A severe car crash or a plane crash
- Hurricanes, tornadoes, and fires

You can start having PTSD symptoms right after the event. Or symptoms can develop months or even years later. These are common of PTSD symptoms:

- Nightmares

- Flashbacks, or feeling like the event is happening again

- Staying away from places and things that remind you of what happened

- Being irritable, angry, or jumpy

- Feeling strong guilt, depression, or worry

- Trouble sleeping

- Feeling "numb"

- Having trouble remembering the event

Women are two to three times more likely to develop PTSD than men. Also, people with ongoing stress in their lives are more likely to develop PTSD after a dangerous event.

How can I help handle my stress?

Everyone has to deal with stress. There are steps you can take to help you handle stress in a positive way and keep it from making you sick. Try these tips to keep stress in check:

Develop a New Attitude

- Become a problem solver. Make a list of the things that cause you stress. From your list, figure out which problems you can solve now and which are beyond your control for the moment. From your list of problems that you can solve now, start with the little ones. Learn how to calmly look at a problem, think of possible solutions, and take action to solve the problem. Being able to solve small problems will give you confidence to tackle the big ones. And feeling confident that you can solve problems will go a long way to helping you feel less stressed.

- Be flexible. Sometimes, it's not worth the stress to argue. Give in once in awhile or meet people halfway.

- Get organized. Think ahead about how you're going to spend your time. Write a to-do list. Figure out what's most important to do and do those things first.

- Set limits. When it comes to things like work and family, figure out what you can really do. There are only so many hours in the day. Set limits for yourself and others. Don't be afraid to say NO to requests for your time and energy.

Relax

- Take deep breaths. If you're feeling stressed, taking a few deep breaths makes you breathe slower and helps your muscles relax.

- Stretch. Stretching can also help relax your muscles and make you feel less tense.

- Massage tense muscles. Having someone massage the muscles in the back of your neck and upper back can help you feel less tense.

- Take time to do something you want to do. We all have lots of things that we have to do. But often we don't take the time to do the things that we really want to do. It could be listening to music, reading a good book, or going to a movie. Think of this as an order from your doctor, so you won't feel guilty!

Take Care of Your Body

- Get enough sleep. Getting enough sleep helps you recover from the stresses of the day. Also, being well-rested helps you think better so that you are prepared to handle problems as they come up. Most adults need seven to nine hours of sleep a night to feel rested.

- Eat right. Try to fuel up with fruits, vegetables, beans, and whole grains. Don't be fooled by the jolt you get from caffeine or high-sugar snack foods. Your energy will wear off, and you could wind up feeling more tired than you did before.

- Get moving. Getting physical activity can not only help relax your tense muscles but improve your mood. Research shows that physical activity can help relieve symptoms of depression and anxiety.

- Don't deal with stress in unhealthy ways. This includes drinking too much alcohol, using drugs, smoking, or overeating.

Connect with Others

- Share your stress. Talking about your problems with friends or family members can sometimes help you feel better. They might also help you see your problems in a new way and suggest solutions that you hadn't thought of.

- Get help from a professional if you need it. If you feel that you can no longer cope, talk to your doctor. She or he may suggest counseling to help you learn better ways to deal with stress. Your doctor may also prescribe medicines, such as antidepressants or sleep aids.

- Help others. Volunteering in your community can help you make new friends and feel better about yourself.

Section 4.3

Controlling Anger

Introduction

We all know what anger is, and we've all felt it: whether as a fleeting annoyance or as full-fledged rage.

Anger is a completely normal, usually healthy, human emotion. But when it gets out of control and turns destructive, it can lead to problems—problems at work, in your personal relationships, and in the overall quality of your life. And it can make you feel as though you're at the mercy of an unpredictable and powerful emotion. This information is meant to help you understand and control anger.

What Is Anger?

The Nature of Anger

Anger is "an emotional state that varies in intensity from mild irritation to intense fury and rage," according to Charles Spielberger, PhD, a psychologist who specializes in the study of anger. Like other emotions, it is accompanied by physiological and biological changes; when you get angry, your heart rate and blood pressure go up, as do the levels of your energy hormones, adrenaline, and noradrenaline.

73

Anger can be caused by both external and internal events. You could be angry at a specific person (such as a coworker or supervisor) or event (a traffic jam, a canceled flight), or your anger could be caused by worrying or brooding about your personal problems. Memories of traumatic or enraging events can also trigger angry feelings.

Expressing Anger

The instinctive, natural way to express anger is to respond aggressively. Anger is a natural, adaptive response to threats; it inspires powerful, often aggressive, feelings and behaviors, which allow us to fight and to defend ourselves when we are attacked. A certain amount of anger, therefore, is necessary to our survival.

On the other hand, we can't physically lash out at every person or object that irritates or annoys us; laws, social norms, and common sense place limits on how far our anger can take us.

People use a variety of both conscious and unconscious processes to deal with their angry feelings. The three main approaches are expressing, suppressing, and calming. Expressing your angry feelings in an assertive—not aggressive—manner is the healthiest way to express anger. To do this, you have to learn how to make clear what your needs are, and how to get them met, without hurting others. Being assertive doesn't mean being pushy or demanding; it means being respectful of yourself and others.

Anger can be suppressed, and then converted or redirected. This happens when you hold in your anger, stop thinking about it, and focus on something positive. The aim is to inhibit or suppress your anger and convert it into more constructive behavior. The danger in this type of response is that if it isn't allowed outward expression, your anger can turn inward—on yourself. Anger turned inward may cause hypertension, high blood pressure, or depression.

Unexpressed anger can create other problems. It can lead to pathological expressions of anger, such as passive-aggressive behavior (getting back at people indirectly, without telling them why, rather than confronting them head-on) or a personality that seems perpetually cynical and hostile. People who are constantly putting others down, criticizing everything, and making cynical comments haven't learned how to constructively express their anger. Not surprisingly, they aren't likely to have many successful relationships.

Finally, you can calm down inside. This means not just controlling your outward behavior, but also controlling your internal responses, taking steps to lower your heart rate, calm yourself down, and let the feelings subside.

As Dr. Spielberger notes, "when none of these three techniques work, that's when someone—or something—is going to get hurt."

Anger Management

The goal of anger management is to reduce both your emotional feelings and the physiological arousal that anger causes. You can't get rid of, or avoid, the things or the people that enrage you, nor can you change them, but you can learn to control your reactions.

Are You Too Angry?

There are psychological tests that measure the intensity of angry feelings, how prone to anger you are, and how well you handle it. But chances are good that if you do have a problem with anger, you already know it. If you find yourself acting in ways that seem out of control and frightening, you might need help finding better ways to deal with this emotion.

Why Are Some People More Angry Than Others?

According to Jerry Deffenbacher, PhD, a psychologist who specializes in anger management, some people really are more "hotheaded" than others are; they get angry more easily and more intensely than the average person does. There are also those who don't show their anger in loud spectacular ways but are chronically irritable and grumpy. Easily angered people don't always curse and throw things; sometimes they withdraw socially, sulk, or get physically ill.

People who are easily angered generally have what some psychologists call a low tolerance for frustration, meaning simply that they feel that they should not have to be subjected to frustration, inconvenience, or annoyance. They can't take things in stride, and they're particularly infuriated if the situation seems somehow unjust: for example, being corrected for a minor mistake.

What makes these people this way? A number of things. One cause may be genetic or physiological: There is evidence that some children are born irritable, touchy, and easily angered, and that these signs are present from a very early age. Another may be sociocultural. Anger is often regarded as negative; we're taught that it's all right to express anxiety, depression, or other emotions but not to express anger. As a result, we don't learn how to handle it or channel it constructively.

Research has also found that family background plays a role. Typically, people who are easily angered come from families that are disruptive, chaotic, and not skilled at emotional communications.

Is It Good to "Let It All Hang Out?"

Psychologists now say that this is a dangerous myth. Some people use this theory as a license to hurt others. Research has found that "letting it rip" with anger actually escalates anger and aggression and does nothing to help you (or the person you're angry with) resolve the situation.

It's best to find out what it is that triggers your anger, and then to develop strategies to keep those triggers from tipping you over the edge.

Strategies to Keep Anger at Bay

Relaxation

Simple relaxation tools, such as deep breathing and relaxing imagery, can help calm down angry feelings. There are books and courses that can teach you relaxation techniques, and once you learn the techniques, you can call upon them in any situation. If you are involved in a relationship where both partners are hot-tempered, it might be a good idea for both of you to learn these techniques.

Some simple steps you can try:

- Breathe deeply, from your diaphragm; breathing from your chest won't relax you. Picture your breath coming up from your "gut."

- Slowly repeat a calm word or phrase such as "relax," "take it easy." Repeat it to yourself while breathing deeply.

- Use imagery; visualize a relaxing experience, from either your memory or your imagination.

- Nonstrenuous, slow yoga-like exercises can relax your muscles and make you feel much calmer.

Practice these techniques daily. Learn to use them automatically when you're in a tense situation.

Cognitive Restructuring

Simply put, this means changing the way you think. Angry people tend to curse, swear, or speak in highly colorful terms that reflect their inner thoughts. When you're angry, your thinking can get very exaggerated and overly dramatic. Try replacing these thoughts with more rational ones. For instance, instead of telling yourself, "oh, it's awful, it's terrible, everything's ruined," tell yourself, "it's frustrating, and it's understandable that I'm upset about it, but it's not the end of the world and getting angry is not going to fix it anyhow."

Be careful of words like "never" or "always" when talking about yourself or someone else. "This !&*%@ machine never works," or "you're always forgetting things" are not just inaccurate, they also serve to make you feel that your anger is justified and that there's no way to solve the problem. They also alienate and humiliate people who might otherwise be willing to work with you on a solution.

Remind yourself that getting angry is not going to fix anything, that it won't make you feel better (and may actually make you feel worse).

Logic defeats anger, because anger, even when it's justified, can quickly become irrational. So use cold hard logic on yourself. Remind yourself that the world is "not out to get you," you're just experiencing some of the rough spots of daily life. Do this each time you feel anger getting the best of you, and it'll help you get a more balanced perspective. Angry people tend to demand things: fairness, appreciation, agreement, willingness to do things their way. Everyone wants these things, and we are all hurt and disappointed when we don't get them, but angry people demand them, and when their demands aren't met, their disappointment becomes anger. As part of their cognitive restructuring, angry people need to become aware of their demanding nature and translate their expectations into desires. In other words, saying, "I would like" something is healthier than saying, "I demand" or "I must have" something. When you're unable to get what you want, you will experience the normal reactions—frustration, disappointment, hurt—but not anger. Some angry people use this anger as a way to avoid feeling hurt, but that doesn't mean the hurt goes away.

Problem Solving

Sometimes, our anger and frustration are caused by very real and inescapable problems in our lives. Not all anger is misplaced, and often it's a healthy, natural response to these difficulties. There is also a cultural belief that every problem has a solution, and it adds to our frustration to find out that this isn't always the case. The best attitude to bring to such a situation, then, is not to focus on finding the solution, but rather on how you handle and face the problem.

Make a plan, and check your progress along the way. Resolve to give it your best, but also not to punish yourself if an answer doesn't come right away. If you can approach it with your best intentions and efforts and make a serious attempt to face it head-on, you will be less likely to lose patience and fall into all-or-nothing thinking, even if the problem does not get solved right away.

Better Communication

Angry people tend to jump to—and act on—conclusions, and some of those conclusions can be very inaccurate. The first thing to do if you're in a heated discussion is slow down and think through your responses. Don't say the first thing that comes into your head, but slow down and think carefully about what you want to say. At the same time, listen carefully to what the other person is saying and take your time before answering.

Listen, too, to what is underlying the anger. For instance, you like a certain amount of freedom and personal space, and your "significant other" wants more connection and closeness. If he or she starts complaining about your activities, don't retaliate by painting your partner as a jailer, a warden, or an albatross around your neck.

It's natural to get defensive when you're criticized, but don't fight back. Instead, listen to what's underlying the words: the message that this person might feel neglected and unloved. It may take a lot of patient questioning on your part, and it may require some breathing space, but don't let your anger—or a partner's—let a discussion spin out of control. Keeping your cool can keep the situation from becoming a disastrous one.

Using Humor

"Silly humor" can help defuse rage in a number of ways. For one thing, it can help you get a more balanced perspective. When you get angry and call someone a name or refer to them in some imaginative phrase, stop and picture what that word would literally look like. If you're at work and you think of a coworker as a "dirt bag" or a "single-cell life form," for example, picture a large bag full of dirt (or an amoeba) sitting at your colleague's desk, talking on the phone, going to meetings. Do this whenever a name comes into your head about another person. If you can, draw a picture of what the actual thing might look like. This will take a lot of the edge off your fury; and humor can always be relied on to help unknot a tense situation.

The underlying message of highly angry people, Dr. Deffenbacher says, is "things oughta go my way!" Angry people tend to feel that they are morally right, that any blocking or changing of their plans is an unbearable indignity and that they should NOT have to suffer this way. Maybe other people do, but not them!

When you feel that urge, he suggests, picture yourself as a god or goddess, a supreme ruler, who owns the streets and stores and office space, striding alone and having your way in all situations while others defer to you. The more detail you can get into your imaginary scenes, the more chances you have to realize that maybe you are being unreasonable; you'll also realize how unimportant the things you're angry about really are. There are two cautions in using humor. First, don't try to just "laugh off" your problems; rather, use humor to help yourself face them more constructively. Second, don't give in to harsh, sarcastic humor; that's just another form of unhealthy anger expression.

What these techniques have in common is a refusal to take yourself too seriously. Anger is a serious emotion, but it's often accompanied by ideas that, if examined, can make you laugh.

Changing Your Environment

Sometimes it's our immediate surroundings that give us cause for irritation and fury. Problems and responsibilities can weigh on you and make you feel angry at the "trap" you seem to have fallen into and all the people and things that form that trap.

Give yourself a break. Make sure you have some "personal time" scheduled for times of the day that you know are particularly stressful. One example is the working mother who has a standing rule that when she comes home from work, for the first 15 minutes "nobody talks to Mom unless the house is on fire." After this brief quiet time, she feels better prepared to handle demands from her kids without blowing up at them.

Some Other Tips for Easing Up on Yourself

Timing: If you and your spouse tend to fight when you discuss things at night—perhaps you're tired, or distracted, or maybe it's just habit—try changing the times when you talk about important matters so these talks don't turn into arguments.

Avoidance: If your child's chaotic room makes you furious every time you walk by it, shut the door. Don't make yourself look at what infuriates you. Don't say, "well, my child should clean up the room so I won't have to be angry!" That's not the point. The point is to keep yourself calm.

Finding alternatives: If your daily commute through traffic leaves you in a state of rage and frustration, give yourself a project—learn or map out a different route, one that's less congested or more scenic. Or find another alternative, such as a bus or commuter train.

Do You Need Counseling?

If you feel that your anger is really out of control, if it is having an impact on your relationships and on important parts of your life, you might consider counseling to learn how to handle it better. A psychologist or other licensed mental health professional can work with you in developing a range of techniques for changing your thinking and your behavior.

When you talk to a prospective therapist, tell her or him that you have problems with anger that you want to work on, and ask about his or her approach to anger management. Make sure this isn't only a course of action designed to "put you in touch with your feelings and express them"—that may be precisely what your problem is. With counseling, psychologists say, a highly angry person can move closer to a middle range of anger in about eight to ten weeks, depending on the circumstances and the techniques used.

What about Assertiveness Training?

It's true that angry people need to learn to become assertive (rather than aggressive), but most books and courses on developing assertiveness are aimed at people who don't feel enough anger. These people are more passive and acquiescent than the average person; they tend to let others walk all over them. That isn't something that most angry people do. Still, these books can contain some useful tactics to use in frustrating situations.

Remember, you can't eliminate anger—and it wouldn't be a good idea if you could. In spite of all your efforts, things will happen that will cause you anger; and sometimes it will be justifiable anger. Life will be filled with frustration, pain, loss, and the unpredictable actions of others. You can't change that; but you can change the way you let such events affect you. Controlling your angry responses can keep them from making you even more unhappy in the long run.

Section 4.4

Coping with a Breakup or Divorce

It's never easy when a marriage or significant relationship ends. Whatever the reason for the split, it can turn your whole world upside down and trigger painful and unsettling feelings. But there are things you can do to get through this difficult time and grow into a stronger, wiser person.

Healing after a Divorce or Breakup

Why do breakups hurt so much, even when the relationship is no longer good? A divorce or breakup is painful because it represents the loss, not just of the relationship, but also of shared dreams and commitments. Romantic relationships begin on a high note of excitement and hope for the future. When these relationships fail, we experience profound disappointment, stress, and grief.

A breakup or divorce launches us into uncharted territory. Everything is disrupted: your routine and responsibilities, your home, your relationships with extended family and friends, and even your identity. A breakup brings uncertainty about the future. What will life be like without your partner? Will you find someone else? Will you end up alone? These unknowns often seem worse than an unhappy relationship.

Recovering from a breakup or divorce is difficult. However, it's important to know (and to keep reminding yourself) that you can and will move on. But healing takes time, so be patient with yourself.

Coping with Separation and Divorce

- Recognize that it's OK to have different feelings. It's normal to feel sad, angry, exhausted, frustrated, and confused—and these feelings can be intense. You also may feel anxious about the future. Accept that reactions like these will lessen over time. Even if the marriage was unhealthy, venturing into the unknown is frightening.

- Give yourself a break. Give yourself permission to feel and to function at a less than optimal level for a period of time. You may not be able to be quite as productive on the job or care for others in exactly the way you're accustomed to for a little while. No one is superman or superwoman; take time to heal, regroup, and re-energize.

- Don't go through this alone. Sharing your feelings with friends and family can help you get through this period. Consider joining a support group where you can talk to others in similar situations. Isolating yourself can raise your stress levels, reduce your concentration, and get in the way of your work, relationships, and overall health. Don't be afraid to get outside help if you need it.

Source: Mental Health America

Allow Yourself to Grieve the Loss of the Relationship

Grief is a natural reaction to loss, and the breakup or divorce of a love relationship involves multiple losses:

- Loss of companionship and shared experiences (which may or may not have been consistently pleasurable)

- Loss of support, be it financial, intellectual, social, or emotional

- Loss of hopes, plans, and dreams (can be even more painful than practical losses)

Allowing yourself to feel the pain of these losses may be scary. You may fear that your emotions will be too intense to bear, or that you'll be stuck in a dark place forever. Just remember that grieving is essential to the healing process. The pain of grief is precisely what helps you let go of the old relationship and move on. And no matter how strong your grief, it won't last forever.

Tips for Grieving after a Breakup or Divorce

- **Don't fight your feelings:** It's normal to have lots of ups and downs, and feel many conflicting emotions, including anger, resentment, sadness, relief, fear, and confusion. It's important to identify and acknowledge these feelings. While these emotions will often be painful, trying to suppress or ignore them will only prolong the grieving process.

- **Talk about how you're feeling:** Even if it is difficult for you to talk about your feelings with other people, it is very important to find a way to do so when you are grieving. Knowing that others are aware of your feelings will make you feel less alone with your pain and will help you heal. Journaling can also be a helpful outlet for your feelings.

- **Remember that moving on is the end goal:** Expressing your feelings will liberate you in a way, but it is important not to dwell on the negative feelings or to over-analyze the situation. Getting stuck in hurtful feelings like blame, anger, and resentment will rob you of valuable energy and prevent you from healing and moving forward.

- **Remind yourself that you still have a future:** When you commit to another person, you create many hopes and dreams. It's hard to let these dreams go. As you grieve the loss of the future you once envisioned, be encouraged by the fact that new hopes and dreams will eventually replace your old ones.

- **Know the difference between a normal reaction to a breakup and depression:** Grief can be paralyzing after a breakup, but after a while, the sadness begins to lift. Day by day, and little by little, you start moving on. However, if you don't feel any forward momentum, you may be suffering from depression.

Reach Out to Others for Support through the Grieving Process

Support from others is critical to healing after a breakup or divorce. You might feel like being alone, but isolating yourself will only make this time more difficult. Don't try to get through this on your own.

Reach out to trusted friends and family members. People who have been through painful breakups or divorces can be especially helpful. They know what it is like and they can assure you that there is hope for healing and new relationships.

- **Spend time with people who support, value, and energize you:** As you consider who to reach out to, choose wisely. Surround yourself with people who are positive and who truly listen to you. It's important that you feel free to be honest about what you're going through, without worrying about being judged, criticized, or told what to do.

- **Get outside help if you need it:** If reaching out to others doesn't come naturally, consider seeing a counselor or joining a support group. The most important thing is that you have at least one place where you feel comfortable opening up.

- **Cultivate new friendships:** If you feel like you have lost your social network along with the divorce or breakup, make an effort to meet new people. Join a networking group or special interest club, take a class, get involved in community activities, or volunteer at a school, place of worship, or other community organization.

Taking Care of Yourself after a Divorce or Relationship Breakup

A divorce is a highly stressful, life-changing event. When you're going through the emotional wringer and dealing with major life changes, it's more important than ever to take care of yourself. The strain and upset of a major breakup can leave you psychologically and physically vulnerable.

Treat yourself like you're getting over the flu. Get plenty of rest, minimize other sources of stress in your life, and reduce your workload if possible.

Learning to take care of yourself can be one of the most valuable lessons you learn following a divorce or breakup. As you feel the emotions of your loss and begin learning from your experience, you can resolve to take better care of yourself and make positive choices going forward.

Self-Care Tips

- **Make time each day to nurture yourself:** Help yourself heal by scheduling daily time for activities you find calming and soothing. Go for a walk in nature, listen to music, enjoy a hot bath, get a massage, read a favorite book, take a yoga class, or savor a warm cup of tea.

- **Pay attention to what you need in any given moment and speak up to express your needs:** Honor what you believe to be right and best for you even though it may be different from what your ex or others want. Say "no" without guilt or angst as a way of honoring what is right for you.

- **Stick to a routine:** A divorce or relationship breakup can disrupt almost every area of your life, amplifying feelings of stress, uncertainty, and chaos. Getting back to a regular routine can provide a comforting sense of structure and normalcy.

- **Take a time out:** Try not to make any major decisions in the first few months after a separation or divorce, like starting a new job or moving to a new city. If you can, wait until you're feeling less emotional so that you can make better decisions.

- **Avoid using alcohol, drugs, or food to cope:** When you're in the middle of a breakup, you may be tempted to do anything to relieve your feelings of pain and loneliness. But using alcohol, drugs, or food as an escape is unhealthy and destructive in the long run. It's essential to find healthier ways of coping with painful feelings.

- **Explore new interests:** A divorce or breakup is a beginning as well as an end. Take the opportunity to explore new interests and activities. Pursuing fun, new activities gives you a chance to enjoy life in the here-and-now, rather than dwelling on the past.

Making Healthy Choices: Eat Well, Sleep Well, and Exercise

When you're going through the stress of a divorce or breakup, healthy habits easily fall by the wayside. You might find yourself not eating at all or overeating your favorite junk foods. Exercise might be harder to fit in because of the added pressures at home and sleep might be elusive. But all of the work you are doing to move forward in a positive way will be pointless if you don't make long-term healthy lifestyle choices.

Learning Important Lessons from a Divorce or Breakup

In times of emotional crisis, there is an opportunity to grow and learn. Just because you are feeling emptiness in your life right now, doesn't mean that nothing is happening or that things will never change. Consider this period a time-out, a time for sowing the seeds for new growth. You can emerge from this experience knowing yourself better and feeling stronger.

In order to fully accept a breakup and move on, you need to understand what happened and acknowledge the part you played. It's important to understand how the choices you made affected the relationship. Learning from your mistakes is the key to not repeating them.

Some Questions to Ask Yourself

- Step back and look at the big picture. How did you contribute to the problems of the relationship?

- Do you tend to repeat the same mistakes or choose the wrong person in relationship after relationship?

- Think about how you react stress and deal with conflict and insecurities. Could you act in a more constructive way?

- Consider whether or not you accept other people the way they are, not the way they could or "should" be.

- Examine your negative feelings as a starting point for change. Are you in control of your feelings, or are they in control of you?

You'll need to be honest with yourself during this part of the healing process. Try not to dwell on who is to blame or beat yourself up over your mistakes. As you look back on the relationship, you have an opportunity to learn more about yourself, how you relate to others, and the problems you need to work on. If you are able to objectively examine your own choices and behavior, including the reasons why you chose your former partner, you'll be able to see where you went wrong and make better choices next time.

Section 4.5

Coping with Grief

"Coping with Grief: When a Loved One Dies," *NIH News in Health*, National Institutes of Health, November 2009.

When someone you love dies, your world changes. You may feel numb, shocked, or frightened. You may feel depressed and have trouble concentrating. You may feel guilty for being the one who is still alive. All of these feelings are normal. There is no right or wrong way to mourn.

Each year, about 2.5 million people die nationwide. Every death leaves behind an average of four or five grieving survivors. For most, extreme feelings of grief begin to fade within six months after the loss. But some bereaved people may continue to struggle for years to move on with their lives.

It's often helpful to talk with family and friends about the person who's gone. People sometimes hesitate to mention a dead person's name or discuss the loss, because they don't want to cause pain. But it can help when people share their feelings.

Researchers have tried for decades to identify different stages of grief. They've found that the grieving process differs for every individual. It's affected by how attached you felt to the person who died; whether you were a parent, child or spouse; how the death occurred; and other factors.

One study found that acceptance of a death comes surprisingly early for most bereaved people, usually within the first month after the loss. The researchers found that in the two years following a death, the most often-reported symptom is yearning for the person who died. Yearning is much more common than depression, anger, and disbelief.

This study and many others have found that if symptoms aren't tapering off by six months after the loss, it may be a sign of a more serious problem, sometimes called complicated grief. People with complicated grief are at risk for major depression, substance abuse, post-traumatic stress disorder, and suicidal thoughts and actions.

"Prolonged grief, or complicated grief, is seen in a small portion of bereaved individuals—about 10% or 20%. Their symptoms are disruptive to their lives and daily functioning," says Dr. Mary-Frances O'Connor, a psychologist at the University of California, Los Angeles. "These people may experience extreme yearning, loneliness, and a feeling that life will never have any meaning. They may have intrusive thoughts and feel ongoing anger or bitterness over the death."

O'Connor's brain imaging studies have found differences in brain activity between bereaved people with complicated grief and those who are coping well with their loss. Both groups showed pain-related brain activity when they looked at photos of their loved ones. But only those with complicated grief showed activation in parts of the brain's reward-processing centers.

"That may seem strange. But other studies have shown that when people are very attached to their loved ones, they feel rewarded when they are with them," O'Connor says. People with complicated grief may still feel very attached, and so feel "rewarded" by seeing photos of their loved ones. Those who adapt well, O'Connor suggests, have somehow accepted the reality that the person is not physically with them anymore. "They still feel sad, but they no longer yearn for the person in the same way," she says.

Complicated grief is difficult to treat. Some evidence suggests that a specialized talk therapy can help people with complicated grief improve faster and better than traditional talk therapy. This experimental therapy, called complicated grief treatment, involves vividly recalling the death with a trained grief counselor and having an imaginary conversation with the person who died. Researchers are now testing whether complicated grief treatment might work even better in combination with antidepressants or other approaches.

Some studies show that people who've been caregivers for a relative with a long-term illness may adapt relatively quickly to the death. Dr. Richard Schulz, a social psychologist at the University of Pittsburgh, studies caregivers for relatives with Alzheimer disease. He and his colleagues found that most did remarkably well after their loved one died. "Their level of depression, which was very high during the caregiving phase before the death, returned to almost normal levels within six months after the death," Schulz says.

People caring for someone with a long-term illness may begin the grieving process while their loved one is still alive. "The death may mark the end of suffering for the caregivers and the patients," Schulz says. "The death also eliminates much of the burden associated with daily care in the home. It frees up time, so the person can now re-engage in social contacts they might have had prior to taking on the caregiver role."

But Schulz's research also found that about one in five caregivers had persistent, severe depression and other troubling symptoms more than six months after the death. Many of those who struggled to adapt were either highly depressed before the death or had positive feelings about their caregiving role.

Treating depression before the death seemed to help caregivers cope afterward. People also did better if they'd participated in a program that helped them cope while their relative was still alive.

"The program provided group support, information about the disease and other resources," says Schulz. "It was not designed to help people after the death, but that was an unexpected benefit. The quality of the caregiving experience may have helped them prepare for the death indirectly."

Some studies have found that when patients, doctors, and family members directly address the prospect of death before it happens, it helps survivors after the death. "If you're in a long-term disease situation where death is likely, it's helpful to engage in end-of-life care planning, to make it easier to deal with the death once it occurs," says Schulz.

Scientists funded by the National Institutes of Health continue to study different aspects of the grieving process and to search for new treatments. Researchers are also looking at how cultural attitudes and beliefs about death can affect grief and mourning.

Remember, although the death of a loved one can feel overwhelming, most people can make it through the grieving process with the support of family and friends. Take care of yourself, accept offers of help or companionship from those around you, and be sure to get additional help or counseling if you need it.

It may take time. The process will be difficult. But you can eventually adjust to life after someone you love has died.

Section 4.6

Pets Are Good for Mental Health

Pets can serve as important sources of social and emotional support for "everyday people," not just individuals facing significant health challenges, according to research published by the American Psychological Association (APA).

And, the study found, pet owners were just as close to key people in their lives as to their animals, indicating no evidence that relationships with pets came at the expense of relationships with other people, or that people relied more on pets when their human social support was poorer.

Psychologists at Miami University and Saint Louis University conducted three experiments to examine the potential benefits of pet ownership among what they called everyday people. The results of the current study were reported in the *Journal of Personality and Social Psychology®*, published online by APA (http://www.apa.org/pubs/journals/psp/index.aspx).

"We observed evidence that pet owners fared better, both in terms of well-being outcomes and individual differences, than non-owners on several dimensions," said lead researcher Allen R. McConnell, PhD, of Miami University in Ohio. "Specifically, pet owners had greater self-esteem, were more physically fit, tended to be less lonely, were more conscientious, were more extraverted, tended to be less fearful, and tended to be less preoccupied than non-owners."

Until now, most research into the benefits of pets has been correlational, meaning it looked at the relationship between two variables but didn't show that one caused the other. For example, prior research showed that elderly Medicare patients with pets had fewer doctor visits than similar patients without pets, or that HIV-positive men with pets were less depressed than those without.

In this study, 217 people (79 percent women, mean age 31, mean annual family income $77,000) answered surveys aimed at determining whether pet owners in the group differed from people who didn't have pets in the areas of well-being, personality type, and attachment style. Several differences between the groups emerged, and in all cases, pet owners were happier, healthier, and better adjusted than were non-owners.

A second experiment, involving 56 dog owners (91 percent of whom were women, with a mean age of 42 and average annual family income of $65,000), examined whether pet owners benefit more when their pet is perceived to fulfill their social needs better. This study found greater well-being among owners whose dogs increased their feelings of belonging, self-esteem, and meaningful existence.

The last study, comprising 97 undergraduates with an average age of 19, found that pets can make people feel better after experiencing rejection. Subjects were asked to write about a time when they felt excluded. Then they were asked to write about their favorite pet, or to write about their favorite friend, or to draw a map of their campus. The researchers found that writing about pets was just as effective as writing about a friend when it came to staving off feelings of rejection.

"[T]he present work presents considerable evidence that pets benefit the lives of their owners, both psychologically and physically, by serving as an important source of social support," the researchers wrote. "Whereas past work has focused primarily on pet owners facing significant health challenges … the present study establishes that there are many positive consequences for everyday people who own pets."

Article: "Friends With Benefits: On the Positive Consequences of Pet Ownership," Allen R. McConnell, PhD, Miami University; Christina M. Brown, PhD, Saint Louis University; Tonya M. Shoda, MA, Laura E. Stayton, BA, and Colleen E. Martin, BA, Miami University; *Journal of Personality and Social Psychology*, Vol. 101, No. 6.

Chapter 5

Mental Health in the Workplace

In the context of workplaces, the phrase "mental health" brings several things to mind:

- On-the-job stress and/or burnout

- The need for conflict resolution between employees

- The emotional fallout from a traumatic event

- Dealing with employee anxiety when there are major changes

Often proactive mental health–friendly practices can prevent or help resolve problematic work situations such as those above.

Mental health and mental illness can be pictured as two points on a continuum with a range of conditions in between. Mental health issues that employers face range from stress to serious mental illnesses such as depression, anxiety disorders, or adult attention deficit/hyperactivity disorder. Mental illnesses are surprisingly common. They affect almost every family and workplace in America.

It has been said that many employers simply do not know how to work productively with employees who have mental illnesses. In fact, many people don't realize that effective treatments are available for mental illnesses and that people recover from mental illnesses and continue to live productive lives.

Excerpted from "Businesses Materials for a Mental Health Friendly Workplace: Executives Booklet," Substance Abuse and Mental Health Services Administration (SAMHSA), August 26, 2008.

Unfortunately, many people with serious mental illnesses do not seek or receive treatment. Common reasons people do not seek treatment include: cost, fear, not knowing where to go for services, and concern about confidentiality and the opinions of coworkers and others in the community. This fear of what people may think—the stigma that surrounds mental illness—is a serious barrier to treatment and recovery.

Benefits to Business

A mental health–friendly workplace makes good business sense. It benefits owners, managers, and employees in ways that affect the bottom line. Consider the following outcomes:

- **Higher productivity and motivation:** Employees feel valued and secure and work more effectively when employers demonstrate a commitment to their well-being.

- **Reduced absenteeism:** Workplace stress is a major cause of absenteeism. Helping employees manage their stress and overall mental health can boost productivity.

- **Health insurance cost containment:** Instituting health and wellness programs can help hold down health insurance rate hikes.

- **Preparedness for disasters:** Assisting employees in times of sudden unexpected trauma with counseling, peer support groups, and links to needed community services can help businesses become productive again sooner.

- **Loyalty and retention:** Businesses with mental health–friendly practices have documented remarkably low turnover rates, along with cost savings in recruitment, new employee orientation, and training.

- **Hiring and promoting the most qualified people:** By openly supporting mental health–friendly policies, employers can increase the pool of qualified applicants.

- **More efficient workplace practices and policies:** The process of thinking about mental health can generate helpful internal policy and benefit reviews, and more effective workplace systems and procedures for employees as a whole.

- **Better workplace relations:** Awareness of and openness to mental health issues help create a positive climate for understanding, conflict resolution, and support.

- Diversity, acceptance, and respect in the workplace: Embracing diversity includes people who live with mental illnesses. In becoming more inclusive, businesses can both thrive and set a standard for others.

The Mental Health–Friendly Workplace

Businesses that value the health of their employees, including their mental health and well-being, have specific practices and policies in place. Such companies can be small, medium, or large. Outstanding examples abound among large corporations in the United States; however, businesses with only a few employees also have found meaningful and innovative ways to be mental health friendly.

Below are specific practices and policies that characterize a mental health–friendly workplace, many of which are found in organizations large and small.

These are characteristics of the mental health–friendly workplace:

- Welcomes all qualified job applicants; diversity is valued

- Includes health care that treats mental illnesses with the same urgency as physical illnesses

- Has programs and practices that promote and support employee health-wellness and/or work-life balance

- Provides training for managers and front-line supervisors in mental health workplace issues, including identification of performance problems that may indicate worker distress and possible need for referral and evaluation

- Safeguards confidentiality of employee health information

- Provides an Employee Assistance Program or other appropriate referral resources to assist managers and employees

- Supports employees who seek treatment or who require hospitalization and disability leave, including planning for return to work

- Ensures exit with dignity as a corporate priority, should it become essential for an employee to leave employment

- Provides all-employee communication regarding equal opportunity employment, the reasonable accommodations policy of the Americans with Disabilities Act, health and wellness programs,

95

and similar topics that promote an accepting, anti-stigmatizing, anti-discriminating climate in the workplace.

Next Steps: Using the Mental Health–Friendly Workplace Resource

First, assess where your company is now and where you want to go:

- Have you noticed excessive absenteeism, low morale, low productivity?

- Could these issues have been dealt with more effectively?

- What elements of a mental health–friendly environment are already in place?

- What additional elements could help you with future issues?

- How will the worth or value to your business of this undertaking be assessed (that is, how will you know that you are achieving the benefits)?

Second, order the free Mental Health–Friendly Resource by calling the National Mental Health Information Center at 800-789-2647 (English/Spanish) or 866-889-2647 (TDD). Or visit www.allmentalhealth. samhsa.gov. Ask for the free Mental Health–Friendly Workplace Resource.

The Resource contains these components:

- Descriptions of Mental Health–Friendly Workplace practices

- Downloadable materials to help in creating Mental Health–Friendly Workplaces

- Training modules for supervisors, including reproducible materials and PowerPoint slides

- Ready-to-use materials for communicating with employees, including a poster, print PSAs, and drop-in articles for in-house communications

The resource is designed for human resource (HR) personnel, or in the absence of HR personnel, for staff members who administer corporate benefits and other personnel policies; communicate health, wellness, and work-life balance information; and coordinate training of supervisory staff.

Myths Surrounding Mental Illnesses

Myth: People with mental illnesses can't hold jobs.

Fact: On the contrary, many are productive employees, business owners, and contributing members of their communities.

Myth: Employees with mental illnesses, even those who have received effective treatment and have recovered, tend to be second-rate workers.

Fact: Employers who have hired these individuals report they are higher than average in attendance and punctuality, and they are as good as or better than other employees in motivation, quality of work, and job tenure. Studies reported by the National Institute of Mental Health (NIMH) and the National Alliance for the Mentally Ill (NAMI) conclude that there are no differences in productivity when compared to other employees.

Myth: There's no hope for people with mental illnesses.

Fact: There are more treatments, strategies, and community supports than ever before, and even more are on the horizon. People with mental illnesses lead active, productive lives.

Myth: People with mental illnesses are violent and unpredictable.

Fact: Chances are you know someone with a mental illness and don't even realize it. In reality, the vast majority of people who have mental illnesses are no more violent than anyone else.

Chapter 6

The Stigma of Mental Illness

Stigmas are negative stereotypes about groups of people. Common stigmas about people who are mentally ill are:

- Individuals who have a mental illness are dangerous.

- Individuals who have a mental illness are irresponsible and can't make life decisions for themselves.

- People who have a mental illness are childlike and must be taken care of by parents or guardians.

- People who have a mental illness should just get over it.

Each of those preconceptions about people who have a mental illness is based on false information. Very few people who have a mental illness are dangerous to society. Most can hold jobs, attend school, and live independently. A person who has a mental illness cannot simply decide to get over it any more than someone who has a different chronic disease such as diabetes, asthma, or heart disease can. A mental illness, like those other diseases, is caused by a physical problem in the body.

Stigmas against individuals who have a mental illness lead to injustices, including discriminatory decisions regarding housing, employment, and education. Overcoming the stigmas commonly associated with mental illness is yet one more challenge that people who have a mental illness must face. Indeed, many people who successfully manage their mental illness report that the stigma they face is in many ways more disabling than the illness itself. The stigmatizing attitudes toward mental illness held by both the public and those who have a mental illness lead to feelings of shame and guilt, loss of self-esteem, social dependence, and a sense of isolation and hopelessness. One of the worst consequences of stigma is that people who are struggling with a mental illness may be reluctant to seek treatment that, in most cases, would significantly relieve their symptoms.

Providing accurate information is one way to reduce stigmas about mental illness. Advocacy groups protest stereotypes imposed upon those who are mentally ill. They demand that the media stop presenting inaccurate views of mental illness and that the public stops believing these negative views. A powerful way of countering stereotypes about mental illness occurs when members of the public meet people who are effectively managing a serious mental illness: holding jobs, providing for themselves, and living as good neighbors in a community. Interaction with people who have mental illnesses challenges a person's assumptions and changes a person's attitudes about mental illness.

Attitudes about mental illness are changing, although there is a long way to go before people accept that mental illness is a disease with a biological basis. A survey by the National Mental Health Association found that 55 percent of people who have never been diagnosed with depression recognize that depression is a disease and not something people should "snap out of." This is a substantial increase over the 38 percent of survey respondents in 1991 who recognized depression as a disease.

The Consequences of Not Treating Mental Illness

Most people don't think twice before going to a doctor if they have an illness such as bronchitis, asthma, diabetes, or heart disease. However, many people who have a mental illness don't get the treatment that would alleviate their suffering. Studies estimate that two-thirds of all young people with mental health problems are not receiving the help they need and that less than one-third of the children under age 18 who have a serious mental health problem receive any mental health services. Mental illness in adults often goes untreated, too. What are the consequences of letting mental illness go untreated?

In September 2000, the U.S. Surgeon General held a conference on children's mental health. The former Surgeon General, Dr. David

Satcher, emphasized the importance of mental health in children by stating, "Children and families are suffering because of missed opportunities for prevention and early identification, fragmented services, and low priorities for resources. Overriding all of this is the issue of stigma, which continues to surround mental illness."

The consequences of mental illness in children and adolescents can be substantial. Many mental health professionals speak of accrued deficits that occur when mental illness in children is not treated. To begin with, mental illness can impair a student's ability to learn. Adolescents whose mental illness is not treated rapidly and aggressively tend to fall further and further behind in school. They are more likely to drop out of school and are less likely to be fully functional members of society when they reach adulthood. We also now know that depressive disorders in young people confer a higher risk for illness and interpersonal and psychosocial difficulties that persist after the depressive episode is over. Furthermore, many adults who suffer from mental disorders have problems that originated in childhood. Depression in youth may predict more severe illness in adult life. Attention deficit hyperactivity disorder, once thought to affect children and adolescents only, may persist into adulthood and may be associated with social, legal, and occupational problems.

The high incidence of mental illness has a great impact on society. Depression alone causes employers to lose over $23 billion each year due to decreased productivity and absenteeism of employees. The Global Burden of Disease Study, conducted by the World Health Organization, assessed the burden of all diseases in units that measure lost years of healthy life due to premature death or disability (disability-adjusted life years, or DALYs). Over 15 percent of the total DALYs were due to mental illness. In 1996, the United States spent more than $69 billion for the direct treatment of mental illnesses. Indirect costs of mental illness due to lost productivity in the workplace, schools, or homes represented a $79 billion loss for the U.S. economy in 1990.

Treatment, including psychotherapy and medication management, is cost-effective for patients, their families, and society. The benefits include fewer visits to other doctors' offices, diagnostic laboratories, and hospitals for physical ailments that are based in psychological distress; reduced need for psychiatric hospitalization; fewer sick days and disability claims; and increased job stability. Conversely, the costs of not treating mental disorders can be seen in ruined relationships, job loss or poor job performance, personal anguish, substance abuse, unnecessary medical procedures, psychiatric hospitalization, and suicide.

Chapter 7

Mental Health Statistics

Understanding the scope of mental health problems and treatment in the United States is central to the National Institute on Mental Health (NIMH)'s mission. Much of what we understand in this area comes from research in the field of epidemiology; the scientific study of patterns of health and illness within a population. Research on psychiatric epidemiology shows that mental disorders are common throughout the United States, affecting tens of millions of people each year and that only a fraction of those affected receive treatment.

Prevalence of Serious Mental Illness

While mental disorders are common in the United States, their burden of illness is particularly concentrated among those who experience disability due to serious mental illness (SMI). The data presented in Figure 7.1 are from the National Survey on Drug Use and Health (NSDUH), which defines SMI as one with these characteristics:

- A mental, behavioral, or emotional disorder (excluding developmental and substance use disorders)

- Diagnosable currently or within the past year

- Of sufficient duration to meet diagnostic criteria specified within the *Diagnostic and Statistical Manual of Mental Disorders*

From "Statistics," National Institute on Mental Health, retrieved June 2012. For additional and updated information, visit http://www.nimh.nih.gov/statistics/index.shtml.

- Resulting in serious functional impairment, which substantially interferes with or limits one or more major life activities

Any Mental Health Disorder

Mental disorders are common in the United States, and in a given year approximately one quarter of adults are diagnosable for one or more disorders. Mental disorders are also common among U.S. children and can be particularly difficult for the children themselves and their caregivers. While mental disorders are widespread in the population, the main burden of illness is concentrated among a much smaller proportion (about six percent, or one in 17) who suffer from a seriously debilitating mental illness.

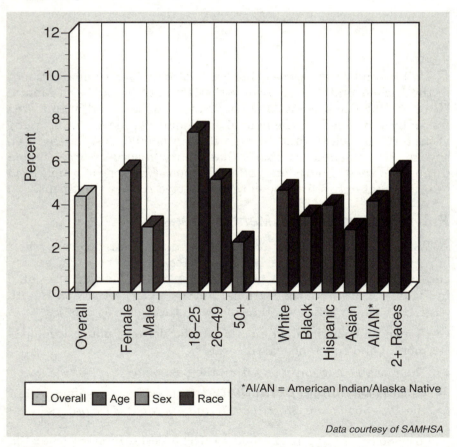

Figure 7.1. Prevalence of Serious Mental Illness among U.S. Adults by Sex, Age, and Race in 2008

- **12-month prevalence:** 26.2% of U.S. adult population; 22.3% of these cases (5.8% of the U.S. adult population) are classified as severe

- **13–18 years old lifetime prevalence:** 46.3% (21.4% of 13 to 18 year olds have a severe disorder)

- **Gender:** Women are no more or less likely than men to experience any mental health disorder over their lifetime.

- **Race:** Non-Hispanic blacks are 30% less likely than non-Hispanic whites to experience any mental health disorder during their lifetime.

- **Average age of onset:** 14 years

Anxiety Disorders

Anxiety is a normal reaction to stress and can actually be beneficial in some situations. For some people, however, anxiety can become excessive, and while the person suffering may realize it is excessive they may also have difficulty controlling it and it may negatively affect their day-to-day living. There are a wide variety of anxiety disorders, including post-traumatic stress disorder, obsessive-compulsive disorder, and specific phobias to name a few. Collectively they are among the most common mental disorders experienced by Americans.

- **12-month prevalence:** 18.1% of U.S. adult population; 22.8% of these cases (that is, 4.1% of U.S. adult population) are classified as severe.

- **13–18 years old lifetime prevalence:** 25.1% (5.9% of 13–18 year olds have a severe anxiety disorder)

- **Gender:** Women are 60% more likely than men to experience an anxiety disorder over their lifetime.

- **Race:** Non-Hispanic blacks are 20% less likely, and Hispanics are 30% less likely, than non-Hispanic whites to experience an anxiety disorder during their lifetime.

Attention Deficit/Hyperactivity Disorder

Attention deficit hyperactivity disorder (ADHD) is one of the most common childhood disorders and can continue through adolescence and into adulthood. Symptoms include difficulty staying focused and paying attention, difficulty controlling behavior, and hyperactivity (over-activity).

105

- **12-month prevalence:** 4.1% of U.S. adult population; 41.3% of these cases (1.7% of the U.S. adult population) are classified as severe.

- **13–18 years old lifetime prevalence:** 9.0% (1.8% of 13–18 year olds have severe ADHD)

- **13–18 years old prevalence by gender:** 12.9% male; 4.9% female

- **Average age of onset:** 7 years old

Autism

Autism is part of a group of disorders called autism spectrum disorders (ASD), which are sometimes also referred to as pervasive developmental disorders. ASD range in severity, with autism being the most debilitating form while other disorders, such as Asperger syndrome, produce milder symptoms. ASD are characterized by deficits in social interaction, verbal and nonverbal communication, and engagement in repetitive behaviors or interests.

Autism Rates, 8-Year Olds

- **Overall:** One in 110
- **Non-Hispanic white:** One in 101
- **Non-Hispanic black:** One in 139
- **Hispanic:** One in 170

Eating Disorders

Anorexia nervosa is characterized by emaciation, a relentless pursuit of thinness, a distortion of body image and intense fear of gaining weight, and extremely disturbed eating behavior. Many people with anorexia see themselves as overweight, even when they are starved or are clearly malnourished. Eating, food, and weight control become obsessions for people with anorexia.

Bulimia nervosa is characterized by recurrent and frequent episodes of eating unusually large amounts of food (for example, binge-eating), and feeling a lack of control over the eating. This binge-eating is followed by a type of behavior that compensates for the binge, such as purging (vomiting, excessive use of laxatives or diuretics), fasting and/or excessive exercise. Unlike anorexia nervosa, people with bulimia can fall within the normal range for their weight. But like people with anorexia, they often fear gaining weight, want desperately to lose weight, and are intensely unhappy with their body size and shape.

Binge-eating disorder is characterized by recurrent binge-eating episodes during which a person feels a loss of control over his or her eating. Unlike bulimia, binge-eating episodes are not followed by purging, excessive exercise or fasting. As a result, people with binge-eating disorder often are overweight or obese. They also experience guilt, shame and/or distress about the binge-eating, which can lead to more binge-eating.

Lifetime Prevalence of Eating Disorders

- **Anorexia nervosa:** 0.6% (female = 0.9%; male = 0.3%)

- **Bulimia nervosa:** 0.6% (female = 0.5%; male = 0.1%)

- **Binge eating disorder:** 2.8% (female = 3.5%; male = 2.0%)

Any Mood Disorder among Adults

Mood disorders represent a category of mental disorders in which the underlying problem primarily affects a person's persistent emotional state (their mood). They include depression, bipolar disorder, and dysthymic disorder.

- **12-month prevalence:** 9.5% of U.S. adult population; 45% of these cases (4.3% of the U.S. adult population) are classified as severe.

- **13–18 years old lifetime prevalence:** 14.0% (4.7% of 13–18 year olds have a severe mood disorder)

- **Gender:** Women are 50% more likely than men to experience a mood disorder over their lifetime.

- **Race:** Non-Hispanic blacks are 40% less likely, and Hispanics are 20% less likely, than non-Hispanic whites to experience a mood disorder during their lifetime.

- **Average age of onset:** 30 years

Personality Disorders

Personality disorders represent "an enduring pattern of inner experience and behavior that deviates markedly from the expectations of the culture of the individual who exhibits it" according to the American Psychiatric Association's *Diagnostic and Statistical Manual on*

Mental Disorders, Fourth Edition (*DSM-IV*). These patterns tend to be fixed and consistent across situations and are typically perceived to be appropriate by the individual even though they may markedly affect their day-to-day life in negative ways. Personality disorders encompass antisocial personality disorder, avoidant personality disorder, and borderline personality disorder.

- **12-month prevalence, any personality disorder:** 9.1% of U.S. adult population (% severe not reported)

  - 12-month prevalence antisocial personality disorder: 1.0%

  - 12-month prevalence avoidant personality disorder: 5.2%

  - 12-month prevalence borderline personality disorder: 1.6%

- **Gender and race:** Sex and race were not found to be associated with personality disorders, however there was a statistical trend for men to be more likely to have antisocial personality disorder than women.

Schizophrenia

Schizophrenia is a chronic, severe, and disabling mental disorder characterized by deficits in thought processes, perceptions, and emotional responsiveness. Schizophrenia's symptoms are typically described as "positive" or "negative." Positive symptoms are those that are found among people with schizophrenia but not present among those who do not have the disorder. These may include delusions, thought disorders, and hallucinations. People with schizophrenia may hear voices other people don't hear, or believe other people are reading their minds, controlling their thoughts, or plotting to harm them. Negative symptoms are those found among people who do not have the disorder but that are missing or lacking among individuals with schizophrenia. These may include avolition (a lack of desire or motivation to accomplish goals), lack of desire to form social relationships, and blunted affect (mood) and emotion. These symptoms make holding a job, forming relationships, and other day-to-day functions especially difficult for people with schizophrenia.

- **12-month prevalence:** 1.1% of U.S. adult population (% severe not reported)

- **12-month healthcare use:** 60% of adults with schizophrenia

Part Two

Mental Illnesses

Chapter 8

Suicide and Mental Illness

Chapter Contents

Section 8.1

Facts about Suicide

"Suicide: Facts at a Glance," Centers for Disease Control
and Prevention (www.cdc.gov), Summer 2010.

Fatal Suicidal Behavior

In 2007:

- Suicide was the eleventh leading cause of death for all ages.

- More than 34,000 suicides occurred in the U.S. This is the equivalent of 94 suicides per day; one suicide every 15 minutes or 11.26 suicides per 100,000 population.

- The National Violent Death Reporting System includes information on the presence of alcohol and other substances at the time of death. For those tested for substances, the findings from the 16 states revealed that one-third of those who died by suicide were positive for alcohol at the time of death and nearly one in five had evidence of opiates, including heroin and prescription pain killers.

Nonfatal Suicidal Thoughts and Behavior

- Among young adults ages 15 to 24 years old, there are approximately 100–200 attempts for every completed suicide.

- Among adults ages 65 years and older, there are approximately four suicide attempts for every completed suicide.

- In 2009, 13.8% of U.S. high school students reported that they had seriously considered attempting suicide during the 12 months preceding the survey; 6.3% of students reported that they had actually attempted suicide one or more times during the same period.

Gender Disparities

- Males take their own lives at nearly four times the rate of females and represent 78.8% of all U.S. suicides.

- During their lifetime, women attempt suicide about two to three times as often as men.

- Suicide is the seventh leading cause of death for males and the fifteenth leading cause for females.

- Suicide rates for males are highest among those aged 75 and older (rate 36.1 per 100,000).

- Suicide rates for females are highest among those aged 45–54 (rate 8.8 per 100,000 population).

- Firearms are the most commonly used method of suicide among males (55.7%).

- Poisoning is the most common method of suicide for females (40.2%).

Racial and Ethnic Disparities

- Among American Indians/Alaska Natives ages 15- to 34-years, suicide is the second leading cause of death.

- Suicide rates among American Indian/Alaskan Native adolescents and young adults ages 15 to 34 (20.0 per 100,000) are 1.8 times higher than the national average for that age group (11.4 per 100,000).

- Hispanic and Black, non-Hispanic female high school students in grades 9–12 reported a higher percentage of suicide attempts (11.1% and 10.4%, respectively) than their White, non-Hispanic counterparts (6.5%).

Age Group Differences

- Suicide is the second leading cause of death among 25–34 year olds and the third leading cause of death among 15- to 24-year olds.

- Among 15- to 24-year olds, suicide accounts for 12.2% of all deaths annually.

- The rate of suicide for adults aged 75 years and older was 16.0 per 100,000.

Nonfatal, Self-Inflicted Injuries

The term "self-inflicted injuries" refers to suicidal and non-suicidal behaviors such as self-mutilation.

- In 2008, 376,306 people were treated in emergency departments for self-inflicted injuries.

- In 2008, 163,489 people were hospitalized due to self-inflicted injury.

- There is one suicide for every 25 attempted suicides.

Suicide-Related Behaviors among U.S. High School Students

In 2009:

- 13.8% of students in grades 9–12 seriously considered suicide in the previous 12 months (17.4% of females and 10.5% of males).

- 6.3% of students reported making at least one suicide attempt in the previous 12 months (8.1% of females and 4.6% of males).

- 1.9% of students had made a suicide attempt that resulted in an injury, poisoning, or an overdose that required medical attention (2.3% of females and 1.6% of males).

Section 8.2

Questions about Suicide Risk

Suicide and Depression

Why do people kill themselves?

Unfortunately, there is no simple answer to this question. People die by suicide for a number of reasons. However, the majority of the people who take their lives (estimated at 90%) were suffering with an underlying mental illness and substance abuse problem at the time of their death. They weren't sick, but their brains were. Too often we think that a person is their brain, that's where their personality or character resides. This is not true. The brain is an organ just like the liver, the kidneys, the gall bladder, etc. When it gets sick too often the appearance of the problem is in the form of a mental illness, as in the case of depression, bipolar disorder, anxiety disorders, or schizophrenia. If the brain is sick too long, it can lead a person to taking their lives. This isn't always the case, as millions of people live with depression and never attempt or die by suicide, but with awareness, education, and treatment, people can be helped so that suicide does not become an option.

Do people attempt suicide to prove something or to get sympathy?

No. A suicide attempt is a cry for help that should never be ignored. It is a warning that something is terribly wrong. Chronic depression can lead to feelings of despair and hopelessness, and a suicide attempt is one way some people choose to express these feelings. Most people who attempt or commit suicide don't really want to die—they just want their pain and suffering to end. A suicide attempt is also not done to gain someone's sympathy, as those that attempt to take their life do it for internal reasons-they simply can't stand the pain they

115

feel emotionally and/or physically. It isn't to try and get someone to feel bad for them, that's the last thing they would want.

A suicide attempt must always be taken seriously. Without intervention and proper treatment, a person who has attempted suicide is at greater risk of another attempt and possible suicide.

What is depression and what are depressive illnesses?

Depression and depressive illnesses are classified as mood disorders in the medical field, including everything from major depression to dysthymia. They have a number of symptoms that affect people socially, occupationally, educationally, interpersonally, etc. How does one become depressed? Basically, here's how it works: the nerves in our brain don't touch each other, but rather pass messages from one to the next through chemicals called neurotransmitters. We need just the right amount of this chemical between the nerves to pass the exact same message to the next nerve. If there isn't enough of that chemical, the message doesn't get passed along correctly and in this case, depression or a depressive illness can result. When it comes to depressive disorders the chemicals most frequently out of balance are serotonin and norepinephrine.

A person living with depression does not always have the same thoughts as a healthy person. This chemical imbalance can lead to the person not understanding the options available to help them relieve their suffering. Many people who suffer from depression report feeling as though they've lost the ability to imagine a happy future, or remember a happy past. Often they don't realize they're suffering from a treatable illness, and seeking help may not even enter their mind. Emotions and even physical pain can become unbearable. They don't want to die, but it's the only way they feel their pain will end. It is a truly irrational choice. Suffering from depression is involuntary, just like cancer or diabetes, but it is a treatable illness that can be managed.

How do alcohol and drugs affect depression?

Alcohol is a depressant, so it can and often does make depression worse. Drug use alone or in combination with alcohol use for someone suffering with depression can be lethal. Too often people attempt to alleviate the symptoms of depression by drinking or using drugs which can increase the risk of suicide by impairing judgment and increasing impulsivity.

116

Can a suicidal person mask their depression?

Sure, they can and sometimes do. But we can all be more aware of the signs and symptoms of depression to help those we care about get the necessary treatment to relieve them of their pain. Plus, because many people who are depressed can not see their symptoms, we have to be their eyes and ears for them to help save their life. Many people suffering from depression and even contemplating suicide hide their feelings and appear to be happy just prior to their suicide attempt. This often confuses the people around them since for so long they had been suffering and appearing depressed, then all of a sudden seem better. However, most of the time a person who is suicidal will give clues as to how desperate they feel. It is critical that you familiarize yourself with the symptoms of depression and the warning signs of suicide, and not be afraid to ask direct questions about feelings of the person you're concerned about—it could be what save's their life!

Is a person at increased risk to attempt suicide if they've been exposed to it in their family or has had a close friend who died by suicide?

Yes, suicide does tend to run in families, but this is generally attributed to the genetic component of depression and related depressive illnesses. A healthy person talking about a suicide or being aware of a suicide among family or friends does not put them at greater risk for attempting suicide. And mere exposure to suicide does not alone put someone at greater risk for suicide. However, when combined with a number of other risk factors, it could increase someone's likelihood of an attempt. Failing to treat or mistreating depressive illness puts a person at increased risk of suicide. It is very important to remember that the vast majority of people living with depression do not have suicidal thoughts or die by suicide.

Why don't people talk about mental illnesses like depression, bipolar disorder and suicide?

Stigma and lack of understanding are the main reasons depression remains a topic we avoid. People suffering from depression fear others will think they're crazy or weak, or somehow a lesser person. Cultural norms are slowly changing, and people are becoming more aware of the nature of depressive illnesses and their impact on a person's well being. Education will help reduce stigma and save lives.

Alcoholism, drug addiction, HIV and AIDS are examples of medical conditions previously attributed to a weakness or character problems. Today, they are widely recognized as medical diseases and people feel comfortable openly discussing the impact of the disease and seeking help through a variety of treatments. The dangers of alcohol and substance abuse have been the subject of major national public health campaigns in the United States, leading to a general public more aware of the value of prevention. Breast cancer is another medical illness that for many years went unspoken, but today receives millions of dollars in research funding, supportive programming and awareness. Issues of medical illnesses in the brain which we call mental illnesses still face huge obstacles to funding, support and awareness, but progress is being made.

Will "talking things out" help treat depression?

Talking does help treat depression. However, research continues to show that a combination of psychotherapy (talk therapy) and antidepressant medication is the most effective way to treat depression. In some cases, well-supported psychotherapies, such as cognitive behavioral therapy or interpersonal therapy can considerably alleviate the symptoms of depression. However, a medical doctor should supervise any course of treatment.

Why do people attempt suicide when they appear to feel better?

Sometimes a severely depressed person contemplating suicide doesn't have enough energy to attempt it. As the disease lifts they may regain some energy but feelings of hopelessness remain, and the increased energy levels contribute to acting on suicidal feelings. Another theory proposes that a person may "give in" to the disease because they can't fight it anymore. This relieves some anxiety, which makes them appear calmer in the period preceding a suicide attempt.

If a person's mind is made up can they still be stopped?

Absolutely! Never give up on someone contemplating suicide. For a person determined to attempt suicide the desire to live is overshadowed by the seeming hopelessness of the disease. The decision to attempt suicide is really a desire to stop suffering. Never give up on someone just because they say they've made up their mind. Depression is a crisis and intervening to help the person regain perspective and aggressively fight the disease can help reverse the downward trend toward suicidal thoughts or attempts.

Is depression the same as the blues?

No. Depression is a medical illness in the brain that can be clinically diagnosed and treated. While it's normal and even expected to feel badly about losing someone you love or experiencing a disappointing or traumatic event, to consistently experience the symptoms of depression for longer than two weeks under normal circumstances may indicate the presence of a diagnosable illness.

Why do depressive illnesses sometimes lead to suicidal thoughts?

As depression deepens and takes over the body and mind, the pain of depression often becomes overwhelming. The chemical imbalance and deep despair can lead the brain to try and find ways to end the pain. This is when suicidal thinking begins. Depressive illnesses can distort thinking such that a person can't think clearly or rationally. The illness can cause thoughts of hopelessness and helplessness, which may lead to suicidal thoughts. Education about the symptoms of depression and the warning signs of suicide help people understand that depression and related depressive illnesses are both preventable and treatable.

What causes a depressive illness?

Depressive illnesses are biological illnesses related to imbalance or disrupted brain chemistry. The brain is an organ of the body and can get sick just like the heart, liver, or kidneys.

A combination of genetic, psychological and environmental factors play a role in how and when a depressive illness manifests, and the same is true for suicide. Because these are illnesses, stress doesn't necessarily have to be present, but can trigger or exacerbate a depression. Although rare, depression can appear out of nowhere when there would be no reason for a person to feel depressed. More commonly depression comes on over a period of time with many factors going on at once in a person's life.

People of all ages, including children, youth and adolescents, can suffer from depressive illnesses. Since they may be genetically predisposed to depression, a person may be at higher risk than someone whose family doesn't have a history of depression. This doesn't however necessarily mean everyone will inherit a depressive illness. They just might have a predisposition or tendency toward it.

What are the different types of depressive illnesses?

Types of depression include:

119

- Seasonal affective disorder
- Major depression
- Dysthymia
- Cyclothymia
- Atypical depression
- Premenstrual syndrome

Can depressive illnesses be treated?

Yes. There are various ways to treat depressive illnesses depending on the type of illness, the severity, and the age of the person being treated. A person suffering with depression should not try to manage the illness on their own. Knowing and recognizing the signs of depressive illness helps avoid needless suffering available through treatment. Depression is a condition like diabetes or high blood pressure that can be effectively managed with the help of mental health professionals including medical doctors, registered nurses, psychologists and therapists, social workers, clergy, family members, and community support.

Research shows a combination of antidepressant medication and psychotherapy to be the quickest, most effective treatment. Often, antidepressant medication is needed to help a person to think more clearly in psychotherapy. There are several types of psychotherapy, but two have proven beneficial in treating depressive illnesses:

- Cognitive therapy focuses on trying to change a person's negative thinking and the inaccurate perceptions they have of themselves and their environment. People are taught to think logically, and to avoid negative self-talk.

- Interpersonal therapy teaches a person how to successfully inter-act with others. Depressive illnesses interfere with how a person treats their family, friends, and co-workers, which affects how they treat them in return. Interpersonal therapy focuses on social skills.

What is an anxiety disorder?

Anxiety is a normal feeling we experience everyday. However, anxi-ety disorders are characterized by feeling excessive fear, nervousness or worry that something bad might happen even though there is no logical or specific reason to be afraid. Many times depressive illnesses and anxiety go hand in hand.

Section 8.3

Suicide Prevention

If you are suicidal or you think someone you know is, we want you to know that help is available and recovery is possible! Start by learning the warning signs, and do whatever you can to get yourself or someone you care about to the help they need so that they can return to living a fully functioning life.

Symptoms and Danger Signs

Warning Signs of Suicide

These signs may mean someone is at risk for suicide. Risk is greater if a behavior is new or has increased and if it seems related to a painful event, loss, or change.

- Talking about wanting to die or to kill oneself.
- Looking for a way to kill oneself, such as searching online or buying a gun.
- Talking about feeling hopeless or having no reason to live.
- Talking about feeling trapped or in unbearable pain.
- Talking about being a burden to others.
- Increasing the use of alcohol or drugs.
- Acting anxious or agitated; behaving recklessly.
- Sleeping too little or too much.
- Withdrawn or feeling isolated.
- Showing rage or talking about seeking revenge.
- Displaying extreme mood swings.

Additional Warning Signs of Suicide

- Preoccupation with death.
- Suddenly happier, calmer.
- Loss of interest in things one cares about.
- Visiting or calling people to say goodbye.
- Making arrangements; setting one's affairs in order.
- Giving things away, such as prized possessions.

A suicidal person urgently needs to see a doctor or mental health professional.

In an emergency, call the National Suicide Prevention Lifeline 1-800-273-TALK (8255).

Common Misconceptions

The following are common misconceptions about suicide:

"People who talk about suicide won't really do it."

Not True: Almost everyone who commits or attempts suicide has given some clue or warning. Do not ignore suicide threats. Statements like "you'll be sorry when I'm dead," "I can't see any way out,"—no matter how casually or jokingly said, may indicate serious suicidal feelings.

"Anyone who tries to kill him/herself must be crazy."

Not True: Most suicidal people are not psychotic or insane. They may be upset, grief-stricken, depressed or despairing. Extreme distress and emotional pain are always signs of mental illness but are not signs of psychosis.

"If a person is determined to kill him/herself, nothing is going to stop him/her."

Not True: Even the most severely depressed person has mixed feelings about death, and most waiver until the very last moment between wanting to live and wanting to end their pain. Most suicidal people do not want to die; they want the pain to stop. The impulse to end it all, however overpowering, does not last forever.

"People who commit suicide are people who were unwilling to seek help."

Not True: Studies of adult suicide victims have shown that more than half had sought medical help within six month before their deaths and a majority had seen a medical professional within one month of their death.

"Talking about suicide may give someone the idea."

Not True: You don't give a suicidal person ideas by talking about suicide. The opposite is true—bringing up the subject of suicide and discussing it openly is one of the most helpful things you can do.

Someone You Know Is Suicidal

Know What to Watch For

- Symptoms of depression
- Warning signs of suicide

Know What to Do

Stigma associated with mental illnesses can prevent people from getting help. Your willingness to talk about mental or emotional issues and suicide with a friend, family member, or co-worker can be the first step in getting them help and preventing suicide.

If You See the Warning Signs of Suicide...

Begin a dialogue by asking questions: Suicidal thoughts are common with some mental illnesses and your willingness to talk about it in a non-judgmental, non-confrontational way can be the help a person needs to seeking professional help. Questions okay to ask:

- "Do you ever feel so badly that you think about suicide?"
- "Do you have a plan to commit suicide or take your life?"
- "Have you thought about when you would do it (today, tomorrow, next week)?"
- "Have you thought about what method you would use?"

Asking these questions will help you to determine if your friend or family members is in immediate danger, and get help if needed. A suicidal person should see a doctor or mental health professional immediately. Calling 911 or going to a hospital emergency room are also good options to prevent a tragic suicide attempt or death. Calling the National Lifeline at 1-800-273-TALK (8255) is also a resource for you or the person you care about for help. Remember, always take thoughts of or plans for suicide seriously.

Never keep a plan for suicide a secret: Don't worry about risking a friendship if you truly feel a life is in danger. You have bigger things to worry about—someone's life might be in danger! It is better to lose a relationship from violating a confidence than it is to go to a funeral. And most of the time they will come back and thank you for saving their life.

Don't try to minimize problems or shame a person into changing their mind: Your opinion of a person's situation is irrelevant. Trying to convince a person suffering with a mental illness that it's not that bad, or that they have everything to live for may only increase their feelings of guilt and hopelessness. Reassure them that help is available, that what they are experiencing is treatable, and that suicidal feelings are temporary. Life can get better!

If you feel the person isn't in immediate danger, acknowledge the pain is legitimate and offer to work together to get help: Make sure you follow through. This is one instance where you must be tenacious in your follow-up. Help find a doctor or a mental health professional, participate in making the first phone call, or go along to the first appointment. If you're in a position to help, don't assume that your persistence is unwanted or intrusive. Risking your feelings to help save a life is a risk worth taking.

Suicidal Thoughts: What to Do

If you have thoughts of suicide, these options are available to you

- Dial: 911
- Dial: 1-800-273-TALK (8255)
- Check yourself into the emergency room.
- Call your local crisis agency.
- Tell someone who can help you find help immediately.
- Stay away from things that might hurt you.

- Most people can be treated with a combination of antidepressant medication and psychotherapy.

If you don't have insurance the following options might be used

- Go to the nearest hospital emergency room.

- Look in your local Yellow Pages under Mental Health and/or Suicide Prevention; then call the mental health organizations/crisis phone lines that are listed. There may be clinics or counseling centers in your area operating on a sliding or no-fee scale.

- Some pharmaceutical companies have "Free Medication Programs" for those who qualify.

Chapter 9

Depressive Disorders

Chapter Contents

Section 9.1

Major Depression

Excerpted from "Depression," National Institute of Mental Health (www.nimh.nih.gov), NIH Publication No. 11-3561, October 4, 2011.

What Is Depression?

Everyone occasionally feels blue or sad. But these feelings are usually short-lived and pass within a couple of days. When you have depression, it interferes with daily life and causes pain for both you and those who care about you. Depression is a common but serious illness.

Many people with a depressive illness never seek treatment. But the majority, even those with the most severe depression, can get better with treatment. Medications, psychotherapies, and other methods can effectively treat people with depression.

What are the different forms of depression?

There are several forms of depressive disorders.

Major depressive disorder, or major depression, is characterized by a combination of symptoms that interfere with a person's ability to work, sleep, study, eat, and enjoy once-pleasurable activities. Major depression is disabling and prevents a person from functioning normally. Some people may experience only a single episode within their lifetime, but more often a person may have multiple episodes.

Dysthymic disorder, or dysthymia, is characterized by long-term (two years or longer) symptoms that may not be severe enough to disable a person but can prevent normal functioning or feeling well. People with dysthymia may also experience one or more episodes of major depression during their lifetimes.

Minor depression is characterized by having symptoms for two weeks or longer that do not meet full criteria for major depression. Without treatment, people with minor depression are at high risk for developing major depressive disorder.

Some forms of depression are slightly different, or they may develop under unique circumstances. However, not everyone agrees on how to characterize and define these forms of depression. They include the following:

- Psychotic depression, which occurs when a person has severe depression plus some form of psychosis, such as having disturbing false beliefs or a break with reality (delusions), or hearing or seeing upsetting things that others cannot hear or see (hallucinations).

- Postpartum depression, which is much more serious than the baby blues that many women experience after giving birth, when hormonal and physical changes and the new responsibility of caring for a newborn can be overwhelming. It is estimated that 10 to 15 percent of women experience postpartum depression after giving birth.

- Seasonal affective disorder (SAD), which is characterized by the onset of depression during the winter months, when there is less natural sunlight. The depression generally lifts during spring and summer. SAD may be effectively treated with light therapy, but nearly half of those with SAD do not get better with light therapy alone. Antidepressant medication and psychotherapy can reduce SAD symptoms, either alone or in combination with light therapy.

Bipolar disorder, also called manic-depressive illness, is not as common as major depression or dysthymia. Bipolar disorder is characterized by cycling mood changes—from extreme highs (mania) to extreme lows (depression).

What are the signs and symptoms of depression?

People with depressive illnesses do not all experience the same symptoms. The severity, frequency, and duration of symptoms vary depending on the individual and his or her particular illness.

Signs and symptoms include the following:

- Persistent sad, anxious, or "empty" feelings
- Feelings of hopelessness or pessimism
- Feelings of guilt, worthlessness, or helplessness
- Irritability, restlessness
- Loss of interest in activities or hobbies once pleasurable, including sex
- Fatigue and decreased energy

- Difficulty concentrating, remembering details, and making decisions
- Insomnia, early-morning wakefulness, or excessive sleeping
- Overeating or appetite loss
- Thoughts of suicide, suicide attempts
- Aches or pains, headaches, cramps, or digestive problems that do not ease even with treatment.

What illnesses often co-exist with depression?

Other illnesses may come on before depression, cause it, or be a consequence of it. But depression and other illnesses interact differently in different people. In any case, co-occurring illnesses need to be diagnosed and treated.

Anxiety disorders, such as post-traumatic stress disorder (PTSD), obsessive-compulsive disorder, panic disorder, social phobia, and generalized anxiety disorder, often accompany depression. PTSD can occur after a person experiences a terrifying event or ordeal, such as a violent assault, a natural disaster, an accident, terrorism, or military combat. People experiencing PTSD are especially prone to having co-existing depression.

In a National Institute of Mental Health (NIMH)–funded study, researchers found that more than 40 percent of people with PTSD also had depression four months after the traumatic event.

Alcohol and other substance abuse or dependence may also co-exist with depression. Research shows that mood disorders and substance abuse commonly occur together.

Depression also may occur with other serious medical illnesses such as heart disease, stroke, cancer, HIV/AIDS, diabetes, and Parkinson disease. People who have depression along with another medical illness tend to have more severe symptoms of both depression and the medical illness, more difficulty adapting to their medical condition, and more medical costs than those who do not have co-existing depression. Treating the depression can also help improve the outcome of treating the co-occurring illness.

What causes depression?

Most likely, depression is caused by a combination of genetic, biological, environmental, and psychological factors.

Depressive illnesses are disorders of the brain. Longstanding theories about depression suggest that important neurotransmitters—chemicals that brain cells use to communicate—are out of balance in depression. But it has been difficult to prove this.

Brain-imaging technologies, such as magnetic resonance imaging (MRI), have shown that the brains of people who have depression look different than those of people without depression. The parts of the brain involved in mood, thinking, sleep, appetite, and behavior appear different. But these images do not reveal why the depression has occurred. They also cannot be used to diagnose depression.

Some types of depression tend to run in families. However, depression can occur in people without family histories of depression too. Scientists are studying certain genes that may make some people more prone to depression. Some genetics research indicates that risk for depression results from the influence of several genes acting together with environmental or other factors. In addition, trauma, loss of a loved one, a difficult relationship, or any stressful situation may trigger a depressive episode. Other depressive episodes may occur with or without an obvious trigger.

How do women experience depression?

Depression is more common among women than among men. Biological, life cycle, hormonal, and psychosocial factors that women experience may be linked to women's higher depression rate. Researchers have shown that hormones directly affect the brain chemistry that controls emotions and mood. For example, women are especially vulnerable to developing postpartum depression after giving birth, when hormonal and physical changes and the new responsibility of caring for a newborn can be overwhelming.

Some women may also have a severe form of premenstrual syndrome (PMS) called premenstrual dysphoric disorder (PMDD). PMDD is associated with the hormonal changes that typically occur around ovulation and before menstruation begins.

During the transition into menopause, some women experience an increased risk for depression. In addition, osteoporosis—bone thinning or loss—may be associated with depression. Scientists are exploring all of these potential connections and how the cyclical rise and fall of estrogen and other hormones may affect a woman's brain chemistry.

Finally, many women face the additional stresses of work and home responsibilities, caring for children and aging parents, abuse, poverty, and relationship strains. It is still unclear, though, why some women faced with enormous challenges develop depression, while others with similar challenges do not.

How do men experience depression?

Men often experience depression differently than women. While women with depression are more likely to have feelings of sadness, worthlessness, and excessive guilt, men are more likely to be very tired, irritable, lose interest in once-pleasurable activities, and have difficulty sleeping.

Men may be more likely than women to turn to alcohol or drugs when they are depressed. They also may become frustrated, discouraged, irritable, angry, and sometimes abusive. Some men throw themselves into their work to avoid talking about their depression with family or friends, or behave recklessly. And although more women attempt suicide, many more men die by suicide in the United States.

How do older adults experience depression?

Depression is not a normal part of aging. Studies show that most seniors feel satisfied with their lives, despite having more illnesses or physical problems. However, when older adults do have depression, it may be overlooked because seniors may show different, less obvious symptoms. They may be less likely to experience or admit to feelings of sadness or grief.

Sometimes it can be difficult to distinguish grief from major depression. Grief after loss of a loved one is a normal reaction to the loss and generally does not require professional mental health treatment. However, grief that is complicated and lasts for a very long time following a loss may require treatment. Researchers continue to study the relationship between complicated grief and major depression.

Older adults also may have more medical conditions such as heart disease, stroke, or cancer, which may cause depressive symptoms. Or they may be taking medications with side effects that contribute to depression. Some older adults may experience what doctors call vascular depression, also called arteriosclerotic depression or subcortical ischemic depression. Vascular depression may result when blood vessels become less flexible and harden over time, becoming constricted. Such hardening of vessels prevents normal blood flow to the body's organs, including the brain. Those with vascular depression may have, or be at risk for, co-existing heart disease or stroke.

Although many people assume that the highest rates of suicide are among young people, older white males age 85 and older actually have the highest suicide rate in the United States. Many have a depressive illness that their doctors are not aware of, even though many of these suicide victims visit their doctors within one month of their deaths.

Most older adults with depression improve when they receive treatment with an antidepressant, psychotherapy, or a combination of both. Research has shown that medication alone and combination treatment are both effective in reducing depression in older adults. Psychotherapy alone also can be effective in helping older adults stay free of depression, especially among those with minor depression. Psychotherapy is particularly useful for those who are unable or unwilling to take antidepressant medication.

How do children and teens experience depression?

Children who develop depression often continue to have episodes as they enter adulthood. Children who have depression also are more likely to have other more severe illnesses in adulthood.

A child with depression may pretend to be sick, refuse to go to school, cling to a parent, or worry that a parent may die. Older children may sulk, get into trouble at school, be negative and irritable, and feel misunderstood. Because these signs may be viewed as normal mood swings typical of children as they move through developmental stages, it may be difficult to accurately diagnose a young person with depression.

Before puberty, boys and girls are equally likely to develop depression. By age 15, however, girls are twice as likely as boys to have had a major depressive episode.

Depression during the teen years comes at a time of great personal change—when boys and girls are forming an identity apart from their parents, grappling with gender issues and emerging sexuality, and making independent decisions for the first time in their lives. Depression in adolescence frequently co-occurs with other disorders such as anxiety, eating disorders, or substance abuse. It can also lead to increased risk for suicide.

How is depression diagnosed and treated?

Depression, even the most severe cases, can be effectively treated. The earlier that treatment can begin, the more effective it is.

The first step to getting appropriate treatment is to visit a doctor or mental health specialist. Certain medications, and some medical conditions such as viruses or a thyroid disorder, can cause the same symptoms as depression. A doctor can rule out these possibilities by doing a physical exam, interview, and lab tests. If the doctor can find no medical condition that may be causing the depression, the next step is a psychological evaluation.

The doctor may refer you to a mental health professional, who should discuss with you any family history of depression or other mental disorder, and get a complete history of your symptoms. You should discuss when your symptoms started, how long they have lasted, how severe they are, and whether they have occurred before and if so, how they were treated. The mental health professional may also ask if you are using alcohol or drugs, and if you are thinking about death or suicide.

Once diagnosed, a person with depression can be treated in several ways. The most common treatments are medication and psychotherapy.

How is medication used in treating depression?

Antidepressants primarily work on brain chemicals called neurotransmitters, especially serotonin and norepinephrine. Other antidepressants work on the neurotransmitter dopamine. Scientists have found that these particular chemicals are involved in regulating mood, but they are unsure of the exact ways that they work. The latest information on medications for treating depression is available on the U.S. Food and Drug Administration (FDA) website (www.fda.gov).

Popular newer antidepressants: Some of the newest and most popular antidepressants are called selective serotonin reuptake inhibitors (SSRIs). Fluoxetine (Prozac), sertraline (Zoloft), escitalopram (Lexapro), paroxetine (Paxil), and citalopram (Celexa) are some of the most commonly prescribed SSRIs for depression. Most are available in generic versions. Serotonin and norepinephrine reuptake inhibitors (SNRIs) are similar to SSRIs and include venlafaxine (Effexor) and duloxetine (Cymbalta).

SSRIs and SNRIs tend to have fewer side effects than older antidepressants, but they sometimes produce headaches, nausea, jitters, or insomnia when people first start to take them. These symptoms tend to fade with time. Some people also experience sexual problems with SSRIs or SNRIs, which may be helped by adjusting the dosage or switching to another medication.

One popular antidepressant that works on dopamine is bupropion (Wellbutrin). Bupropion tends to have similar side effects as SSRIs and SNRIs, but it is less likely to cause sexual side effects. However, it can increase a person's risk for seizures.

Tricyclics: Tricyclics are older antidepressants. Tricyclics are powerful, but they are not used as much today because their potential side effects are more serious. They may affect the heart in people with heart conditions. They sometimes cause dizziness, especially in older adults. They also may cause drowsiness, dry mouth, and weight gain. These side effects can usually be corrected by changing the dosage or switching to another medication. However, tricyclics may be especially dangerous if taken in overdose. Tricyclics include imipramine and nortriptyline.

MAOIs: Monoamine oxidase inhibitors (MAOIs) are the oldest class of antidepressant medications. They can be especially effective in cases of atypical depression, such as when a person experiences increased appetite and the need for more sleep rather than decreased appetite and sleep. They also may help with anxious feelings or panic and other specific symptoms.

However, people who take MAOIs must avoid certain foods and beverages (including cheese and red wine) that contain a substance called tyramine. Certain medications, including some types of birth control pills, prescription pain relievers, cold and allergy medications, and herbal supplements, also should be avoided while taking an MAOI. These substances can interact with MAOIs to cause dangerous increases in blood pressure. The development of a new MAOI skin patch may help reduce these risks. If you are taking an MAOI, your doctor should give you a complete list of foods, medicines, and substances to avoid.

MAOIs can also react with SSRIs to produce a serious condition called serotonin syndrome, which can cause confusion, hallucinations, increased sweating, muscle stiffness, seizures, changes in blood pressure or heart rhythm, and other potentially life-threatening conditions. MAOIs should not be taken with SSRIs.

Are antidepressants safe?

Despite the relative safety and popularity of SSRIs and other antidepressants, studies have suggested that they may have unintentional effects on some people, especially adolescents and young adults. In 2004, the Food and Drug Administration (FDA) conducted a thorough review of published and unpublished controlled clinical trials of antidepressants that involved nearly 4,400 children and adolescents. The review revealed that four percent of those taking antidepressants thought about or attempted suicide (although no suicides occurred), compared to two percent of those receiving placebos.

This information prompted the FDA, in 2005, to adopt a black box warning label on all antidepressant medications to alert the public about the potential increased risk of suicidal thinking or attempts in children and adolescents taking antidepressants. In 2007, the FDA proposed that makers of all antidepressant medications extend the warning to include young adults up through age 24. A black box warning is the most serious type of warning on prescription drug labeling.

The warning emphasizes that patients of all ages taking antidepressants should be closely monitored, especially during the initial weeks of treatment. Possible side effects to look for are worsening depression, suicidal thinking or behavior, or any unusual changes in behavior such as sleeplessness, agitation, or withdrawal from normal social situations. The warning adds that families and caregivers should also be told of the need for close monitoring and report any changes to the doctor. The latest information from the FDA can be found on their website (www.fda.gov).

Results of a comprehensive review of pediatric trials conducted between 1988 and 2006 suggested that the benefits of antidepressant medications likely outweigh their risks to children and adolescents with major depression and anxiety disorders. The study was funded in part by NIMH.

Also, the FDA issued a warning that combining an SSRI or SNRI antidepressant with one of the commonly used "triptan" medications for migraine headache could cause a life-threatening "serotonin syndrome," marked by agitation, hallucinations, elevated body temperature, and rapid changes in blood pressure. Although most dramatic in the case of the MAOIs, newer antidepressants may also be associated with potentially dangerous interactions with other medications.

What about St. John's wort?

The extract from the herb St. John's wort (*Hypericum perforatum*) has been used for centuries in many folk and herbal remedies. In an eight-week trial involving 340 patients diagnosed with major depression, St. John's wort was compared to a common SSRI and a placebo (sugar pill). The trial found that St. John's wort was no more effective than the placebo in treating major depression. However, use of St. John's wort for minor or moderate depression may be more effective. Its use in the treatment of depression remains under study.

In 2000, the FDA issued a Public Health Advisory letter stating that the herb may interfere with certain medications used to treat heart disease, depression, seizures, certain cancers, and those used to prevent organ transplant rejection. The herb also may interfere with the effectiveness of oral contraceptives. Consult with your doctor before taking any herbal supplement.

How is psychotherapy used in treating depression?

Several types of psychotherapy—or talk therapy—can help people with depression.

Two main types of psychotherapies—cognitive-behavioral therapy (CBT) and interpersonal therapy (IPT)—are effective in treating depression. CBT helps people with depression restructure negative thought patterns. Doing so helps people interpret their environment and interactions with others in a positive and realistic way. It may also help you recognize things that may be contributing to the depression and help you change behaviors that may be making the depression worse. IPT helps people understand and work through troubled relationships that may cause their depression or make it worse.

For mild to moderate depression, psychotherapy may be the best option. However, for severe depression or for certain people, psychotherapy may not be enough. For teens, a combination of medication and psychotherapy may be the most effective approach to treating major depression and reducing the chances of it coming back. Another study looking at depression treatment among older adults found that people who responded to initial treatment of medication and IPT were less likely to have recurring depression if they continued their combination treatment for at least two years.

What are electroconvulsive therapy and other brain stimulation therapies?

For cases in which medication and/or psychotherapy does not help relieve a person's treatment-resistant depression, electroconvulsive therapy (ECT) may be useful. ECT, formerly known as shock therapy, once had a bad reputation. But in recent years, it has greatly improved and can provide relief for people with severe depression who have not been able to feel better with other treatments. [For more information about ECT and other brain stimulation therapies, see Chapter 24—Brain Stimulation Therapies.]

How can I help a loved one who is depressed?

If you know someone who is depressed, it affects you too. The most important thing you can do is help your friend or relative get a diagnosis and treatment. You may need to make an appointment and go with him or her to see the doctor. Encourage your loved one to stay in treatment, or to seek different treatment if no improvement occurs after six to eight weeks.

Here are some suggestions you can follow to help your friend or relative:

- Offer emotional support, understanding, patience, and encouragement.

- Talk to him or her, and listen carefully.

- Never dismiss feelings, but point out realities and offer hope.

- Never ignore comments about suicide, and report them to your loved one's therapist or doctor.

- Invite your loved one out for walks, outings and other activities. Keep trying if he or she declines, but don't push him or her to take on too much too soon.

- Provide assistance in getting to the doctor's appointments.

- Remind your loved one that with time and treatment, the depression will lift.

How can I help myself if I am depressed?

If you have depression, you may feel exhausted, helpless, and hopeless. It may be extremely difficult to take any action to help yourself. But as you begin to recognize your depression and begin treatment, you will start to feel better.

Here are some suggestions you can try to help yourself:

- Do not wait too long to get evaluated or treated. There is research showing the longer one waits, the greater the impairment can be down the road. Try to see a professional as soon as possible.

- Try to be active and exercise. Go to a movie, a ballgame, or another event or activity that you once enjoyed.

- Set realistic goals for yourself.

- Break up large tasks into small ones, set some priorities and do what you can as you can.

- Try to spend time with other people and confide in a trusted friend or relative. Try not to isolate yourself, and let others help you.

- Expect your mood to improve gradually, not immediately. Do not expect to suddenly snap out of your depression. Often during treatment for depression, sleep and appetite will begin to improve before your depressed mood lifts.

- Postpone important decisions, such as getting married or divorced or changing jobs, until you feel better. Discuss decisions with others who know you well and have a more objective view of your situation.

- Remember that positive thinking will replace negative thoughts as your depression responds to treatment.

- Continue to educate yourself about depression.

Where can I go for help?

If you are unsure where to go for help, ask your family doctor. Others who can help include mental health specialists, such as psychiatrists, psychologists, social workers, or mental health counselors, health maintenance organizations, community mental health centers, and hospital psychiatry departments and outpatient clinics. Mental health programs at universities or medical schools and state hospital outpatient clinics can also be helpful resources. In addition, consider turning to family services, social agencies, clergy, peer support groups, private clinics and facilities, employee assistance programs, or local medical and/or psychiatric societies. You can also check the phone book under "mental health," "health," "social services," "hotlines," or "physicians" for phone numbers and addresses. An emergency room doctor also can provide temporary help and can tell you where and how to get further help.

What if I or someone I know is in crisis?

If you are thinking about harming yourself, or know someone who is, tell someone who can help immediately.

- Do not leave your friend or relative alone, and do not isolate yourself.

- Call your doctor.

- Call 911 or go to a hospital emergency room to get immediate help, or ask a friend or family member to help you do these things.

- Call the toll-free, 24-hour hotline of the National Suicide Prevention Lifeline at 800-273-TALK (800-273-8255); TTY: 800-799-4TTY (4889) to talk to a trained counselor.

Section 9.2

Dysthymia

From "Dysthymia," © 2012 A.D.A.M. Inc. Reprinted with permission.

Dysthymia is a chronic type of depression in which a person's moods are regularly low. However, symptoms are not as severe as with major depression.

Causes, Incidence, and Risk Factors

The exact cause of dysthymia is unknown. It tends to run in families. Dysthymia occurs more often in women than in men and affects up to 5% of the general population.

Many people with dysthymia have a long-term medical problem or another mental health disorder, such as anxiety, alcohol abuse, or drug addiction. About half of people with dysthymia will also have an episode of major depression at some point in their lives.

Dysthymia in the elderly is often caused by:

- Difficulty caring for themselves
- Isolation
- Mental decline
- Medical illnesses

Symptoms

The main symptom of dysthymia is a low, dark, or sad mood on most days for at least two years. In children and adolescents, the mood can be irritable instead of depressed and may last for at least one year.

In addition, two or more of the following symptoms will be present almost all of the time that the person has dysthymia:

- Feelings of hopelessness
- Too little or too much sleep
- Low energy or fatigue

- Low self-esteem
- Poor appetite or overeating
- Poor concentration

People with dysthymia will often take a negative or discouraging view of themselves, their future, other people, and life events. Problems often seem more difficult to solve.

Signs and Tests

Your health care provider will take a history of your mood and other mental health symptoms. The health care provider may also check your blood and urine to rule out medical causes of depression.

Treatment

Treatment for dysthymia includes antidepressant drug therapy, along with some type of talk therapy.

Medications often do not work as well for dysthymia as they do for major depression. It also may take longer after starting medication for you to feel better.

The following medications are used to treat dysthymia:

- Selective serotonin reuptake inhibitors (SSRIs) are the drugs most commonly used for dysthymia. They include: fluoxetine (Prozac), sertraline (Zoloft), paroxetine (Paxil), fluvoxamine (Luvox), citalopram (Celexa), and escitalopram (Lexapro).

- Other antidepressants used to treat dysthymia include: serotonin norepinephrine reuptake inhibitors (SNRIs), bupropion (Wellbutrin), tricyclic antidepressants, and monoamine oxidase inhibitors (MAOIs).

People with dysthymia often benefit from some type of talk therapy. Talk therapy is a good place to talk about feelings and thoughts, and most importantly, to learn ways to deal with them. Types of talk therapy include:

- Cognitive behavioral therapy (CBT) teaches depressed people ways of correcting negative thoughts. People can learn to be more aware of their symptoms, learn what seems to make depression worse, and learn problem-solving skills.

- Insight-oriented or psychodynamic psychotherapy can help someone with depression understand the psychological factors that may be behind their depressive behaviors, thoughts, and feelings.

- Joining a support group of people who are experiencing problems like yours can also help. Ask your therapist or health care provider for a recommendation.

Expectations (Prognosis)

Dysthymia is a chronic condition that lasts many years. Though some people completely recover, others continue to have some symptoms, even with treatment.

Although it is not as severe as major depression, dysthymia symptoms can affect a person's ability to function in their family, and at work.

Dysthymia also increases the risk for suicide.

Complications

If it is not treated, dysthymia can turn into a major depressive episode. This is known as double depression.

Calling Your Health Care Provider

Call for an appointment with your health care provider if:

- You regularly feel depressed or low
- Your symptoms are getting worse

Call for help immediately if you or someone you know develops these symptoms, which are signs of a suicide risk:

- Giving away belongings, or talking about going away and the need to get affairs in order
- Performing self-destructive behaviors, such as injuring themselves
- Suddenly changing behaviors, especially being calm after a period of anxiety
- Talking about death or suicide, or even stating the desire to harm themselves
- Withdrawing from friends or being unwilling to go out anywhere

Section 9.3

Seasonal Affective Disorder

Maggie started off her junior year of high school with great energy. She had no trouble keeping up with her schoolwork and was involved in several after-school activities. But after the Thanksgiving break, she began to have difficulty getting through her assigned reading and had to work harder to apply herself. She couldn't concentrate in class, and after school all she wanted to do was sleep.

Maggie's grades began to drop and she rarely felt like socializing. Even though Maggie was always punctual before, she began to have trouble getting up on time and was absent or late from school many days during the winter.

At first, Maggie's parents thought she was slacking off. They were upset with her, but figured it was just a phase—especially since her energy finally seemed to return in the spring. But when the same thing happened the following November, they took Maggie to the doctor, who diagnosed her with a type of depression called seasonal affective disorder.

What Is Seasonal Affective Disorder?

Seasonal affective disorder (SAD) is a form of depression that appears at the same time each year. With SAD, a person typically has symptoms of depression and unexplained fatigue as winter approaches and daylight hours become shorter. When spring returns and days become longer again, people with SAD experience relief from their symptoms, returning to their usual mood and energy level.

Did you know?

In rare cases, SAD has a reverse seasonal pattern, with depression occurring only during the summer months.

What Causes SAD?

Experts believe that, with SAD, depression is somehow triggered by the brain's response to decreased daylight exposure. No one really understands how and why this happens. Current theories about what causes SAD focus on the role that sunlight might play in the brain's production of key chemicals.

Experts think that two specific chemicals in the brain, melatonin and serotonin may be involved in SAD. These two chemicals help regulate a person's sleep-wake cycles, energy, and mood. Shorter days and longer hours of darkness in fall and winter may cause increased levels of melatonin and decreased levels of serotonin, creating the biological conditions for depression.

Melatonin is linked to sleep. The body produces it in greater quantities when it's dark or when days are shorter. This increased production of melatonin can cause a person to feel sleepy and lethargic.

With serotonin, it's the reverse—serotonin production goes up when a person is exposed to sunlight, so it's likely that a person will have lower levels of serotonin during the winter when the days are shorter. Low levels of serotonin are associated with depression, whereas increasing the availability of serotonin helps to combat depression.

What Are the Symptoms of SAD?

Someone with SAD will show several particular changes from the way he or she normally feels and acts. These changes occur in a predictable seasonal pattern. The symptoms of SAD are the same as symptoms of depression, and a person with SAD may notice several or all of these symptoms:

- **Changes in mood:** A person may feel sad or be in an irritable mood most of the time for at least 2 weeks during a specific time of year. During that time, a guy or girl may feel a sense of hopelessness or worthlessness. As part of the mood change that goes with SAD, people can be self-critical; they may also be more sensitive than usual to criticism and cry or get upset more often or more easily.

- **Lack of enjoyment:** Someone with SAD may lose interest in things he or she normally likes to do and may seem unable to enjoy things as before. People with SAD can also feel like they no longer do certain tasks as well as they used to, and they may have feelings of dissatisfaction or guilt. A person with SAD may seem to lose interest in friends and may stop participating in social activities.

- **Low energy:** Unusual tiredness or unexplained fatigue is also part of SAD and can cause people to feel low on energy.

- **Changes in sleep:** A person may sleep much more than usual. Excessive sleeping can make it impossible for a student to get up and get ready for school in the morning.

- **Changes in eating:** Changes in eating and appetite related to SAD may include cravings for simple carbohydrates (think comfort foods and sugary foods) and the tendency to overeat. Because of this change in eating, SAD can result in weight gain during the winter months.

- **Difficulty concentrating:** SAD can affect concentration, too, interfering with a person's school performance and grades. A student may have more trouble than usual completing assignments on time or seem to lack his or her usual motivation. Someone with SAD may notice that his or her grades may drop, and teachers may comment that the student seems less motivated or is making less effort in school.

- **Less time socializing:** People with SAD may spend less time with friends, in social activities, or in extracurricular activities.

The problems caused by SAD, such as lower-than-usual grades or less energy for socializing with friends, can affect self-esteem and leave a person feeling disappointed, isolated, and lonely—especially if he or she doesn't realize what's causing the changes in energy, mood, and motivation.

Like other forms of depression, the symptoms of SAD can be mild, severe, or anywhere in between. Milder symptoms interfere less with someone's ability to participate in everyday activities, but stronger symptoms can interfere much more. It's the seasonal pattern of SAD—the fact that symptoms occur only for a few months each winter (for at least 2 years in a row) but not during other seasons—that distinguishes SAD from other forms of depression.

Who Gets SAD?

SAD can affect adults, teens, and children. It's estimated that about 6 in every 100 people (6%) experience SAD.

The number of people with SAD varies from region to region. One study of SAD in the United States found the rates of SAD were seven times higher among people in New Hampshire than in Florida, suggesting that the farther people live from the equator, the more likely they are to develop SAD.

Interestingly, when people who get SAD travel to areas far south of the equator that have longer daylight hours during winter months, they do not get their seasonal symptoms. This supports the theory that SAD is related to light exposure.

Most people don't get seasonal depression, even if they live in areas where days are shorter during winter months. Experts don't fully understand why certain people are more likely to experience SAD than others. It may be that they're more sensitive than others to variations in light, and therefore may experience more dramatic shifts in hormone production according to their exposure to light.

Like other forms of depression, females are about four times more likely than males to develop SAD. People with relatives who have experienced depression are also more likely to develop it. Individual biology, brain chemistry, family history, environment, and life experiences may also make certain individuals more prone to SAD and other forms of depression.

Researchers are continuing to investigate what leads to SAD, as well as why some people are more likely than others to experience it.

How Is SAD Diagnosed and Treated?

Doctors and mental health professionals make a diagnosis of SAD after a careful evaluation. A medical checkup is also important to make sure that symptoms aren't due to a medical condition that needs treatment. Tiredness, fatigue, and low energy could be a sign of another medical condition such as hypothyroidism, hypoglycemia, or mononucleosis. Other medical conditions can cause appetite changes, sleep changes, or extreme fatigue.

Once a person's been diagnosed with SAD, doctors may recommend one of several treatments:

Increased light exposure: Because the symptoms of SAD are triggered by lack of exposure to light, and they tend to go away on their own when available light increases, treatment for SAD often involves increased exposure to light during winter months. For someone with mild symptoms, it may be enough to spend more time outside during the daylight hours, perhaps by exercising outdoors or taking a daily walk. Full spectrum (daylight) lightbulbs that fit in regular lamps can help bring a bit more daylight into your home in winter months and might help with mild symptoms.

Light therapy: Stronger symptoms of SAD may be treated with light therapy (also called phototherapy). Light therapy involves the use of a special light that simulates daylight. A special light box or panel is placed on a tabletop or desk, and the person sits in front of the light for a short period of time every day (45 minutes a day or so, usually in the morning). The person should occasionally glance at the light (the light has to be absorbed through the retinas in order to work), but not stare into it for long periods. Symptoms tend to improve within a few days in some cases or within a few weeks in others. Generally, doctors recommend the use of light therapy until enough sunlight is available outdoors.

Like any medical treatment, light treatment should only be used under the supervision of a doctor. People who have another type of depressive disorder, skin that's sensitive to light, or medical conditions that may make the eyes vulnerable to light damage should use light therapy with caution. The lights that are used for SAD phototherapy must filter out harmful UV rays. Tanning beds or booths should not be used to alleviate symptoms of SAD. Some mild side effects of phototherapy might include headache or eyestrain.

Talk therapy: Talk therapy (psychotherapy) is also used to treat people with SAD. Talk therapy focuses on revising the negative thoughts and feelings associated with depression and helps ease the sense of isolation or loneliness that people with depression often feel. The support and guidance of a professional therapist can be helpful for someone experiencing SAD. Talk therapy can also help someone to learn about and understand their condition as well as learn what to do to prevent or minimize future bouts of seasonal depression.

Medication: Doctors may also prescribe medications for teens with SAD. Antidepressant medications help to regulate the balance of serotonin and other neurotransmitters in the brain that affect mood and energy. Medications need to be prescribed and monitored by a doctor. If your doctor prescribes medication for SAD or another form of depression, be sure to let him or her know about any other medications or remedies you may be taking, including over-the-counter or herbal medicines. These can interfere with prescription medications.

Dealing with SAD

When symptoms of SAD first develop, it can be confusing, both for the person with SAD and family and friends. Some parents or teachers may mistakenly think that teens with SAD are slacking off or not trying their best. If you think you're experiencing some of the symptoms of SAD, talk to a parent, guidance counselor, or other trusted adult about what you're feeling.

If you've been diagnosed with SAD, there are a few things you can do to help:

- Follow your doctor's recommendations for treatment.

- Learn all you can about SAD and explain the condition to others so they can work with you.

- Get plenty of exercise, especially outdoors. Exercise can be a mood lifter.

- Spend time with friends and loved ones who understand what you're going through—they can help provide you with personal contact and a sense of connection.

- Be patient. Don't expect your symptoms to go away immediately.

- Ask for help with homework and other assignments if you need it. If you feel you can't concentrate on things, remember that it's part of the disorder and that things will get better again. Talk to your teachers and work out a plan to get your assignments done.

- Eat right. It may be hard, but avoiding simple carbohydrates and sugary snacks and concentrating on plenty of whole grains, vegetables, and fruits can help you feel better in the long term.

- Develop a sleep routine. Regular bedtimes can help you reap the mental health benefits of daytime light.

Depression in any form can be serious. If you think you have symptoms of any type of depression, talk to someone who can help you get treatment.

Chapter 10

Bipolar Disorder

Chapter Contents

Section 10.1

Facts about Bipolar Disorder

Excerpted from "Bipolar Disorders," National Institute of Mental Health (NIMH), September 28, 2011. The complete text, including references, can be found online at http://www.nimh.nih.gov/health/publications/bipolar-disorder/complete-index.shtml.

What is bipolar disorder?

Bipolar disorder, also known as manic-depressive illness, is a brain disorder that causes unusual shifts in mood, energy, activity levels, and the ability to carry out day-to-day tasks. Symptoms of bipolar disorder are severe. They are different from the normal ups and downs that everyone goes through from time to time. Bipolar disorder symptoms can result in damaged relationships, poor job or school performance, and even suicide. But bipolar disorder can be treated, and people with this illness can lead full and productive lives.

Bipolar disorder often develops in a person's late teens or early adult years. At least half of all cases start before age 25. Some people have their first symptoms during childhood, while others may develop symptoms late in life.

Bipolar disorder is not easy to spot when it starts. The symptoms may seem like separate problems, not recognized as parts of a larger problem. Some people suffer for years before they are properly diagnosed and treated. Like diabetes or heart disease, bipolar disorder is a long-term illness that must be carefully managed throughout a person's life.

What are the symptoms of bipolar disorder?

People with bipolar disorder experience unusually intense emotional states that occur in distinct periods called mood episodes. An overly joyful or overexcited state is called a manic episode, and an extremely sad or hopeless state is called a depressive episode. Sometimes, a mood episode includes symptoms of both mania and depression. This is called a mixed state. People with bipolar disorder also may be explosive and irritable during a mood episode.

Extreme changes in energy, activity, sleep, and behavior go along with these changes in mood. It is possible for someone with bipolar disorder to experience a long-lasting period of unstable moods rather than discrete episodes of depression or mania.

A person may be having an episode of bipolar disorder if he or she has a number of manic or depressive symptoms for most of the day, nearly every day, for at least one or two weeks. Sometimes symptoms are so severe that the person cannot function normally at work, school, or home.

Symptoms of mania or a manic episode include mood changes and behavioral changes.

- **Mood changes:** A long period of feeling "high," or an overly happy or outgoing mood; extremely irritable mood, agitation, feeling "jumpy" or "wired."

- **Behavioral changes:** Talking very fast, jumping from one idea to another, having racing thoughts; being easily distracted; increasing goal-directed activities, such as taking on new projects; being restless; sleeping little; having an unrealistic belief in one's abilities; behaving impulsively and taking part in a lot of pleasurable, high-risk behaviors, such as spending sprees, impulsive sex, and impulsive business investments.

Symptoms of depression or a depressive episode also include mood changes and behavioral changes.

- **Mood changes:** A long period of feeling worried or empty; loss of interest in activities once enjoyed, including sex.

- **Behavioral changes:** Feeling tired or slowed down; having problems concentrating, remembering, and making decisions; being restless or irritable; changing eating, sleeping, or other habits; thinking of death or suicide, or attempting suicide.

In addition to mania and depression, bipolar disorder can cause a range of moods, as shown in Figure 10.1.

One side of the scale includes severe depression, moderate depression, and mild low mood. Moderate depression may cause less extreme symptoms, and mild low mood is called dysthymia when it is chronic or long-term. In the middle of the scale is normal or balanced mood.

At the other end of the scale are hypomania and severe mania. Some people with bipolar disorder experience hypomania. During hypomanic episodes, a person may have increased energy and activity levels that

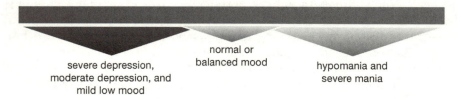

Figure 10.1. *Scale of Severe Depression, Moderate Depression, and Mild Low Mood*

are not as severe as typical mania, or he or she may have episodes that last less than a week and do not require emergency care. A person having a hypomanic episode may feel very good, be highly productive, and function well. This person may not feel that anything is wrong even as family and friends recognize the mood swings as possible bipolar disorder. Without proper treatment, however, people with hypomania may develop severe mania or depression.

During a mixed state, symptoms often include agitation, trouble sleeping, major changes in appetite, and suicidal thinking. People in a mixed state may feel very sad or hopeless while feeling extremely energized.

Sometimes, a person with severe episodes of mania or depression has psychotic symptoms too, such as hallucinations or delusions. The psychotic symptoms tend to reflect the person's extreme mood. For example, psychotic symptoms for a person having a manic episode may include believing he or she is famous, has a lot of money, or has special powers. In the same way, a person having a depressive episode may believe he or she is ruined and penniless, or has committed a crime. As a result, people with bipolar disorder who have psychotic symptoms are sometimes wrongly diagnosed as having schizophrenia, another severe mental illness that is linked with hallucinations and delusions.

People with bipolar disorder may also have behavioral problems. They may abuse alcohol or substances, have relationship problems, or perform poorly in school or at work. At first, it's not easy to recognize these problems as signs of a major mental illness.

How does bipolar disorder affect someone over time?

Bipolar disorder usually lasts a lifetime. Episodes of mania and depression typically come back over time. Between episodes, many people with bipolar disorder are free of symptoms, but some people may have lingering symptoms.

Doctors usually diagnose mental disorders using guidelines from the *Diagnostic and Statistical Manual of Mental Disorders*, or *DSM*. According to the *DSM*, there are four basic types of bipolar disorder:

1. Bipolar I disorder is mainly defined by manic or mixed episodes that last at least seven days, or by manic symptoms that are so severe that the person needs immediate hospital care. Usually, the person also has depressive episodes, typically lasting at least two weeks. The symptoms of mania or depression must be a major change from the person's normal behavior.

2. Bipolar II disorder is defined by a pattern of depressive episodes shifting back and forth with hypomanic episodes, but no full-blown manic or mixed episodes.

3. Bipolar disorder not otherwise specified (BP-NOS) is diagnosed when a person has symptoms of the illness that do not meet diagnostic criteria for either bipolar I or II. The symptoms may not last long enough, or the person may have too few symptoms, to be diagnosed with bipolar I or II. However, the symptoms are clearly out of the person's normal range of behavior.

4. Cyclothymic disorder, or cyclothymia, is a mild form of bipolar disorder. People who have cyclothymia have episodes of hypomania that shift back and forth with mild depression for at least two years. However, the symptoms do not meet the diagnostic requirements for any other type of bipolar disorder.

Some people may be diagnosed with rapid-cycling bipolar disorder. This is when a person has four or more episodes of major depression, mania, hypomania, or mixed symptoms within a year. Some people experience more than one episode in a week, or even within one day. Rapid cycling seems to be more common in people who have severe bipolar disorder and may be more common in people who have their first episode at a younger age. One study found that people with rapid cycling had their first episode about four years earlier, during mid to late teen years, than people without rapid cycling bipolar disorder. Rapid cycling affects more women than men.

Bipolar disorder tends to worsen if it is not treated. Over time, a person may suffer more frequent and more severe episodes than when the illness first appeared. Also, delays in getting the correct diagnosis and treatment make a person more likely to experience personal, social, and work-related problems.

Proper diagnosis and treatment helps people with bipolar disorder lead healthy and productive lives. In most cases, treatment can help reduce the frequency and severity of episodes.

What illnesses often co-exist with bipolar disorder?

Substance abuse is very common among people with bipolar disorder, but the reasons for this link are unclear. Some people with bipolar disorder may try to treat their symptoms with alcohol or drugs. However, substance abuse may trigger or prolong bipolar symptoms, and the behavioral control problems associated with mania can result in a person drinking too much.

Anxiety disorders, such as post-traumatic stress disorder (PTSD) and social phobia, also co-occur often among people with bipolar disorder. Bipolar disorder also co-occurs with attention deficit hyperactivity disorder (ADHD), which has some symptoms that overlap with bipolar disorder, such as restlessness and being easily distracted.

People with bipolar disorder are also at higher risk for thyroid disease, migraine headaches, heart disease, diabetes, obesity, and other physical illnesses. These illnesses may cause symptoms of mania or depression. They may also result from treatment for bipolar disorder.

Other illnesses can make it hard to diagnose and treat bipolar disorder. People with bipolar disorder should monitor their physical and mental health. If a symptom does not get better with treatment, they should tell their doctors.

What are the risk factors for bipolar disorder?

Scientists are learning about the possible causes of bipolar disorder. Most scientists agree that there is no single cause. Rather, many factors likely act together to produce the illness or increase risk.

Genetics: Bipolar disorder tends to run in families, so researchers are looking for genes that may increase a person's chance of developing the illness. Genes are the building blocks of heredity. They help control how the body and brain work and grow. Genes are contained inside a person's cells that are passed down from parents to children.

Children with a parent or sibling who has bipolar disorder are four to six times more likely to develop the illness, compared with children who do not have a family history of bipolar disorder. However, most children with a family history of bipolar disorder will not develop the illness.

Genetic research on bipolar disorder is being helped by advances in technology. This type of research is now much quicker and more far-reaching than in the past. One example is the launch of the Bipolar Disorder Phenome Database, funded in part by National Institute of Mental Health (NIMH). Using the database, scientists will be able to link visible signs of the disorder with the genes that may influence them. So far, researchers using this database found that most people with bipolar disorder had these characteristics:

- Missed work because of their illness

- Other illnesses at the same time, especially alcohol and/or substance abuse and panic disorders

- Been treated or hospitalized for bipolar disorder

The researchers also identified certain traits, such as the following, that appeared to run in families:

- History of psychiatric hospitalization

- Co-occurring obsessive-compulsive disorder (OCD)

- Age at first manic episode

- Number and frequency of manic episodes.

Scientists continue to study these traits, which may help them find the genes that cause bipolar disorder some day. But genes are not the only risk factor for bipolar disorder. Studies of identical twins have shown that the twin of a person with bipolar illness does not always develop the disorder. This is important because identical twins share all of the same genes. The study results suggest factors besides genes are also at work. Rather, it is likely that many different genes and a person's environment are involved. However, scientists do not yet fully understand how these factors interact to cause bipolar disorder.

Brain structure and functioning: Brain-imaging studies are helping scientists learn what happens in the brain of a person with bipolar disorder. Newer brain-imaging tools, such as functional magnetic resonance imaging (fMRI) and positron emission tomography (PET), allow researchers to take pictures of the living brain at work. These tools help scientists study the brain's structure and activity.

Some imaging studies show how the brains of people with bipolar disorder may differ from the brains of healthy people or people with other mental disorders. For example, one study using MRI found that the pattern of brain development in children with bipolar disorder was similar to that in children with multidimensional impairment, a disorder that causes symptoms that overlap somewhat with bipolar disorder and schizophrenia. This suggests that the common pattern of brain development may be linked to general risk for unstable moods.

Learning more about these differences, along with information gained from genetic studies, helps scientists better understand bipolar disorder. Someday scientists may be able to predict which types of treatment will work most effectively. They may even find ways to prevent bipolar disorder.

How is bipolar disorder diagnosed?

The first step in getting a proper diagnosis is to talk to a doctor, who may conduct a physical examination, an interview, and lab tests. Bipolar disorder cannot currently be identified through a blood test or a brain scan, but these tests can help rule out other contributing factors, such as a stroke or brain tumor. If the problems are not caused by other illnesses, the doctor may conduct a mental health evaluation. The doctor may also provide a referral to a trained mental health professional, such as a psychiatrist, who is experienced in diagnosing and treating bipolar disorder.

The doctor or mental health professional should conduct a complete diagnostic evaluation. He or she should discuss any family history of bipolar disorder or other mental illnesses and get a complete history of symptoms. The doctor or mental health professionals should also talk to the person's close relatives or spouse and note how they describe the person's symptoms and family medical history.

People with bipolar disorder are more likely to seek help when they are depressed than when experiencing mania or hypomania. Therefore, a careful medical history is needed to assure that bipolar disorder is not mistakenly diagnosed as major depressive disorder, which is also called unipolar depression. Unlike people with bipolar disorder, people who have unipolar depression do not experience mania. Whenever possible, previous records and input from family and friends should also be included in the medical history.

How is bipolar disorder treated?

To date, there is no cure for bipolar disorder. But proper treatment helps most people with bipolar disorder gain better control of their mood swings and related symptoms. This is also true for people with the most severe forms of the illness.

Because bipolar disorder is a lifelong and recurrent illness, people with the disorder need long-term treatment to maintain control of bipolar symptoms. An effective maintenance treatment plan includes medication and psychotherapy for preventing relapse and reducing symptom severity.

How are medications used to treat bipolar disorder?

Bipolar disorder can be diagnosed and medications prescribed by people with an M.D. (doctor of medicine). Usually, bipolar medications are prescribed by a psychiatrist. In some states, clinical psychologists, psychiatric nurse practitioners, and advanced psychiatric nurse specialists can also prescribe medications. Check with your state's licensing agency to find out more.

Not everyone responds to medications in the same way. Several different medications may need to be tried before the best course of treatment is found.

Keeping a chart of daily mood symptoms, treatments, sleep patterns, and life events can help the doctor track and treat the illness most effectively. Sometimes this is called a daily life chart. If a person's symptoms change or if side effects become serious, the doctor may switch or add medications.

Some of the types of medications generally used to treat bipolar disorder are listed below. Information on medications can change. For the most up to date information on use and side effects contact the U.S. Food and Drug Administration (FDA) via their website (www.fda.gov).

Mood stabilizing medications are usually the first choice to treat bipolar disorder. In general, people with bipolar disorder continue treatment with mood stabilizers for years. Except for lithium, many of these medications are anticonvulsants. Anticonvulsant medications are usually used to treat seizures, but they also help control moods. These medications are commonly used as mood stabilizers in bipolar disorder:

- Lithium (sometimes known as Eskalith or Lithobid) was the first mood-stabilizing medication approved by the U.S. Food and Drug Administration (FDA) in the 1970s for treatment of mania. It is often very effective in controlling symptoms of mania and preventing the recurrence of manic and depressive episodes.

- Valproic acid or divalproex sodium (Depakote), approved by the FDA in 1995 for treating mania, is a popular alternative to lithium for bipolar disorder. It is generally as effective as lithium for treating bipolar disorder. Valproic acid may increase levels of testosterone (a male hormone) in teenage girls and lead to polycystic ovary syndrome (PCOS) in women who begin taking the medication before age 20. PCOS causes a woman's eggs to develop into cysts, or fluid filled sacs that collect in the ovaries instead of being released by monthly periods. This condition can cause obesity, excess body hair, disruptions in the menstrual cycle, and other serious symptoms. Most of these symptoms will improve after stopping treatment with valproic acid. Young girls and women taking valproic acid should be monitored carefully by a doctor.

- More recently, the anticonvulsant lamotrigine (Lamictal) received FDA approval for maintenance treatment of bipolar disorder.

- Other anticonvulsant medications, including gabapentin (Neurontin) topiramate (Topamax), and oxcarbazepine (Trileptal) are sometimes prescribed. No large studies have shown that these medications are more effective than mood stabilizers.

Valproic acid, lamotrigine, and other anticonvulsant medications have an FDA warning. The warning states that their use may increase the risk of suicidal thoughts and behaviors. People taking anticonvulsant medications for bipolar or other illnesses should be closely monitored for new or worsening symptoms of depression, suicidal thoughts or behavior, or any unusual changes in mood or behavior. People taking these medications should not make any changes without talking to their health care professional.

People with bipolar disorder often have thyroid gland problems. Lithium treatment may also cause low thyroid levels in some people. Low thyroid function, called hypothyroidism, has been associated with rapid cycling in some people with bipolar disorder, especially women.

Because too much or too little thyroid hormone can lead to mood and energy changes, it is important to have a doctor check thyroid levels carefully. A person with bipolar disorder may need to take thyroid medication, in addition to medications for bipolar disorder, to keep thyroid levels balanced.

Atypical antipsychotic medications are sometimes prescribed to treat symptoms of bipolar disorder. Often, these medications are taken with other medications. Atypical antipsychotic medications are called *atypical* to set them apart from earlier medications, which are called *conventional* or *first-generation* antipsychotics.

- Olanzapine (Zyprexa), when given with an antidepressant medication, may help relieve symptoms of severe mania or psychosis. Olanzapine is also available in an injectable form, which quickly treats agitation associated with a manic or mixed episode. Olanzapine can be used for maintenance treatment of bipolar disorder as well, even when a person does not have psychotic symptoms. However, some studies show that people taking olanzapine may gain weight and have other side effects that can increase their risk for diabetes and heart disease. These side effects are more likely in people taking olanzapine when compared with people prescribed other atypical antipsychotics.

- Aripiprazole (Abilify), like olanzapine, is approved for treatment of a manic or mixed episode. Aripiprazole is also used for maintenance treatment after a severe or sudden episode. As with olanzapine, aripiprazole also can be injected for urgent treatment of symptoms of manic or mixed episodes of bipolar disorder.

- Quetiapine (Seroquel) relieves the symptoms of severe and sudden manic episodes. In that way, quetiapine is like almost all antipsychotics. In 2006, it became the first atypical antipsychotic to also receive FDA approval for the treatment of bipolar depressive episodes.

- Risperidone (Risperdal) and ziprasidone (Geodon) are other atypical antipsychotics that may also be prescribed for controlling manic or mixed episodes.

Antidepressant medications are sometimes used to treat symptoms of depression in bipolar disorder. People with bipolar disorder who take antidepressants often take a mood stabilizer too. Doctors usually require this because taking only an antidepressant can increase a person's risk of switching to mania or hypomania, or of developing rapid cycling symptoms. To prevent this switch, doctors who prescribe antidepressants for treating bipolar disorder also usually require the person to take a mood-stabilizing medication at the same time.

Recently, a large-scale, NIMH-funded study showed that for many people, adding an antidepressant to a mood stabilizer is no more effective in treating the depression than using only a mood stabilizer.

- Fluoxetine (Prozac), paroxetine (Paxil), sertraline (Zoloft), and bupropion (Wellbutrin) are examples of antidepressants that may be prescribed to treat symptoms of bipolar depression.

Some medications are better at treating one type of bipolar symptoms than another. For example, lamotrigine (Lamictal) seems to be helpful in controlling depressive symptoms of bipolar disorder.

Are antidepressants safe?

Antidepressants are safe and popular, but some studies have suggested that they may have unintentional effects on some people, especially in adolescents and young adults. The FDA warning says that patients of all ages taking antidepressants should be watched closely, especially during the first few weeks of treatment. Possible side effects to look for are depression that gets worse, suicidal thinking or behavior, or any unusual changes in behavior such as trouble sleeping, agitation, or withdrawal from normal social situations. Families and caregivers should report any changes to the doctor. For the latest information visit the FDA website (www.fda.gov).

What are the side effects of medications used to treat bipolar disorders?

Before starting a new medication, people with bipolar disorder should talk to their doctor about the possible risks and benefits.

The psychiatrist prescribing the medication or pharmacist can also answer questions about side effects. Over the last decade, treatments have improved, and some medications now have fewer or more tolerable side effects than earlier treatments. However, everyone responds differently to medications. In some cases, side effects may not appear until a person has taken a medication for some time.

If the person with bipolar disorder develops any severe side effects from a medication, he or she should talk to the doctor who prescribed it as soon as possible. The doctor may change the dose or prescribe a different medication. People being treated for bipolar disorder should not stop taking a medication without talking to a doctor first. Suddenly stopping a medication may lead to "rebound," or worsening of bipolar disorder symptoms. Other uncomfortable or potentially dangerous withdrawal effects are also possible.

The following sections describe some common side effects of the different types of medications used to treat bipolar disorder. These medications may also be linked with rare but serious side effects. Talk with the treating doctor or a pharmacist to make sure you understand signs of serious side effects for the medications you're taking.

Mood Stabilizers

In some cases, lithium can cause side effects such as restlessness, dry mouth, bloating or indigestion, acne, unusual discomfort to cold temperatures, joint or muscle pain, or brittle nails or hair. Lithium also causes side effects not listed here. If extremely bothersome or unusual side effects occur, tell your doctor as soon as possible.

If a person with bipolar disorder is being treated with lithium, it is important to make regular visits to the treating doctor. The doctor needs to check the levels of lithium in the person's blood, as well as kidney and thyroid function.

Common side effects of other mood stabilizing medications include drowsiness, dizziness, headache, diarrhea, constipation, heartburn, mood swings, and a stuffed or runny nose, or other cold-like symptoms.

Atypical Antipsychotics

Some people have side effects when they start taking atypical antipsychotics. Most side effects go away after a few days and often can be managed successfully. People who are taking antipsychotics should not drive until they adjust to their new medication. Side effects of many antipsychotics include drowsiness, dizziness when changing positions, blurred vision, rapid heartbeat, sensitivity to the sun, skin rashes, and for women, menstrual problems.

Atypical antipsychotic medications can cause major weight gain and changes in a person's metabolism. This may increase a person's risk of getting diabetes and high cholesterol. A person's weight, glucose levels, and lipid levels should be monitored regularly by a doctor while taking these medications.

In rare cases, long-term use of atypical antipsychotic drugs may lead to a condition called tardive dyskinesia (TD). The condition causes muscle movements that commonly occur around the mouth. A person with TD cannot control these moments. TD can range from mild to severe, and it cannot always be cured. Some people with TD recover partially or fully after they stop taking the drug.

Antidepressants

The antidepressants most commonly prescribed for treating symptoms of bipolar disorder can also cause mild side effects that usually do not last long. These can include the following:

- Headache, which usually goes away within a few days

- Nausea (feeling sick to your stomach), which usually goes away within a few days

- Sleep problems, such as sleeplessness or drowsiness. This may happen during the first few weeks but then go away. To help lessen these effects, sometimes the medication dose can be reduced, or the time of day it is taken can be changed.

- Agitation (feeling jittery)

- Sexual problems, which can affect both men and women. These include reduced sex drive and problems having and enjoying sex.

Some antidepressants are more likely to cause certain side effects than other types. Your doctor or pharmacist can answer questions about these medications. Any unusual reactions or side effects should be reported to a doctor immediately.

Should women who are pregnant or may become pregnant take medication for bipolar disorder?

Women with bipolar disorder who are pregnant or may become pregnant face special challenges. The mood stabilizing medications in use today can harm a developing fetus or nursing infant. But stopping medications, either suddenly or gradually, greatly increases the risk that bipolar symptoms will recur during pregnancy.

Scientists are not sure yet, but lithium is likely the preferred mood-stabilizing medication for pregnant women with bipolar disorder. However, lithium can lead to heart problems in the fetus. Women need to know that most bipolar medications are passed on through breast milk. Pregnant women and nursing mothers should talk to their doctors about the benefits and risks of all available treatments.

How is psychotherapy used to treat bipolar disorders?

In addition to medication, psychotherapy, or talk therapy, can be an effective treatment for bipolar disorder. It can provide support, education, and guidance to people with bipolar disorder and their families. Some psychotherapy treatments used to treat bipolar disorder include:

- Cognitive behavioral therapy (CBT) helps people with bipolar disorder learn to change harmful or negative thought patterns and behaviors.

- Family-focused therapy includes family members. It helps enhance family coping strategies, such as recognizing new episodes early and helping their loved one. This therapy also improves communication and problem-solving.

- Interpersonal and social rhythm therapy helps people with bipolar disorder improve their relationships with others and manage their daily routines. Regular daily routines and sleep schedules may help protect against manic episodes.

- Psychoeducation teaches people with bipolar disorder about the illness and its treatment. This treatment helps people recognize signs of relapse so they can seek treatment early, before a full-blown episode occurs. Usually done in a group, psychoeducation may also be helpful for family members and caregivers.

A licensed psychologist, social worker, or counselor typically provides these therapies. This mental health professional often works with the psychiatrist to track progress. The number, frequency, and type of sessions should be based on the treatment needs of each person. As with medication, following the doctor's instructions for any psychotherapy will provide the greatest benefit.

Recently, NIMH funded a clinical trial called the Systematic Treatment Enhancement Program for Bipolar Disorder (STEP-BD). This was the largest treatment study ever conducted for bipolar disorder. In a study on psychotherapies, STEP-BD researchers compared people in two groups. The first group was treated with collaborative care (three sessions of psychoeducation over six weeks). The second group was treated with medication and intensive psychotherapy (30 sessions over nine months of CBT, interpersonal and social rhythm therapy, or family-focused therapy). Researchers found that the second group had fewer relapses, lower hospitalization rates, and were better able to stick with their treatment plans. They were also more likely to get well faster and stay well longer.

Are there other treatments for bipolar disorder?

Electroconvulsive therapy (ECT): For cases in which medication and/or psychotherapy does not work, electroconvulsive therapy (ECT) may be useful. ECT, formerly known as shock therapy, once had a bad reputation. But in recent years, it has greatly improved and can provide relief for people with severe bipolar disorder who have not been able to feel better with other treatments. [For more information about ECT, see Chapter 24—Brain Stimulation Therapies.]

Sleep medications: People with bipolar disorder who have trouble sleeping usually sleep better after getting treatment for bipolar disorder. However, if sleeplessness does not improve, the doctor may suggest a change in medications. If the problems still continue, the doctor may prescribe sedatives or other sleep medications.

People with bipolar disorder should tell their doctor about all prescription drugs, over-the-counter medications, or supplements they are taking. Certain medications and supplements taken together may cause unwanted or dangerous effects.

Herbal supplements: In general, there is not much research about herbal or natural supplements. Little is known about their effects on bipolar disorder. An herb called St. John's wort (*Hypericum perforatum*), often marketed as a natural antidepressant, may cause a switch to mania in some people with bipolar disorder. St. John's wort can also make other medications less effective, including some antidepressant and anticonvulsant medications. Scientists are also researching omega-3 fatty acids (most commonly found in fish oil) to measure their usefulness for long-term treatment of bipolar disorder. Study results have been mixed. It is important to talk with a doctor before taking any herbal or natural supplements because of the serious risk of interactions with other medications.

What can people with bipolar disorder expect from treatment?

Bipolar disorder has no cure, but can be effectively treated over the long-term. It is best controlled when treatment is continuous, rather than on and off. In the STEP-BD study, a little more than half of the people treated for bipolar disorder recovered over one year's time. For this study, recovery meant having two or fewer symptoms of the disorder for at least eight weeks.

However, even with proper treatment, mood changes can occur. In the STEP-BD study, almost half of those who recovered still had lingering symptoms. These people experienced a relapse or recurrence that was usually a return to a depressive state. If a person had a mental illness in addition to bipolar disorder, he or she was more likely to experience a relapse. Scientists are unsure, however, how these other illnesses or lingering symptoms increase the chance of relapse. For some people, combining psychotherapy with medication may help to prevent or delay relapse.

Treatment may be more effective when people work closely with a doctor and talk openly about their concerns and choices. Keeping track of mood changes and symptoms with a daily life chart can help a doctor assess a person's response to treatments. Sometimes the doctor needs to change a treatment plan to make sure symptoms are controlled most effectively. A psychiatrist should guide any changes in type or dose of medication.

How can I help a friend or relative who has bipolar disorder?

If you know someone who has bipolar disorder, it affects you too. The first and most important thing you can do is help him or her get the right diagnosis and treatment. You may need to make the appointment and go with him or her to see the doctor. Encourage your loved one to stay in treatment.

To help a friend or relative, offer emotional support, understanding, patience, and encouragement. Learn about bipolar disorder so you can understand what your friend or relative is experiencing. Talk to your friend or relative and listen carefully. Listen to feelings your friend or relative expresses—be understanding about situations that may trigger bipolar symptoms. Invite your friend or relative out for positive distractions, such as walks, outings, and other activities, and remind your friend or relative that, with time and treatment, he or she can get better.

Never ignore comments about your friend or relative harming himself or herself. Always report such comments to his or her therapist or doctor.

Is support for caregivers important?

Like other serious illnesses, bipolar disorder can be difficult for spouses, family members, friends, and other caregivers. Relatives and friends often have to cope with the person's serious behavioral problems, such as wild spending sprees during mania, extreme withdrawal during depression, or poor work or school performance. These behaviors can have lasting consequences.

Caregivers usually take care of the medical needs of their loved ones. The caregivers have to deal with how this affects their own health. The stress that caregivers are under may lead to missed work or lost free time, strained relationships with people who may not understand the situation, and physical and mental exhaustion.

Stress from caregiving can make it hard to cope with a loved one's bipolar symptoms. One study shows that if a caregiver is under a lot of stress, his or her loved one has more trouble following the treatment plan, which increases the chance for a major bipolar episode. It is important that people caring for those with bipolar disorder also take care of themselves.

How can I help myself if I have bipolar disorder?

It may be very hard to take that first step to help yourself. It may take time, but you can get better with treatment. To help yourself follow these suggestions:

- Talk to your doctor about treatment options and progress.

- Keep a regular routine, such as eating meals at the same time every day and going to sleep at the same time every night.

- Try to get enough sleep.

- Stay on your medication.

- Learn about warning signs signaling a shift into depression or mania.

- Expect your symptoms to improve gradually, not immediately.

Where can I go for help?

If you are unsure where to go for help, ask your family doctor. Mental health specialists, such as psychiatrists, psychologists, social workers, or mental health counselors may also be able to help you. Other resources include health maintenance organizations, community mental health centers, hospital psychiatry departments and outpatient clinics, mental health programs at universities or medical schools, and state hospital outpatient clinics. Family services, social agencies, clergy, peer support groups, private clinics and facilities, employee assistance programs, and local medical and/or psychiatric societies are other places you can turn to for help.

You can also check the phone book under "mental health," "health," "social services," "hotlines," or "physicians" for phone numbers and addresses. An emergency room doctor can also provide temporary help and can tell you where and how to get further help.

What if I or someone I know is in crisis?

If you are thinking about harming yourself, or know someone who is, tell someone who can help immediately.

- Call your doctor.

- Call 911 or go to a hospital emergency room to get immediate help or ask a friend or family member to help you do these things.

- Call the toll-free, 24-hour hotline of the National Suicide Prevention Lifeline at 800-273-TALK (800-273-8255); TTY: 800-799-4TTY (4889) to talk to a trained counselor.

Make sure you or the suicidal person is not left alone.

Section 10.2

Cyclothymic Disorder

Cyclothymic disorder is a mild form of bipolar disorder (manic depressive illness) in which a person has mood swings over a period of years that go from mild depression to euphoria and excitement.

Causes

The causes of cyclothymic disorder are unknown. Major depression, bipolar disorder, and cyclothymia often occur together in families. This suggests that these mood disorders share similar causes.

Cyclothymia usually begins early in life. It appears to be equally common in men and women.

Symptoms

- Episodes of hypomania and mild depression occur for at least two years (one or more years in children and adolescents)

- Mood swings are less severe than in bipolar disorder, major depression, or mania

- Symptoms are persistent, with no more than two symptom-free months in a row

Exams and Tests

Your description of your mood history usually leads to diagnosis of the disorder. Your health care providers may order blood and urine tests to rule out medical causes of mood swings.

Treatment

Mood stabilizing medication, antidepressants, talk therapy, or some combination of these three therapies may be used to treat cyclothymic disorder.

Some of the more commonly used mood stabilizers are:

- **Lithium:** Lithium has been used for years in patients with bipolar disorder, and it may also help patients with cyclothymic disorder.

- **Antiseizure drugs:** Valproic acid (Depakote), carbamazepine (Tegretol), oxcarbazepine (Trileptal), and lamotrigine (Lamictal) are the most established mood stabilizing antiseizure drugs.

People with cyclothymia may not respond to medications as strongly as patients with bipolar disorder.

Support Groups

As with other illnesses, you can ease the stress of living with cyclothymia by joining a support group whose members share common experiences and problems.

Outlook (Prognosis)

Less than half of people with cyclothymic disorder will eventually develop bipolar disorder. In other people, cyclothymia will continue as a chronic condition or disappear with time.

Possible Complications

The condition can progress to bipolar disorder.

When to Contact a Medical Professional

Call a mental health professional if you or a loved one has persistent alternating periods of depression and excitement that negatively affect work, school, or social life. Seek immediate help if you or a loved one is having thoughts of suicide.

Chapter 11

Anxiety Disorders

Chapter Contents

Section 11.1

Panic Disorder

From "Panic Disorder: When Fear Overwhelms," National Institute of
Mental Health (www.nimh.nih.gov), June 30, 2011.

Do you sometimes have sudden attacks of fear that last for several minutes? Do you feel like you are having a heart attack or can't breathe? Do these attacks occur at unpredictable times causing you to worry about the possibility of having another one at any time? If so, you may have a type of anxiety disorder called panic disorder.

What is panic disorder?

People with panic disorder have sudden and repeated attacks of fear that last for several minutes. Sometimes symptoms may last longer. These are called panic attacks. Panic attacks are characterized by a fear of disaster or of losing control even when there is no real danger. A person may also have a strong physical reaction during a panic attack. It may feel like having a heart attack. Panic attacks can occur at any time, and many people with panic disorder worry about and dread the possibility of having another attack.

A person with panic disorder may become discouraged and feel ashamed because he or she cannot carry out normal routines like going to the grocery store or driving. Having panic disorder can also interfere with school or work.

Panic disorder often begins in the late teens or early adulthood. More women than men have panic disorder. But not everyone who experiences panic attacks will develop panic disorder.

What are the signs and symptoms of panic disorder?

- Sudden and repeated attacks of fear
- A feeling of being out of control during a panic attack
- An intense worry about when the next attack will happen
- A fear or avoidance of places where panic attacks have occurred in the past

- Physical symptoms during an attack, such as a pounding or racing heart, sweating, breathing problems, weakness or dizziness, feeling hot or a cold chill, tingly or numb hands, chest pain, or stomach pain

What causes panic disorder?

Panic disorder sometimes runs in families, but no one knows for sure why some people have it while others don't. Researchers have found that several parts of the brain are involved in fear and anxiety. By learning more about fear and anxiety in the brain, scientists may be able to create better treatments. Researchers are also looking for ways in which stress and environmental factors may play a role.

How is panic disorder treated?

First, talk to your doctor about your symptoms. Your doctor should do an exam to make sure that another physical problem isn't causing the symptoms. The doctor may refer you to a mental health specialist.

Panic disorder is generally treated with psychotherapy, medication, or both. Some people do better with cognitive behavior therapy, while others do better with medication. Still others do best with a combination of the two. Talk with your doctor about the best treatment for you.

Psychotherapy: A type of psychotherapy called cognitive behavior therapy is especially useful for treating panic disorder. It teaches a person different ways of thinking, behaving, and reacting to situations that help him or her feel less anxious and fearful.

Medication: Doctors also may prescribe medication to help treat panic disorder. The most commonly prescribed medications for panic disorder are anti-anxiety medications and antidepressants. Anti-anxiety medications are powerful and there are different types. Many types begin working right away, but they generally should not be taken for long periods.

Antidepressants are used to treat depression, but they also are helpful for panic disorder. They may take several weeks to start working. Some of these medications may cause side effects such as headache, nausea, or difficulty sleeping. These side effects are usually not a problem for most people, especially if the dose starts off low and is increased slowly over time. Talk to your doctor about any side effects you may have.

It's important to know that although antidepressants can be safe and effective for many people, they may be risky for some, especially children,

171

teens, and young adults. A "black box"—the most serious type of warning that a prescription drug can have—has been added to the labels of antidepressant medications. These labels warn people that antidepressants may cause some people to have suicidal thoughts or make suicide attempts. Anyone taking antidepressants should be monitored closely, especially when they first start treatment with medications.

Another type of medication called beta-blockers can help control some of the physical symptoms of panic disorder such as excessive sweating, a pounding heart, or dizziness. Although beta blockers are not commonly prescribed, they may be helpful in certain situations that bring on a panic attack.

Section 11.2

Obsessive-Compulsive Disorder

From "Obsessive-Compulsive Disorder: When Unwanted Thoughts Take Over," National Institute of Mental Health (www.nimh.nih.gov), 2010.

Do you feel the need to check and re-check things over and over? Do you have the same thoughts constantly? Do you feel a very strong need to perform certain rituals repeatedly and feel like you have no control over what you are doing? If so, you may have a type of anxiety disorder called obsessive-compulsive disorder (OCD).

What is OCD?

Everyone double checks things sometimes. For example, you might double check to make sure the stove or iron is turned off before leaving the house. But people with OCD feel the need to check things repeatedly, or have certain thoughts or perform routines and rituals over and over. The thoughts and rituals associated with OCD cause distress and get in the way of daily life.

The frequent upsetting thoughts are called obsessions. To try to control them, a person will feel an overwhelming urge to repeat certain rituals or behaviors called compulsions. People with OCD can't control these obsessions and compulsions.

For many people, OCD starts during childhood or the teen years. Most people are diagnosed by about age 19. Symptoms of OCD may come and go and be better or worse at different times.

What are the signs and symptoms of OCD?

People with OCD generally have these experiences:

- Have repeated thoughts or images about many different things, such as fear of germs, dirt, or intruders; acts of violence; hurting loved ones; sexual acts; conflicts with religious beliefs; or being overly tidy

- Do the same rituals over and over such as washing hands, locking and unlocking doors, counting, keeping unneeded items, or repeating the same steps again and again

- Can't control the unwanted thoughts and behaviors

- Don't get pleasure when performing the behaviors or rituals, but get brief relief from the anxiety the thoughts cause

- Spend at least one hour a day on the thoughts and rituals, which cause distress and get in the way of daily life.

What causes OCD?

OCD sometimes runs in families, but no one knows for sure why some people have it, while others don't. Researchers have found that several parts of the brain are involved in fear and anxiety. By learning more about fear and anxiety in the brain, scientists may be able to create better treatments. Researchers are also looking for ways in which stress and environmental factors may play a role.

How is OCD treated?

First, talk to your doctor about your symptoms. Your doctor should do an exam to make sure that another physical problem isn't causing the symptoms. The doctor may refer you to a mental health specialist.

OCD is generally treated with psychotherapy, medication, or both. Some people with OCD do better with cognitive behavior therapy, especially exposure and response prevention. Others do better with medication. Still others do best with a combination of the two. Talk with your doctor about the best treatment for you.

Psychotherapy: A type of psychotherapy called cognitive behavior therapy is especially useful for treating OCD. It teaches a person different ways of thinking, behaving, and reacting to situations that help him or her feel less anxious or fearful without having obsessive thoughts or acting compulsively. One type of therapy called exposure and response prevention is especially helpful in reducing compulsive behaviors in OCD.

Medication: Doctors also may prescribe medication to help treat OCD. The most commonly prescribed medications for OCD are anti-anxiety medications and antidepressants. Anti-anxiety medications are powerful and there are different types. Many types begin working right away, but they generally should not be taken for long periods.

Antidepressants are used to treat depression, but they are also particularly helpful for OCD, probably more so than anti-anxiety medications. They may take several weeks—10 to 12 weeks for some—to start working. Some of these medications may cause side effects such as headache, nausea, or difficulty sleeping. These side effects are usually not a problem for most people, especially if the dose starts off low and is increased slowly over time. Talk to your doctor about any side effects you may have.

It's important to know that although antidepressants can be safe and effective for many people, they may be risky for some, especially children, teens, and young adults. A "black box"—the most serious type of warning that a prescription drug can have—has been added to the labels of antidepressant medications. These labels warn people that antidepressants may cause some people to have suicidal thoughts or make suicide attempts. Anyone taking antidepressants should be monitored closely, especially when they first start treatment with medications.

Section 11.3

Compulsive Hoarding

What is compulsive hoarding?

Compulsive hoarding is a common and potentially disabling problem, characterized by the accumulation of excessive clutter, to the point that parts of one's home can no longer be used for their intended purpose.

Compulsive hoarding, which may affect up to two million people in the United States, is often found in patients with other diseases, including dementia, Alzheimer's, schizophrenia, and anorexia. It's most often seen in patients with obsessive-compulsive disorder (OCD). Researchers aren't certain whether compulsive hoarding is a subtype of OCD or a separate disorder.

Questions and Answers about Compulsive Hoarding

Is hoarding a kind of obsessive-compulsive disorder?

Right now, compulsive hoarding is considered by many researchers to be a type of obsessive-compulsive disorder. However, for some people, compulsive hoarding may also be related to:

- Impulse control disorders (such as impulsive buying or stealing)
- Depression
- Social anxiety
- Bipolar disorder
- Certain personality traits

How common is compulsive hoarding? What are its features?

- We don't know exactly. Some researchers have guessed that about half of one percent of the population suffers from compulsive hoarding, but the actual number may be much higher.

- People usually start hoarding during childhood or early adolescence, although the problem usually does not become severe until the person is an adult.

- Compulsive hoarding may run in families.

- Many people with compulsive hoarding do not recognize how bad the problem really is; often it is a family member who is most bothered by the clutter.

What causes compulsive hoarding?

Compulsive hoarding is thought to result from problems in one or more of these areas:

- **Information processing:** People with compulsive hoarding often have problems such as:

  - Difficulty categorizing their possessions (for example, deciding what is valuable and what is not)

  - Difficulty making decisions about what to do with possessions

  - Trouble remembering where things are (and so they often want to keep everything in sight so they don't forget)

- **Beliefs about possessions:** People with compulsive hoarding often:

  - Feel a strong sense of emotional attachment toward their possessions (for example, an object might be felt to be very special, or a part of them)

  - Feel a need to stay in control of their possessions (and so they don't want anyone touching or moving their possessions)

  - Worry about forgetting things (and use their possessions as visual reminders)

- **Emotional distress about discarding:** People with compulsive hoarding often:

  - Feel very anxious or upset when they have to make a decision about discarding things

- Feel distressed when they see something they want and think they can't feel better until they acquire that object

- Control their uncomfortable feelings by avoiding making the decision or putting it off until later

Treatment for Compulsive Hoarding

There is no "cure" for compulsive hoarding, meaning there is no treatment that will make the problem go away completely and never come back at all. However, some treatments may help people to manage the symptoms more effectively.

Medications: Research studies using antidepressant medications (that increase the level of serotonin activity in the brain) show that some people with compulsive hoarding respond well to these medications, however, many do not. People with compulsive hoarding do not appear to respond as well to medications as do people with other kinds of obsessive-compulsive symptoms.

Cognitive-behavioral therapy: Cognitive-behavioral therapy is a form of counseling that goes beyond "just talking". In this form of treatment, the therapist often visits the person's home and helps them learn how to make decisions and think clearly about their possessions. There have not been as many studies of this kind of treatment, therefore it's hard to say with certainty how effective it is for hoarding. However, the available evidence suggests that cognitive-behavioral therapy is effective for many people with compulsive hoarding, perhaps more so than medications.

When a Loved One Hoards

In our hoarding clinic and research program, one of the most common inquiries we get is: "My [mother, father, sibling, friend, spouse, etc.] has a terrible hoarding problem. But he/she doesn't seem to recognize that it's a problem and isn't interested in doing anything about it. How can I make him/her see that this is a problem and get the help he/she so badly needs?"

The short answer: In most cases, you can't. That is, assuming that your loved one is an adult who is legally competent to manage his/her own affairs (meaning he/she has not been declared incompetent by a judge and appointed a legal guardian), and the clutter is not immediately life-threatening, he/she has the right to hoard, even though the hoarding might have terrible consequences for his/her quality of life.

The long answer: Even though in most cases you can't make the person do anything, you can alter your approach to minimize the likelihood of getting a defensive or "stubborn" reaction. Often, it's tempting to start arguing with the person, trying to persuade them to see things the way you do. This kind of direct confrontation rarely works.

We find that the best way to help people increase their motivation to work on the problem is to start with three key assumptions:

- Ambivalence is normal.

- People have a right to make their own choices.

- Nothing will happen until the person is ready to change.

Here are some general principles to guide your conversations:

- **Show empathy:** Showing empathy doesn't necessarily mean that you agree with everything the person says. But it does mean you are willing to listen and to try to see things from the other person's perspective.

- **Don't argue:** There is simply no point in arguing about hoarding. The harder you argue, the more the person is likely to argue back. The only solution is to get out of the argument.

- **Respect autonomy:** Remember, most of you are dealing with an adult who has freedom of choice about his or her own possessions. Try to engage your loved one in a discussion (rather than an argument) about the home and his or her behavior. Ask your loved one what he or she wants to do, rather than just telling him or her what you want: "What do you think you would like to do about the clutter in the home?"; "How do you suggest we proceed?"

Help the person recognize that his/her actions are inconsistent with his/her greater goals or values. Ask the person about his or her goals and values: "What's really important to you in life?"; "How would you like your life to be five years from now?"; "What are your hopes and goals in life?" Discuss whether or not the person's acquiring, or difficulty organizing, or getting rid of things fit with those goals and values. This is most effective if you ask, rather than tell: "How does the condition of your home fit with your desire to be a good grandmother?"; " You've told me that friendships are very important to you, how well can you pursue that goal, given the way things are right now?"

If you have been accustomed to arguing, threatening, and blaming, your new approaches will surprise your loved one and it may take a little time before the person begins to trust you. Try these methods in several conversations and notice whether the balance seems to be tilting in the right direction. If so, be patient and keep up the good work.

Section 11.4

Social Anxiety Disorder

From "Social Phobia (Social Anxiety Disorder): Always Embarrassed," National Institute of Mental Health (www.nimh.nih.gov), June 30, 2011.

Are you afraid of being judged by others or of being embarrassed all the time? Do you feel extremely fearful and unsure around other people most of the time? Do these worries make it hard for you to do everyday tasks like run errands, or talk to people at work or school? If so, you may have a type of anxiety disorder called social phobia, also called social anxiety disorder.

What is social phobia?

Social phobia is a strong fear of being judged by others and of being embarrassed. This fear can be so strong that it gets in the way of going to work or school or doing other everyday things.

Everyone has felt anxious or embarrassed at one time or another. For example, meeting new people or giving a public speech can make anyone nervous. But people with social phobia worry about these and other things for weeks before they happen.

People with social phobia are afraid of doing common things in front of other people. For example, they might be afraid to sign a check in front of a cashier at the grocery store, or they might be afraid to eat or drink in front of other people, or use a public restroom. Most people who have social phobia know that they shouldn't be as afraid as they are, but they can't control their fear. Sometimes, they end up staying away from places or events where they think they might have to do something that will embarrass them. For some people, social phobia is a problem only in certain situations, while others have symptoms in almost any social situation.

Social phobia usually starts during youth. A doctor can tell that a person has social phobia if the person has had symptoms for at least six months. Without treatment, social phobia can last for many years or a lifetime.

What are the signs and symptoms of social phobia?

People with social phobia tend to have these experiences:

- Be very anxious about being with other people and have a hard time talking to them, even though they wish they could

- Be very self-conscious in front of other people and feel embarrassed

- Be very afraid that other people will judge them

- Worry for days or weeks before an event where other people will be

- Stay away from places where there are other people

- Have a hard time making friends and keeping friends

- Blush, sweat, or tremble around other people

- Feel nauseous or sick to their stomach when with other people.

What causes social phobia?

Social phobia sometimes runs in families, but no one knows for sure why some people have it, while others don't. Researchers have found that several parts of the brain are involved in fear and anxiety. By learning more about fear and anxiety in the brain, scientists may be able to create better treatments. Researchers are also looking for ways in which stress and environmental factors may play a role.

How is social phobia treated?

First, talk to your doctor about your symptoms. Your doctor should do an exam to make sure that another physical problem isn't causing the symptoms. The doctor may refer you to a mental health specialist.

Social phobia is generally treated with psychotherapy, medication, or both. Some people do better with cognitive behavior therapy, while others do better with medication. Still others do best with a combination of the two. Talk with your doctor about the best treatment for you.

Psychotherapy: A type of psychotherapy called cognitive behavior therapy is especially useful for treating social phobia. It teaches a person different ways of thinking, behaving, and reacting to situations that help him or her feel less anxious and fearful. It can also help people learn and practice social skills.

Medication: Doctors also may prescribe medication to help treat social phobia. The most commonly prescribed medications for social phobia are anti-anxiety medications and antidepressants. Anti-anxiety medications are powerful and there are different types. Many types begin working right away, but they generally should not be taken for long periods.

Antidepressants are used to treat depression, but they are also helpful for social phobia. They are probably more commonly prescribed for social phobia than anti-anxiety medications. Antidepressants may take several weeks to start working. Some may cause side effects such as headache, nausea, or difficulty sleeping. These side effects are usually not a problem for most people, especially if the dose starts off low and is increased slowly over time. Talk to your doctor about any side effects you may have.

A type of antidepressant called monoamine oxidase inhibitors (MAOIs) is especially effective in treating social phobia. However, they are rarely used as a first line of treatment because when MAOIs are combined with certain foods or other medicines, dangerous side effects can occur.

It's also important to know that although antidepressants can be safe and effective for many people, they may be risky for some, especially children, teens, and young adults. A "black box"—the most serious type of warning that a prescription drug can have—has been added to the labels of antidepressant medications. These labels warn people that antidepressants may cause some people to have suicidal thoughts or make suicide attempts.

Anyone taking antidepressants should be monitored closely, especially when they first start treatment with medications.

Another type of medication called beta-blockers can help control some of the physical symptoms of social phobia such as excessive sweating, shaking, or a racing heart. They are most commonly prescribed when the symptoms of social phobia occur in specific situations, such as stage fright.

Section 11.5

Generalized Anxiety Disorder

From "Generalized Anxiety Disorder (GAD): When Worry
Gets Out of Control," National Institute of Mental Health
(www.nimh.nih.gov), September 8, 2011.

Are you extremely worried about everything in your life, even if
there is little or no reason to worry? Are you very anxious about just
getting through the day? Are you afraid that everything will always
go badly? If so, you may have an anxiety disorder called generalized
anxiety disorder (GAD).

What is GAD?

All of us worry about things like health, money, or family problems.
But people with GAD are extremely worried about these and many
other things, even when there is little or no reason to worry about
them. They are very anxious about just getting through the day. They
think things will always go badly. At times, worrying keeps people with
GAD from doing everyday tasks.

GAD develops slowly. It often starts during the teen years or young
adulthood. Symptoms may get better or worse at different times, and
often are worse during times of stress.

People with GAD may visit a doctor many times before they find
out they have this disorder. They ask their doctors to help them with
headaches or trouble falling asleep, which can be symptoms of GAD
but they don't always get the help they need right away. It may take
doctors some time to be sure that a person has GAD instead of something else.

What are the signs and symptoms of GAD?

- Worry very much about everyday things
- Have trouble controlling their constant worries
- Know that they worry much more than they should
- Not be able to relax

- Have a hard time concentrating
- Be easily startled
- Have trouble falling asleep or staying asleep
- Feel tired all the time
- Have headaches, muscle aches, stomach aches, or unexplained pains
- Have a hard time swallowing
- Tremble or twitch
- Be irritable, sweat a lot, and feel light-headed or out of breath
- Have to go to the bathroom a lot.

What causes GAD?

GAD sometimes runs in families, but no one knows for sure why some people have it, while others don't. Researchers have found that several parts of the brain are involved in fear and anxiety. By learning more about fear and anxiety in the brain, scientists may be able to create better treatments. Researchers are also looking for ways in which stress and environmental factors may play a role.

How is GAD treated?

First, talk to your doctor about your symptoms. Your doctor should do an exam to make sure that another physical problem isn't causing the symptoms. The doctor may refer you to a mental health specialist.

GAD is generally treated with psychotherapy, medication, or both. Some people do better with cognitive behavior therapy, while others do better with medication. Still others do best with a combination of the two. Talk with your doctor about the best treatment for you.

Psychotherapy: A type of psychotherapy called cognitive behavior therapy is especially useful for treating GAD. It teaches a person different ways of thinking, behaving, and reacting to situations that help him or her feel less anxious and worried.

Medication: Doctors also may prescribe medication to help treat GAD. Two types of medications are commonly used to treat GAD—anti-anxiety medications and antidepressants. Anti-anxiety medications are powerful and there are different types. Many types begin working right away, but they generally should not be taken for long periods.

Antidepressants are used to treat depression, but they also are helpful for GAD. They may take several weeks to start working. These medications may cause side effects such as headache, nausea, or difficulty sleeping. These side effects are usually not a problem for most people, especially if the dose starts off low and is increased slowly over time. Talk to your doctor about any side effects you may have.

It's important to know that although antidepressants can be safe and effective for many people, they may be risky for some, especially children, teens, and young adults. A "black box"—the most serious type of warning that a prescription drug can have—has been added to the labels of antidepressant medications. These labels warn people that antidepressants may cause some people to have suicidal thoughts or make suicide attempts. Anyone taking antidepressants should be monitored closely, especially when they first start treatment with medications.

Chapter 12

Phobias and Fears

Almost everyone has an irrational fear or two. But, when fears become so severe that they interfere with your normal life they are called phobias. Phobias can be managed and cured. Self-help strategies and therapy can help you overcome your anxiety and fears and get on with your life.

What Is a Phobia?

A phobia is an intense fear of something that, in reality, poses little or no actual danger. Common phobias and fears include closed-in places, heights, highway driving, flying insects, snakes, and needles. However, we can develop phobias of virtually anything. Most phobias develop in childhood, but they can also develop in adults.

If you have a phobia, you probably realize that your fear is unreasonable, yet you still can't control your feelings. Just thinking about the feared object or situation may make you anxious. And when you're actually exposed to the thing you fear, the terror is automatic and overwhelming.

"Phobias and Fears," by Melinda Smith, M.A., Robert Segal, M.A., and Jeanne Segal, Ph.D., updated April 2012. © 2012 Helpguide.org. All rights reserved. Reprinted with permission. Helpguide provides a detailed list of references and resources for this article, with links to related Helpguide topics and information from other websites. For a complete list of these resources, go to http://helpguide .org/mental/phobia_symptoms_types_treatment.htm.

The experience is so nerve-wracking that you may go to great lengths to avoid it—inconveniencing yourself or even changing your lifestyle. If you have claustrophobia, for example, you might turn down a lucrative job offer if you have to ride the elevator to get to the office. If you have a fear of heights, you might drive an extra twenty miles in order to avoid a tall bridge.

Understanding your phobia is the first step to overcoming it. It's important to know that phobias are common. Having a phobia doesn't mean you're crazy! It also helps to know that phobias are highly treatable. You can overcome your anxiety and fear, no matter how out of control it feels.

Barbara's Fear of Flying

Barbara is terrified of flying. Unfortunately, she has to travel a lot for work, and this traveling takes a terrible toll. For weeks before every trip, she has a knot in her stomach and a feeling of anxiety that won't go away. On the day of the flight, she wakes up feeling like she's going to throw up. Once she's on the plane, her heart pounds, she feels lightheaded, and she starts to hyperventilate. Every time it gets worse and worse.

Barbara's fear of flying has gotten so bad that she finally told her boss she can only travel to places within driving distance. Her boss was not happy about this, and Barbara's not sure what will happen at work. She's afraid she'll be demoted or lose her job altogether. But better that, she tells herself, than getting on a plane again.

"Normal" Fear vs. Phobias

It is normal and even helpful to experience fear in dangerous situations. Fear is an adaptive human response. It serves a protective purpose, activating the automatic "fight-or-flight" response. With our bodies and minds alert and ready for action, we are able to respond quickly and protect ourselves.

But with phobias the threat is greatly exaggerated or nonexistent. For example, it is only natural to be afraid of a snarling Doberman, but it is irrational to be terrified of a friendly poodle on a leash, as you might be if you have a dog phobia.

Normal Fears in Children

Many childhood fears are natural and tend to develop at specific ages. For example, many young children are afraid of the dark and may need a nightlight to sleep. That doesn't mean they have a phobia. In most cases, they will grow out of this fear as they get older.

If your child's fear is not interfering with his or her daily life or causing him or a her a great deal of distress, then there's little cause for undue concern. However, if the fear is interfering with your child's social activities, school performance, or sleep, you may want to see a qualified child therapist.

Table 12.1. The Difference Between Normal Fear and a Phobia

Normal fear	Phobia
Feeling anxious when flying through turbulence or taking off during a storm	Not going to your best friend's island wedding because you'd have to fly there
Experiencing butterflies when peering down from the top of a skyscraper or climbing a tall ladder	Turning down a great job because it's on the 10th floor of the office building
Getting nervous when you see a pit bull or a Rottweiler	Steering clear of the park because you might see a dog
Feeling a little queasy when getting a shot or when your blood is being drawn	Avoiding necessary medical treatments or doctor's checkups because you're terrified of needles

Which of my child's fears are normal? According to the Child Anxiety Network, the following fears are extremely common and considered normal:

- **0–2 years:** Loud noises, strangers, separation from parents, large objects.

- **3–6 years:** Imaginary things such as ghosts, monsters, the dark, sleeping alone, strange noises.

- **7–16 years:** More realistic fears such as injury, illness, school performance, death, natural disasters.

Common Types of Phobias and Fears

There are four general types of phobias and fears:

- **Animal phobias:** Examples include fear of snakes, fear of spiders, fear of rodents, and fear of dogs.

- **Natural environment phobias:** Examples include fear of heights, fear of storms, fear of water, and fear of the dark.

- **Situational phobias (fears triggered by a specific situation):** Examples include fear of enclosed spaces (claustrophobia), fear of flying, fear of driving, fear of tunnels, and fear of bridges.

- **Blood-injection-injury phobia:** The fear of blood, fear or injury, or a fear of needles or other medical procedures.

Common Phobias and Fears

- Fear of spiders

- Fear of snakes

- Fear of heights

- Fear or closed spaces

- Fear of storms

- Fear of needles and injections

- Fear of public speaking

- Fear of flying

- Fear of germs

- Fear of illness or death

Some phobias don't fall into one of the four common categories. Such phobias include fear of choking, fear of getting a disease such as cancer, and fear of clowns.

Social Phobia and Fear of Public Speaking

Social phobia, also called social anxiety disorder, is fear of social situations where you may be embarrassed or judged. If you have social phobia you may be excessively self-conscious and afraid of humiliating yourself in front of others. Your anxiety over how you will look and what others will think may lead you to avoid certain social situations you'd otherwise enjoy.

Fear of public speaking, an extremely common phobia, is a type of social phobia. Other fears associated with social phobia include fear of eating or drinking in public, talking to strangers, taking exams, mingling at a party, and being called on in class.

Agoraphobia (Fear of Open Spaces)

Agoraphobia is another phobia that doesn't fit neatly into any of the four categories. Traditionally thought to involve a fear of public places and open spaces, it is now believed that agoraphobia develops as a complication of panic attacks.

Afraid of having another panic attack, you become anxious about being in situations where escape would be difficult or embarrassing, or where help wouldn't be immediately available. For example, you are likely to avoid crowded places such as shopping malls and movie theaters. You may also avoid cars, airplanes, subways, and other forms of travel. In more severe cases, you might only feel safe at home.

Signs and Symptoms of Phobias

The symptoms of a phobia can range from mild feelings of apprehension and anxiety to a full-blown panic attack. Typically, the closer you are to the thing you're afraid of, the greater your fear will be. Your fear will also be higher if getting away is difficult.

Physical Signs and Symptoms of a Phobia

- Difficulty breathing
- Racing or pounding heart
- Chest pain or tightness
- Trembling or shaking
- Feeling dizzy or lightheaded
- A churning stomach
- Hot or cold flashes; tingling sensations
- Sweating

Emotional Signs and Symptoms of a Phobia

- Feeling of overwhelming anxiety or panic
- Feeling an intense need to escape
- Feeling "unreal" or detached from yourself
- Fear of losing control or going crazy
- Feeling like you're going to die or pass out

189

- Knowing that you're overreacting, but feeling powerless to control your fear

Symptoms of Blood-Injection-Injury Phobia

The symptoms of blood-injection-injury phobia are slightly different from other phobias. When confronted with the sight of blood or a needle, you experience not only fear but disgust.

Like other phobias, you initially feel anxious as your heart speeds up. However, unlike other phobias, this acceleration is followed by a quick drop in blood pressure, which leads to nausea, dizziness, and fainting. Although a fear of fainting is common in all specific phobias, blood-injection-injury phobia is the only phobia where fainting can actually occur.

When to Seek Help for Phobias and Fears

Although phobias are common, they don't always cause considerable distress or significantly disrupt your life. For example, if you have a snake phobia, it may cause no problems in your everyday activities if you live in a city where you are not likely to run into one. On the other hand, if you have a severe phobia of crowded spaces, living in a big city would pose a problem.

If your phobia doesn't really impact your life that much, it's probably nothing to be concerned about. But if avoidance of the object, activity, or situation that triggers your phobia interferes with your normal functioning or keeps you from doing things you would otherwise enjoy, it's time to seek help.

Consider Treatment for Your Phobia If

- It causes intense and disabling fear, anxiety, and panic.
- You recognize that your fear is excessive and unreasonable.
- You avoid certain situations and places because of your phobia.
- Your avoidance interferes with your normal routine or causes significant distress.
- You've had the phobia for at least six months.

Self-Help or Therapy for Phobias: Which Treatment Is Best?

When it comes to treating phobias, self-help strategies and therapy can both be effective. What's best for you depends on a number of factors, including the severity of your phobia, your insurance coverage, and the amount of support you need.

As a general rule, self-help is always worth a try. The more you can do for yourself, the more in control you'll feel—which goes a long way when it comes to phobias and fears. However, if your phobia is so severe that it triggers panic attacks or uncontrollable anxiety, you may want to get additional support.

The good news is that therapy for phobias has a great track record. Not only does it work extremely well, but you tend to see results very quickly—sometimes in as a little as one to four sessions.

However, support doesn't have to come in the guise of a professional therapist. Just having someone to hold your hand or stand by your side as you face your fears can be extraordinarily helpful.

Phobia Treatment Tip 1: Face Your Fears, One Step at a Time

It's only natural to want to avoid the thing or situation you fear. But when it comes to conquering phobias, facing your fears is the key. While avoidance may make you feel better in the short-term, it prevents you from learning that your phobia may not be as frightening or overwhelming as you think. You never get the chance to learn how to cope with your fears and experience control over the situation. As a result, the phobia becomes increasingly scarier and more daunting in your mind.

Exposure: Gradually and Repeatedly Facing Your Fears

The most effective way to overcome a phobia is by gradually and repeatedly exposing yourself to what you fear in a safe and controlled way. During this exposure process, you'll learn to ride out the anxiety and fear until it inevitably passes.

Through repeated experiences facing your fear, you'll begin to realize that the worst isn't going to happen; you're not going to die or "lose it". With each exposure, you'll feel more confident and in control. The phobia begins to lose its power.

Successfully facing your fears takes planning, practice, and patience. The following tips will help you get the most out of the exposure process.

Climbing up the "Fear Ladder"

If you've tried exposure in the past and it didn't work, you may have started with something too scary or overwhelming. It's important to begin with a situation that you can handle, and work your way up from there, building your confidence and coping skills as you move up the "fear ladder."

Make a list: Make a list of the frightening situations related to your phobia. If you're afraid of flying, your list (in addition to the obvious, such as taking a flight or getting through takeoff) might include booking your ticket, packing your suitcase, driving to the airport, watching planes take off and land, going through security, boarding the plane, and listening to the flight attendant present the safety instructions.

Build your fear ladder: Arrange the items on your list from the least scary to the most scary. The first step should make you slightly anxious, but not so frightening that you're too intimidated to try it. When creating the ladder, it can be helpful to think about your end goal (for example, to be able to be near dogs without panicking) and then break down the steps needed to reach that goal.

Work your way up the ladder: Start with the first step (in this example, looking at pictures of dogs) and don't move on until you start to feel more comfortable doing it. If at all possible, stay in the situation long enough for your anxiety to decrease. The longer you expose yourself to the thing you're afraid of, the more you'll get used to it and the less anxious you'll feel when you face it the next time. If the situation itself is short (for example, crossing a bridge), do it over and over again until your anxiety starts to lessen. Once you've done a step on several separate occasions without feeling too much anxiety, you can move on to the next step. If a step is too hard, break it down into smaller steps or go slower.

Practice: It's important to practice regularly. The more often you practice, the quicker your progress will be. However, don't rush. Go at a pace that you can manage without feeling overwhelmed. And remember: you will feel uncomfortable and anxious as you face your fears, but the feelings are only temporary. If you stick with it, the anxiety will fade. Your fears won't hurt you.

Facing a Fear of Dogs: A Sample Fear Ladder

- **Step 1:** Look at pictures of dogs.
- **Step 2:** Watch a video with dogs in it.
- **Step 3:** Look at a dog through a window.
- **Step 4:** Stand across the street from a dog on a leash.

- **Step 5:** Stand 10 feet away from a dog on a leash.
- **Step 6:** Stand 5 feet away from a dog on a leash.
- **Step 7:** Stand beside a dog on a leash.
- **Step 8:** Pet a small dog that someone is holding.
- **Step 9:** Pet a larger dog on a leash.
- **Step 10:** Pet a larger dog off leash.

If You Start to Feel Overwhelmed

While it's natural to feel scared or anxious as you face your phobia, you should never feel overwhelmed by these feelings. If you start to feel overwhelmed, immediately back off. You may need to spend more time learning to control feelings of anxiety (see the relaxation techniques below), or you may feel more comfortable working with a therapist.

Phobia Treatment Tip 2: Learn Relaxation Techniques

As you'll recall, when you're afraid or anxious, you experience a variety of uncomfortable physical symptoms, such as a racing heart and a suffocating feeling. These physical sensations can be frightening themselves—and a large part of what makes your phobia so distressing. However, by learning and practicing relaxation techniques, you can become more confident in your ability to tolerate these uncomfortable sensations and calm yourself down quickly.

Relaxation techniques such as deep breathing, meditation, and muscle relaxation are powerful antidotes to anxiety, panic, and fear. With regular practice, they can improve your ability to control the physical symptoms of anxiety, which will make facing your phobia less intimidating. Relaxation techniques will also help you cope more effectively with other sources of stress and anxiety in your life.

A Simple Deep Breathing Relaxation Exercise

When you're anxious, you tend to take quick, shallow breaths (also known as hyperventilating), which actually adds to the physical feelings of anxiety. By breathing deeply from the abdomen, you can reverse these physical sensations. You can't be upset when you're breathing slowly, deeply, and quietly. Within a few short minutes of deep breathing, you'll feel less tense, short of breath, and anxious.

- Sit or stand comfortably with your back straight. Put one hand on your chest and the other on your stomach.

193

- Take a slow breath in through your nose, counting to four. The hand on your stomach should rise. The hand on your chest should move very little.

- Hold your breath for a count of seven.

- Exhale through your mouth to a count of eight, pushing out as much air as you can while contracting your abdominal muscles. The hand on your stomach should move in as you exhale, but your other hand should move very little.

- Inhale again, repeating the cycle until you feel relaxed and centered.

Try practicing this deep breathing technique for five minutes twice day. You don't need to feel anxious to practice. In fact, it's best to practice when you're feeling calm until you're familiar and comfortable with the exercise. Once you're comfortable with this deep breathing technique, you can start to use it when you're facing your phobia or in other stressful situations.

Phobia Treatment Tip 3: Challenge Negative Thoughts

Learning to challenge unhelpful thoughts is an important step in overcoming your phobia. When you have a phobia, you tend to over-estimate how bad it will be if you're exposed to the situation you fear. At the same time, you underestimate your ability to cope.

The anxious thoughts that trigger and fuel phobias are usually negative and unrealistic. It can help to put these thoughts to the test. Begin by writing down any negative thoughts you have when confronted with your phobia. Many times, these thoughts fall into the following categories:

- **Fortune telling:** For example, "This bridge is going to collapse;" "I'll make a fool of myself for sure;" "I will definitely lose it when the elevator doors close."

- **Overgeneralization:** "I fainted once while getting a shot. I'll never be able to get a shot again without passing out;" "That pit bull lunged at me. All dogs are dangerous."

- **Catastrophizing:** "The captain said we're going through turbulence. The plane is going to crash!" "The person next to me coughed. Maybe it's the swine flu. I'm going to get very sick!"

Once you've identified your negative thoughts, evaluate them. Use the following example to get started.

- **Negative thought:** "The elevator will break down and I'll get trapped and suffocate." Is there any evidence that contradicts this thought?

  - "I see many people using the elevator and it has never broken down."

  - "I cannot remember ever hearing of anyone dying from suffocation in an elevator."

  - "I have never actually been in an elevator that has broken down."

  - "There are air vents in an elevator which will stop the air running out."

- **Could you do anything to resolve this situation if it does occur?**

  - "I guess I could press the alarm button or use the telephone to call for assistance."

- **Are you making a thinking error?**

  - "Yes. I'm fortune telling, as I have no evidence to suggest that the elevator will break down."

- **What would you say to a friend who has this fear?**

  - "I would probably say that the chances of it happening are very slim as you don't see or hear about it very often."

Source: Mood Juice

It's also helpful to come up with some positive coping statements that you can tell yourself when facing your phobia. For example:

- "I've felt this way before and nothing terrible happened. It may be unpleasant, but it won't harm me."

- "If the worst happens and I have a panic attack while I'm driving, I'll simply pull over and wait for it to pass."

- "I've flown many times and the plane has never crashed. In fact, I don't know anyone who's ever been in a plane crash. Statistically, flying is very safe."

195

Chapter 13

Posttraumatic Stress Disorder

What is posttraumatic stress disorder, or PTSD?

PTSD is an anxiety disorder that some people get after seeing or living through a dangerous event. When in danger, it's natural to feel afraid. This fear triggers many split-second changes in the body to prepare to defend against the danger or to avoid it. This fight-or-flight response is a healthy reaction meant to protect a person from harm. But in PTSD, this reaction is changed or damaged. People who have PTSD may feel stressed or frightened even when they're no longer in danger.

Anyone can get PTSD at any age. This includes war veterans and survivors of physical and sexual assault, abuse, accidents, disasters, and many other serious events. Not everyone with PTSD has been through a dangerous event. Some people get PTSD after a friend or family member experiences danger or is harmed. The sudden, unexpected death of a loved one can also cause PTSD.

What are the symptoms of PTSD?

PTSD can cause many symptoms. These symptoms can be grouped into three categories:

1. **Re-experiencing symptoms:** Flashbacks—reliving the trauma over and over, including physical symptoms like a racing heart

---

Excerpted from "Post-Traumatic Stress Disorder (PTSD)," National Institute of Mental Health (www.nimh.nih.gov), August 31, 2010.

or sweating; bad dreams; frightening thoughts. Re-experiencing symptoms may cause problems in a person's everyday routine. They can start from the person's own thoughts and feelings. Words, objects, or situations that are reminders of the event can also trigger re-experiencing.

2. **Avoidance symptoms:** Staying away from places, events, or objects that are reminders of the experience; feeling emotionally numb; feeling strong guilt, depression, or worry; losing interest in activities that were enjoyable in the past; having trouble remembering the dangerous event. Things that remind a person of the traumatic event can trigger avoidance symptoms. These symptoms may cause a person to change his or her personal routine. For example, after a bad car accident, a person who usually drives may avoid driving or riding in a car.

3. **Hyperarousal symptoms:** Being easily startled; feeling tense or on edge; having difficulty sleeping, and/or having angry outbursts. Hyperarousal symptoms are usually constant, instead of being triggered by things that remind one of the traumatic event. They can make the person feel stressed and angry. These symptoms may make it hard to do daily tasks, such as sleeping, eating, or concentrating.

It's natural to have some of these symptoms after a dangerous event. Sometimes people have very serious symptoms that go away after a few weeks. This is called acute stress disorder, or ASD. When the symptoms last more than a few weeks and become an ongoing problem, they might be PTSD. Some people with PTSD don't show any symptoms for weeks or months.

Do children react differently than adults?

Children and teens can have extreme reactions to trauma, but their symptoms may not be the same as adults. In very young children, these symptoms can include bedwetting, when they'd learned how to use the toilet before; forgetting how or being unable to talk; acting out the scary event during playtime; and being unusually clingy with a parent or other adult.

Older children and teens usually show symptoms more like those seen in adults. They may also develop disruptive, disrespectful, or destructive behaviors. Older children and teens may feel guilty for not preventing injury or deaths. They may also have thoughts of revenge.

How is PTSD detected?

A doctor who has experience helping people with mental illnesses, such as a psychiatrist or psychologist, can diagnose PTSD. The diagnosis is made after the doctor talks with the person who has symptoms of PTSD.

To be diagnosed with PTSD, a person must have all of the following for at least one month:

- At least one re-experiencing symptom
- At least three avoidance symptoms
- At least two hyperarousal symptoms
- Symptoms that make it hard to go about daily life, go to school or work, be with friends, and take care of important tasks

Why do some people get PTSD and other people do not?

It is important to remember that not everyone who lives through a dangerous event gets PTSD. In fact, most will not get the disorder.

Many factors play a part in whether a person will get PTSD. Some of these are risk factors that make a person more likely to get PTSD. Other factors, called resilience factors, can help reduce the risk of the disorder. Some of these risk and resilience factors are present before the trauma and others become important during and after a traumatic event.

Risk factors for PTSD include the following:

- Living through dangerous events and traumas
- Having a history of mental illness
- Getting hurt
- Seeing people hurt or killed
- Feeling horror, helplessness, or extreme fear
- Having little or no social support after the event
- Dealing with extra stress after the event, such as loss of a loved one, pain and injury, or loss of a job or home.

Resilience factors such as the following may reduce the risk of PTSD:

- Seeking out support from other people, such as friends and family

- Finding a support group after a traumatic event

- Feeling good about one's own actions in the face of danger

- Having a coping strategy, or a way of getting through the bad event and learning from it

- Being able to act and respond effectively despite feeling fear

Researchers are studying the importance of various risk and resilience factors. With more study, it may be possible someday to predict who is likely to get PTSD and prevent it.

How is PTSD treated?

The main treatments for people with PTSD are psychotherapy (talk therapy), medications, or both. Everyone is different, so a treatment that works for one person may not work for another. It is important for anyone with PTSD to be treated by a mental health care provider who is experienced with PTSD. Some people with PTSD need to try different treatments to find what works for their symptoms.

If someone with PTSD is going through an ongoing trauma, such as being in an abusive relationship, both of the problems need to be treated. Other ongoing problems can include panic disorder, depression, substance abuse, and feeling suicidal.

How is psychotherapy used to treat PTSD?

Psychotherapy is talk therapy. It involves talking with a mental health professional to treat a mental illness. Psychotherapy can occur one-on-one or in a group. Talk therapy treatment for PTSD usually lasts 6 to 12 weeks, but can take more time. Research shows that support from family and friends can be an important part of therapy.

Many types of psychotherapy can help people with PTSD. Some types target the symptoms of PTSD directly. Other therapies focus on social, family, or job-related problems. The doctor or therapist may combine different therapies depending on each person's needs.

One helpful therapy is called cognitive behavioral therapy, or CBT. There are several parts to CBT:

- **Exposure therapy:** This therapy helps people face and control their fear. It exposes them to the trauma they experienced in a safe way. It uses mental imagery, writing, or visits to the place where the event happened. The therapist uses these tools to help people with PTSD cope with their feelings.

- **Cognitive restructuring:** This therapy helps people make sense of the bad memories. Sometimes people remember the event differently than how it happened. They may feel guilt or shame about what is not their fault. The therapist helps people with PTSD look at what happened in a realistic way.

- **Stress inoculation training:** This therapy tries to reduce PTSD symptoms by teaching a person how to reduce anxiety. Like cognitive restructuring, this treatment helps people look at their memories in a healthy way.

Other types of treatment can also help people with PTSD. People with PTSD should talk about all treatment options with their therapist.

How are medications used to treat PTSD?

The U.S. Food and Drug Administration (FDA) has approved two medications for treating adults with PTSD: Sertraline (Zoloft) and Paroxetine (Paxil). Both of these medications are antidepressants, which are also used to treat depression. They may help control PTSD symptoms such as sadness, worry, anger, and feeling numb inside. Taking these medications may make it easier to go through psychotherapy.

Sometimes people taking these medications have side effects. The effects can be annoying, but they usually go away. However, medications affect everyone differently. Any side effects or unusual reactions should be reported to a doctor immediately.

The most common side effects of antidepressants like sertraline and paroxetine are:

- Headache, which usually goes away within a few days.

- Nausea (feeling sick to your stomach), which usually goes away within a few days.

- Sleeplessness or drowsiness, which may occur during the first few weeks but then goes away. Sometimes the medication dose needs to be reduced or the time of day it is taken needs to be adjusted to help lessen these side effects.

- Agitation (feeling jittery).

- Sexual problems, which can affect both men and women, including reduced sex drive, and problems having and enjoying sex.

Doctors may also prescribe other types of medications, such as the ones listed below. There is little information on how well these work for people with PTSD.

Benzodiazepines: These medications may be given to help people relax and sleep. People who take benzodiazepines may have memory problems or become dependent on the medication.

Antipsychotics: These medications are usually given to people with other mental disorders, like schizophrenia. People who take antipsychotics may gain weight and have a higher chance of getting heart disease and diabetes.

Other antidepressants: Like sertraline and paroxetine, the antidepressants fluoxetine (Prozac) and citalopram (Celexa) can help people with PTSD feel less tense or sad. For people with PTSD who also have other anxiety disorders or depression, antidepressants may be useful in reducing symptoms of these co-occurring illnesses.

Are antidepressants safe?

Despite the relative safety and popularity of SSRIs and other antidepressants, some studies have suggested that they may have unintentional effects on some people, especially adolescents and young adults. In 2004, the Food and Drug Administration (FDA) conducted a thorough review of published and unpublished controlled clinical trials of antidepressants that involved nearly 4,400 children and adolescents. The review revealed that 4% of those taking antidepressants thought about or attempted suicide (although no suicides occurred), compared to 2% of those receiving placebos.

This information prompted the FDA, in 2005, to adopt a black box warning label on all antidepressant medications to alert the public about the potential increased risk of suicidal thinking or attempts in children and adolescents taking antidepressants. In 2007, the FDA proposed that makers of all antidepressant medications extend the warning to include young adults up through age 24. A black box warning is the most serious type of warning on prescription drug labeling.

The warning emphasizes that patients of all ages taking antidepressants should be closely monitored, especially during the initial weeks of treatment. Possible side effects to look for are worsening depression, suicidal thinking or behavior, or any unusual changes in behavior such as sleeplessness, agitation, or withdrawal from normal social situations. The warning adds that families and caregivers should also be told of the need for close monitoring and report any changes to the physician. The latest information can be found on the FDA website (www.fda.gov).

Results of a comprehensive review of pediatric trials conducted between 1988 and 2006 suggested that the benefits of antidepressant medications likely outweigh their risks to children and adolescents with major depression and anxiety disorders. The study was funded in part by the National Institute of Mental Health.

How can I help a friend or relative who has PTSD?

If you know someone who has PTSD, it affects you too. The first and most important thing you can do to help a friend or relative is to help him or her get the right diagnosis and treatment. You may need to make an appointment for your friend or relative and go with him or her to see the doctor. Encourage him or her to stay in treatment, or to seek different treatment if his or her symptoms don't get better after six to eight weeks.

To help a friend or relative, you can try these suggestions:

- Offer emotional support, understanding, patience, and encouragement.

- Learn about PTSD so you can understand what your friend or relative is experiencing.

- Talk to your friend or relative, and listen carefully.

- Listen to feelings your friend or relative expresses and be understanding of situations that may trigger PTSD symptoms.

- Invite your friend or relative out for positive distractions such as walks, outings, and other activities.

- Remind your friend or relative that, with time and treatment, he or she can get better.

Never ignore comments about your friend or relative harming him or herself, and report such comments to your friend's or relative's therapist or doctor.

How can I help myself?

It may be very hard to take that first step to help yourself. It is important to realize that although it may take some time, with treatment, you can get better.

To help yourself, take the following steps:

- Talk to your doctor about treatment options.

- Engage in mild activity or exercise to help reduce stress.

- Set realistic goals for yourself.

- Break up large tasks into small ones, set some priorities, and do what you can as you can.

- Try to spend time with other people and confide in a trusted friend or relative. Tell others about things that may trigger symptoms.

- Expect your symptoms to improve gradually, not immediately.

- Identify and seek out comforting situations, places, and people.

What if I or someone I know is in crisis?

If you are thinking about harming yourself, or know someone who is, tell someone who can help immediately:

- Call your doctor.

- Call 911 or go to a hospital emergency room to get immediate help or ask a friend or family member to help you do these things.

- Call the toll-free, 24-hour hotline of the National Suicide Prevention Lifeline at 800-273-TALK (800-273-8255); TTY: 800-799-4TTY (4889) to talk to a trained counselor.

- Make sure you or the suicidal person is not left alone.

Chapter 14

Psychotic Disorders

Chapter Contents

Section 14.1

Psychosis

Psychosis is a loss of contact with reality, usually including false beliefs about what is taking place or who one is (delusions) and seeing or hearing things that aren't there (hallucinations).

Causes

A number of substances and medical conditions can cause psychosis, including:

- Alcohol and certain illegal drugs, both during use and during withdrawal

- Brain tumors or cysts

- Dementia (including Alzheimer's disease)

- Degenerative brain diseases, such as Parkinson's disease, Huntington's disease, and certain chromosomal disorders

- HIV and other infections that affect the brain

- Some prescription drugs, such as steroids and stimulants

- Some types of epilepsy

- Stroke

Psychosis is also part of a number of psychiatric disorders, including:

- Bipolar disorder (manic or depressed)

- Delusional disorder

- Depression with psychotic features

- Personality disorders (schizotypal, shizoid, paranoid, and sometimes borderline)

- Schizoaffective disorder

- Schizophrenia

Symptoms

Psychotic symptoms may include:

- Disorganized thought and speech

- False beliefs that are not based in reality (delusions), especially unfounded fear or suspicion

- Hearing, seeing, or feeling things that are not there (hallucinations)

- Thoughts that "jump" between unrelated topics (disordered thinking)

Exams and Tests

Psychiatric evaluation and testing are used to diagnose the cause of the psychosis.

Laboratory testing and brain scans may not be needed, but sometimes can help pinpoint the diagnosis. Tests may include:

- Blood tests for abnormal electrolyte and hormone levels

- Blood tests for syphilis and other infections

- Drug screens

- MRI of the brain

Treatment

Treatment depends on the cause of the psychosis. Care in a hospital is often needed to ensure the patient's safety.

Antipsychotic drugs, which reduce hallucinations and delusions and improve thinking and behavior are helpful, whether the cause is a medical or psychiatric disorder.

How well a person does depends on the cause of the psychosis. If the cause can be corrected, the outlook is often good, and treatment with antipsychotic medication may be brief.

Some chronic conditions, such as schizophrenia, may need life-long treatment with antipsychotic medications to control symptoms.

Possible Complications

Psychosis can prevent people from functioning normally and caring for themselves. If the condition is left untreated, people can sometimes harm themselves or others.

When to Contact a Medical Professional

Call your health care provider or mental health professional if you or a member of your family is losing contact with reality. If there is any concern about safety, immediately take the person to the nearest emergency room to be seen by a doctor.

Prevention

Prevention depends on the cause. For example, avoiding alcohol abuse prevents alcohol-induced psychosis.

Section 14.2

Schizophrenia

Excerpted from "Schizophrenia," National Institute of Mental Health (www.nimh.nih.gov), November 21, 2011.

Schizophrenia is a chronic, severe, and disabling brain disorder that has affected people throughout history. About one percent of Americans have this illness.

Symptoms

The symptoms of schizophrenia fall into three broad categories: positive symptoms, negative symptoms, and cognitive symptoms.

Positive Symptoms

Positive symptoms are psychotic behaviors not seen in healthy people. People with positive symptoms often lose touch with reality.

These symptoms can come and go. Sometimes they are severe and at other times hardly noticeable, depending on whether the individual is receiving treatment. They include the following:

Hallucinations: Hallucinations are things a person sees, hears, smells, or feels that no one else can see, hear, smell, or feel. "Voices" are the most common type of hallucination in schizophrenia. Many people with the disorder hear voices. The voices may talk to the person about his or her behavior, order the person to do things, or warn the person of danger. Sometimes the voices talk to each other. People with schizophrenia may hear voices for a long time before family and friends notice the problem.

Other types of hallucinations include seeing people or objects that are not there, smelling odors that no one else detects, and feeling things like invisible fingers touching their bodies when no one is near.

Delusions: Delusions are false beliefs that are not part of the person's culture and do not change. The person believes delusions even after other people prove that the beliefs are not true or logical. People with schizophrenia can have delusions that seem bizarre, such as believing that neighbors can control their behavior with magnetic waves. They may also believe that people on television are directing special messages to them, or that radio stations are broadcasting their thoughts aloud to others. Sometimes they believe they are someone else, such as a famous historical figure. They may have paranoid delusions and believe that others are trying to harm them, such as by cheating, harassing, poisoning, spying on, or plotting against them or the people they care about. These beliefs are called delusions of persecution.

Thought disorders: Thought disorders are unusual or dysfunctional ways of thinking. One form of thought disorder is called disorganized thinking. This is when a person has trouble organizing his or her thoughts or connecting them logically. They may talk in a garbled way that is hard to understand. Another form is called thought blocking. This is when a person stops speaking abruptly in the middle of a thought. When asked why he or she stopped talking, the person may say that it felt as if the thought had been taken out of his or her head. Finally, a person with a thought disorder might make up meaningless words, or neologisms.

Movement disorders: Movement disorders may appear as agitated body movements. A person with a movement disorder may repeat certain motions over and over. In the other extreme, a person may become catatonic. Catatonia is a state in which a person does not move and does not respond to others. Catatonia is rare today, but it was more common when treatment for schizophrenia was not available.

Negative Symptoms

Negative symptoms are associated with disruptions to normal emotions and behaviors. These symptoms are harder to recognize as part of the disorder and can be mistaken for depression or other conditions. These symptoms include the following:

- Flat affect (a person's face does not move or he or she talks in a dull or monotonous voice)

- Lack of pleasure in everyday life

- Lack of ability to begin and sustain planned activities

- Speaking little, even when forced to interact

People with negative symptoms need help with everyday tasks. They often neglect basic personal hygiene. This may make them seem lazy or unwilling to help themselves, but the problems are symptoms caused by the schizophrenia.

Cognitive Symptoms

Cognitive symptoms are subtle. Like negative symptoms, cognitive symptoms may be difficult to recognize as part of the disorder. Often, they are detected only when other tests are performed. Cognitive symptoms include the following:

- Poor executive functioning (the ability to understand information and use it to make decisions)

- Trouble focusing or paying attention

- Problems with working memory (the ability to use information immediately after learning it).

Cognitive symptoms often make it hard to lead a normal life and earn a living. They can cause great emotional distress.

Schizophrenia and Violence

People with schizophrenia are not usually violent. In fact, most violent crimes are not committed by people with schizophrenia. However, some symptoms are associated with violence, such as delusions of persecution. Substance abuse may also increase the chance a person will become violent. If a person with schizophrenia becomes violent, the violence is usually directed at family members and tends to take place at home.

The risk of violence among people with schizophrenia is small. But people with the illness attempt suicide much more often than others. About ten percent (especially young adult males) die by suicide. It is hard to predict which people with schizophrenia are prone to suicide. If you know someone who talks about or attempts suicide, help him or her find professional help right away.

Schizophrenia and Substance Abuse

Some people who abuse drugs show symptoms similar to those of schizophrenia. Therefore, people with schizophrenia may be mistaken for people who are affected by drugs. Most researchers do not believe that substance abuse causes schizophrenia. However, people who have schizophrenia are much more likely to have a substance or alcohol abuse problem than the general population.

Substance abuse can make treatment for schizophrenia less effective. Some drugs, like marijuana and stimulants such as amphetamines or cocaine, may make symptoms worse. In fact, research has found increasing evidence of a link between marijuana and schizophrenia symptoms. In addition, people who abuse drugs are less likely to follow their treatment plan.

Schizophrenia and Smoking

Addiction to nicotine is the most common form of substance abuse in people with schizophrenia. They are addicted to nicotine at three times the rate of the general population (75 to 90 percent vs. 25 to 30 percent).

The relationship between smoking and schizophrenia is complex. People with schizophrenia seem to be driven to smoke, and researchers are exploring whether there is a biological basis for this need. In addition to its known health hazards, several studies have found that smoking may make antipsychotic drugs less effective.

Quitting smoking may be very difficult for people with schizophrenia because nicotine withdrawal may cause their psychotic symptoms to get worse for a while. Quitting strategies that include nicotine replacement methods may be easier for patients to handle. Doctors who treat people with schizophrenia should watch their patients' response to antipsychotic medication carefully if the patient decides to start or stop smoking.

Causes of Schizophrenia

Experts think schizophrenia is caused by several factors.

Genes and Environment

Scientists have long known that schizophrenia runs in families. The illness occurs in one percent of the general population, but it occurs in ten percent of people who have a first-degree relative with the disorder, such as a parent, brother, or sister. People who have second-degree relatives (aunts, uncles, grandparents, or cousins) with the disease also develop schizophrenia more often than the general population. The risk is highest for an identical twin of a person with schizophrenia. He or she has a 40 to 65 percent chance of developing the disorder.

We inherit our genes from both parents. Scientists believe several genes are associated with an increased risk of schizophrenia, but that no gene causes the disease by itself. In fact, recent research has found that people with schizophrenia tend to have higher rates of rare genetic mutations. These genetic differences involve hundreds of different genes and probably disrupt brain development.

Other recent studies suggest that schizophrenia may result in part when a certain gene that is key to making important brain chemicals malfunctions. This problem may affect the part of the brain involved in developing higher functioning skills. Research into this gene is on-going, so it is not yet possible to use the genetic information to predict who will develop the disease.

Different Brain Chemistry and Structure

Scientists think that an imbalance in the complex, interrelated chemical reactions of the brain involving the neurotransmitters dopamine and glutamate, and possibly others, plays a role in schizophrenia. Neurotransmitters are substances that allow brain cells to communicate with each other. Scientists are learning more about brain chemistry and its link to schizophrenia.

Also, in small ways the brains of people with schizophrenia look different than those of healthy people. For example, fluid-filled cavities at the center of the brain, called ventricles, are larger in some people with schizophrenia. The brains of people with the illness also tend to have less gray matter, and some areas of the brain may have less or more activity.

Studies of brain tissue after death also have revealed differences in the brains of people with schizophrenia. Scientists found small changes in the distribution or characteristics of brain cells that likely occurred before birth. Some experts think problems during brain development before birth may lead to faulty connections. The problem may not show up in a person until puberty. The brain undergoes major changes during puberty, and these changes could trigger psychotic symptoms. Scientists have learned a lot about schizophrenia, but more research is needed to help explain how it develops.

Treatment

Because the causes of schizophrenia are still unknown, treatments focus on eliminating the symptoms of the disease. Treatments include antipsychotic medications and various psychosocial treatments.

Antipsychotic Medications

Antipsychotic medications have been available since the mid-1950s. The older types are called conventional or *typical* antipsychotics. Some of the more commonly used typical medications include:

- Chlorpromazine (Thorazine)

- Haloperidol (Haldol)

- Perphenazine (Etrafon, Trilafon)

- Fluphenazine (Prolixin).

In the 1990s, new antipsychotic medications were developed. These new medications are called second generation, or *atypical* antipsychotics.

One of these medications, clozapine (Clozaril) is an effective medication that treats psychotic symptoms, hallucinations, and breaks with reality. But clozapine can sometimes cause a serious problem called agranulocytosis, which is a loss of the white blood cells that help a person fight infection. People who take clozapine must get their white blood cell counts checked every week or two. This problem and the cost of blood tests make treatment with clozapine difficult for many people. But clozapine is potentially helpful for people who do not respond to other antipsychotic medications.

Other atypical antipsychotics were also developed. None cause agranulocytosis. Examples include the following:

- Risperidone (Risperdal)

- Olanzapine (Zyprexa)

- Quetiapine (Seroquel)

- Ziprasidone (Geodon)

- Aripiprazole (Abilify)

- Paliperidone (Invega).

When a doctor says it is okay to stop taking a medication, it should be gradually tapered off, never stopped suddenly.

Side Effects

Some people have side effects when they start taking these medications. Most side effects go away after a few days and often can be managed successfully. People who are taking antipsychotics should not drive until they adjust to their new medication. Side effects of many antipsychotics include drowsiness, dizziness when changing positions, blurred vision, rapid heartbeat, sensitivity to the sun, skin rashes, and menstrual problems for women.

Atypical antipsychotic medications can cause major weight gain and changes in a person's metabolism. This may increase a person's risk of getting diabetes and high cholesterol. A person's weight, glucose levels, and lipid levels should be monitored regularly by a doctor while taking an atypical antipsychotic medication.

Typical antipsychotic medications can cause side effects related to physical movement, such as rigidity, persistent muscle spasms, tremors, and restlessness.

Long-term use of typical antipsychotic medications may lead to a condition called tardive dyskinesia (TD). TD causes muscle movements a person can't control. The movements commonly happen around the mouth. TD can range from mild to severe, and in some people the problem cannot be cured. Sometimes people with TD recover partially or fully after they stop taking the medication.

TD happens to fewer people who take the atypical antipsychotics, but some people may still get TD. People who think that they might have TD should check with their doctor before stopping their medication.

Antipsychotics and Interactions with Other Medications

Antipsychotics can produce unpleasant or dangerous side effects when taken with certain medications. For this reason, all doctors treating a patient need to be aware of all the medications that person is taking. Doctors need to know about prescription and over-the-counter medicine, vitamins, minerals, and herbal supplements. People also need to discuss any alcohol or other drug use with their doctor.

Psychosocial Treatments

Psychosocial treatments can help people with schizophrenia who are already stabilized on antipsychotic medication. Psychosocial treatments help these patients deal with the everyday challenges of the illness, such as difficulty with communication, self-care, work, and forming and keeping relationships. Learning and using coping mechanisms to address these problems allow people with schizophrenia to socialize and attend school and work.

Patients who receive regular psychosocial treatment also are more likely to keep taking their medication, and they are less likely to have relapses or be hospitalized. A therapist can help patients better understand and adjust to living with schizophrenia. The therapist can provide education about the disorder, common symptoms or problems patients may experience, and the importance of staying on medications.

Illness management skills: People with schizophrenia can take an active role in managing their own illness. Once patients learn basic facts about schizophrenia and its treatment, they can make informed decisions about their care. If they know how to watch for the early warning signs of relapse and make a plan to respond, patients can learn to prevent relapses. Patients can also use coping skills to deal with persistent symptoms.

Integrated treatment for co-occurring substance abuse: Substance abuse is the most common co-occurring disorder in people with schizophrenia. But ordinary substance abuse treatment programs usually do not address this population's special needs. When schizophrenia treatment programs and drug treatment programs are used together, patients get better results.

Rehabilitation: Rehabilitation emphasizes social and vocational training to help people with schizophrenia function better in their communities. Because schizophrenia usually develops in people during the critical career-forming years of life (ages 18 to 35), and because the disease makes normal thinking and functioning difficult, most patients do not receive training in the skills needed for a job.

Rehabilitation programs can include job counseling and training, money management counseling, help in learning to use public transportation, and opportunities to practice communication skills. Rehabilitation programs work well when they include both job training and specific therapy designed to improve cognitive or thinking skills. Programs like this help patients hold jobs, remember important details, and improve their functioning.

Family education: People with schizophrenia are often discharged from the hospital into the care of their families. So it is important that family members know as much as possible about the disease. With the help of a therapist, family members can learn coping strategies and problem-solving skills. In this way the family can help make sure their loved one sticks with treatment and stays on his or her medication. Families should learn where to find outpatient and family services.

Cognitive behavioral therapy: Cognitive behavioral therapy (CBT) is a type of psychotherapy that focuses on thinking and behavior. CBT helps patients with symptoms that do not go away even when they take medication. The therapist teaches people with schizophrenia how to test the reality of their thoughts and perceptions, how to "not listen" to their voices, and how to manage their symptoms overall. CBT can help reduce the severity of symptoms and reduce the risk of relapse.

Self-help groups: Self-help groups for people with schizophrenia and their families are becoming more common. Professional therapists usually are not involved, but group members support and comfort each other. People in self-help groups know that others are facing the same problems, which can help everyone feel less isolated. The networking that takes place in self-help groups can also prompt families to work together to advocate for research and more hospital and community treatment programs. Also, groups may be able to draw public attention to the discrimination many people with mental illnesses face.

Once patients learn basic facts about schizophrenia and its treatment, they can make informed decisions about their care.

Helping a Person with Schizophrenia

People with schizophrenia can get help from professional case managers and caregivers at residential or day programs. However, family members usually are a patient's primary caregivers.

People with schizophrenia often resist treatment. They may not think they need help because they believe their delusions or hallucinations are real. In these cases, family and friends may need to take action to keep their loved one safe. Laws vary from state to state, and it can be difficult to force a person with a mental disorder into treatment or hospitalization. But when a person becomes dangerous to himself or herself, or to others, family members or friends may have to call the police to take their loved one to the hospital.

Treatment at the hospital: In the emergency room, a mental health professional will assess the patient and determine whether a voluntary or involuntary admission is needed. For a person to be admitted involuntarily, the law states that the professional must witness psychotic behavior and hear the person voice delusional thoughts. Family and friends can provide needed information to help a mental health professional make a decision.

After a loved one leaves the hospital: Family and friends can help their loved ones get treatment and take their medication once they go home. If patients stop taking their medication or stop going to follow-up appointments, their symptoms likely will return. Sometimes symptoms become severe for people who stop their medication and treatment. This is dangerous, since they may become unable to care for themselves. Some people end up on the street or in jail, where they rarely receive the kind of help they need.

Family and friends can also help patients set realistic goals and learn to function in the world. Each step toward these goals should be small and taken one at a time. The patient will need support during this time. When people with a mental illness are pressured and criticized, they usually do not get well. Often, their symptoms may get worse. Telling them when they are doing something right is the best way to help them move forward.

It can be difficult to know how to respond to someone with schizophrenia who makes strange or clearly false statements. Remember that these beliefs or hallucinations seem very real to the person. It is not helpful to say they are wrong or imaginary. But going along with the delusions is not helpful, either. Instead, calmly say that you see things differently. Tell them that you acknowledge that everyone has the right to see things his or her own way. In addition, it is important to understand that schizophrenia is a biological illness. Being respectful, supportive, and kind without tolerating dangerous or inappropriate behavior is the best way to approach people with this disorder.

Section 14.3

Schizoaffective Disorder

What is schizoaffective disorder?

Some psychiatric disorders are very difficult to diagnose accurately. One of the most confusing conditions is schizoaffective disorder.

This relatively rare disorder is defined as "the presence of psychotic symptoms in the absence of mood changes for at least two weeks in a patient who has a mood disorder." The diagnosis is used when an individual does not fit diagnostic standards for either schizophrenia or "affective" (mood) disorders such as depression and bipolar disorder (manic depression).

Some people may have symptoms of both a depressive disorder and schizophrenia at the same time, or they may have symptoms of schizophrenia without mood symptoms.

Many individuals with schizoaffective disorder are originally diagnosed with manic depression. If the person experiences delusions or hallucinations that go away in less than two weeks when the mood is "normal," bipolar disorder may be the proper diagnosis. Someone who experiences psychosis for three or four weeks while in a manic phase does not have schizoaffective disorder.

However, if delusions or hallucinations continue after the mood has stabilized and are accompanied by other symptoms of schizophrenia such as catatonia, paranoia, bizarre behavior, or thought disorders, a diagnosis of schizoaffective disorder may be appropriate. Accurate diagnosis is easier once the acute psychotic episode is under control.

Distinguishing between bipolar disorder and schizophrenia can be particularly difficult in an adolescent, since at that age psychotic features are especially common during manic periods.

Because schizoaffective disorder is so complicated, misdiagnosis is common. Some people may be misdiagnosed as having schizophrenia. Others may be misdiagnosed as having bipolar disorder. And those diagnosed as having schizoaffective disorder may actually have schizophrenia with prominent mood symptoms. Or they may have a mood disorder with symptoms similar to those of schizophrenia.

What is the treatment for this disorder?

Psychiatrists often treat this disorder with an antipsychotic medication and lithium, or with carbamazepine (an anticonvulsant medication) and lithium.

As a practical matter, differentiating between schizophrenia, bipolar disorder, and schizoaffective disorder is not absolutely critical, since antipsychotic medication is recommended for all three. If a mood problem is suspected, lithium or an antidepressant should be added.

What is the prognosis for those with this disorder?

The prognosis for individuals diagnosed with schizoaffective disorder is generally better than for those diagnosed with schizophrenia, but not quite as good for those diagnosed with a mood disorder. (Schizophrenia is a chronic brain disorder interfering with a persons' ability to think clearly, manage emotions, make decisions, and relate to others. Persons with schizophrenia may experience hallucinations and delusions. Mood disorders, including depression and bipolar disorder, are chronic illnesses in which the person's mood may return to "normal" between depressive or manic episodes.) Those with schizoaffective disorder generally respond to lithium better than those with schizophrenia, but not as well as those with mood disorders.

More research is needed to fully understand this illness and why it resists conventional treatment. New medications may be developed to treat this disorder more effectively.

Section 14.4

Schizophreniform Disorder

Schizophreniform is a psychiatric disorder which has many similarities with schizophrenia.

The two primary differences between schizophrenia and schizophreniform disorder are:

- The disturbance lasts for at least a month but less than the six months required for a diagnosis of schizophrenia.

- The person doesn't necessarily have difficulties functioning socially, or at work or school.

Like schizophrenia, however, at least two of the following symptoms must be present:

- Delusions (firmly held beliefs which are not based in reality, and are maintained despite evidence which disproves the belief or even when practically no one else ascribes to the same belief)

- Hallucinations (e.g. seeing or hearing things which aren't really there)

- Speech which is disorganized (e.g. the person can't stay on one topic, gives irrelevant responses, or his/her words make no sense at all)

- Extremely disorganized or catatonic behavior (e.g., is extremely unkempt, dresses bizarrely, is unresponsive to his/her surroundings, has a rigid posture, or exhibits bizarre or overly excited movements)

- "Negative" symptoms, such as lack of emotional expression or response, or significantly impaired thinking, or is unable to initiate or carry out basic tasks)

(The patient needs to meet only one (rather than two) of the above criterion if the delusions are bizarre, or the person is hearing at least two voices talking to each other, or is hearing a voice which is giving an ongoing commentary on the person's activities or thoughts.)

Also, the symptoms must not be due to schizoaffective disorder or a mood disorder with psychosis, and must not be due to a health condition or the effects of a substance.

Some of the people who are initially diagnosed with schizophreniform disorder will recover from the illness before the six month period is up. However, the majority will not recover and will end up being diagnosed with either schizophrenia or schizoaffective disorder.

Treatment

Treatment for schizophreniform is generally the same as for schizophrenia. Antipsychotic medication is usually prescribed to minimize or alleviate the symptoms. Supportive psychosocial interventions involving the family and the patient can also be very helpful.

Chapter 15

Personality Disorders

Chapter Contents

Section 15.1

Borderline Personality Disorder

Excerpted from "Borderline Personality Disorder," National Institute of
Mental Health, March 2012. The complete text of this document, including references, can be found online at http://www.nimh.nih.gov/health/
publications/borderline-personality-disorder/index.shtml.

What is borderline personality disorder?

Borderline personality disorder is a serious mental illness marked
by unstable moods, behavior, and relationships. Because some people
with severe borderline personality disorder have brief psychotic episodes, experts originally thought of this illness as atypical, or borderline, versions of other mental disorders. While mental health experts
now generally agree that the name "borderline personality disorder"
is misleading, a more accurate term does not exist yet.

Most people who have borderline personality disorder suffer from
problems with regulating emotions and thoughts, impulsive and reckless behavior, and unstable relationships with other people. People with
this disorder also have high rates of co-occurring disorders, such as
depression, anxiety disorders, substance abuse, and eating disorders,
along with self-harm, suicidal behaviors, and completed suicides.

To be diagnosed with borderline personality disorder, a person must
show an enduring pattern of behavior that includes at least five of the
following symptoms:

- Extreme reactions—including panic, depression, rage, or frantic
  actions—to abandonment, whether real or perceived

- A pattern of intense and stormy relationships with family,
  friends, and loved ones, often veering from extreme closeness
  and love (idealization) to extreme dislike or anger (devaluation)

- Distorted and unstable self-image or sense of self, which can result in sudden changes in feelings, opinions, values, or plans and
  goals for the future (such as school or career choices)

- Impulsive and often dangerous behaviors, such as spending sprees,
  unsafe sex, substance abuse, reckless driving, and binge eating

- Recurring suicidal behaviors or threats or self-harming behavior, such as cutting

- Intense and highly changeable moods, with each episode lasting from a few hours to a few days

- Chronic feelings of emptiness and/or boredom

- Inappropriate, intense anger or problems controlling anger

- Having stress-related paranoid thoughts or severe dissociative symptoms, such as feeling cut off from oneself, observing oneself from outside the body, or losing touch with reality.

Seemingly mundane events may trigger symptoms. For example, people with borderline personality disorder may feel angry and distressed over minor separations—such as vacations, business trips, or sudden changes of plans—from people to whom they feel close. Studies show that people with this disorder may see anger in an emotionally neutral face and have a stronger reaction to words with negative meanings than people who do not have the disorder.

Are people with personality disorders at increased risk for self-injurious behaviors?

Self-injurious behavior includes suicide and suicide attempts, as well as self-harming behaviors. As many as 80 percent of people with borderline personality disorder have suicidal behaviors, and about 4 to 9 percent commit suicide.

Suicide is one of the most tragic outcomes of any mental illness. Some treatments can help reduce suicidal behaviors in people with borderline personality disorder. For example, one study showed that dialectical behavior therapy (DBT) reduced suicide attempts in women by half compared with other types of psychotherapy, or talk therapy. DBT also reduced use of emergency room and inpatient services and retained more participants in therapy, compared to other approaches to treatment.

Unlike suicide attempts, self-harming behaviors do not stem from a desire to die. However, some self-harming behaviors may be life threatening. Self-harming behaviors linked with borderline personality disorder include cutting, burning, hitting, head banging, hair pulling, and other harmful acts. People with borderline personality disorder may self-harm to help regulate their emotions, to punish themselves, or to express their pain. They do not always see these behaviors as harmful.

How is borderline personality disorder treated?

Borderline personality disorder can be treated with psychotherapy, or "talk" therapy. In some cases, a mental health professional may also recommend medications to treat specific symptoms. When a person is under more than one professional's care, it is essential for the professionals to coordinate with one another on the treatment plan.

The treatments described below are just some of the options that may be available to a person with borderline personality disorder. However, the research on treatments is still in very early stages. More studies are needed to determine the effectiveness of these treatments, who may benefit the most, and how best to deliver treatments.

Psychotherapy: Psychotherapy is usually the first treatment for people with borderline personality disorder. Current research suggests psychotherapy can relieve some symptoms, but further studies are needed to better understand how well psychotherapy works.

It is important that people in therapy get along with and trust their therapist. The very nature of borderline personality disorder can make it difficult for people with this disorder to maintain this type of bond with their therapist.

Types of psychotherapy used to treat borderline personality disorder include the following:

- **Cognitive behavioral therapy (CBT):** CBT can help people with borderline personality disorder identify and change core beliefs and/or behaviors that underlie inaccurate perceptions of themselves and others and problems interacting with others. CBT may help reduce a range of mood and anxiety symptoms and reduce the number of suicidal or self-harming behaviors.

- **Dialectical behavior therapy (DBT):** This type of therapy focuses on the concept of mindfulness, or being aware of and attentive to the current situation. DBT teaches skills to control intense emotions, reduces self-destructive behaviors, and improves relationships. This therapy differs from CBT in that it seeks a balance between changing and accepting beliefs and behaviors.

- **Schema-focused therapy:** This type of therapy combines elements of CBT with other forms of psychotherapy that focus on reframing schemas, or the ways people view themselves. This approach is based on the idea that borderline personality disorder stems from a dysfunctional self-image—possibly brought on by negative childhood experiences—that affects how people react to their environment, interact with others, and cope with problems or stress.

Therapy can be provided one-on-one between the therapist and the patient or in a group setting. Therapist-led group sessions may help teach people with borderline personality disorder how to interact with others and how to express themselves effectively.

One type of group therapy, Systems Training for Emotional Predictability and Problem Solving (STEPPS), is designed as a relatively brief treatment consisting of 20 two-hour sessions led by an experienced social worker. Scientists funded by NIMH reported that STEPPS, when used with other types of treatment (medications or individual psychotherapy), can help reduce symptoms and problem behaviors of borderline personality disorder, relieve symptoms of depression, and improve quality of life. The effectiveness of this type of therapy has not been extensively studied.

Families of people with borderline personality disorder may also benefit from therapy. The challenges of dealing with an ill relative on a daily basis can be very stressful, and family members may unknowingly act in ways that worsen their relative's symptoms.

Some therapies, such as DBT-family skills training (DBT-FST), include family members in treatment sessions. These types of programs help families develop skills to better understand and support a relative with borderline personality disorder. Other therapies, such as Family Connections, focus on the needs of family members. More research is needed to determine the effectiveness of family therapy in borderline personality disorder. Studies with other mental disorders suggest that including family members can help in a person's treatment.

Medications: No medications have been approved by the U.S. Food and Drug Administration to treat borderline personality disorder. Only a few studies show that medications are necessary or effective for people with this illness. However, many people with borderline personality disorder are treated with medications in addition to psychotherapy. While medications do not cure borderline personality disorder, some medications may be helpful in managing specific symptoms. For some people, medications can help reduce symptoms such as anxiety, depression, or aggression. Often, people are treated with several medications at the same time, but there is little evidence that this practice is necessary or effective.

Medications can cause different side effects in different people. People who have borderline personality disorder should talk with their prescribing doctor about what to expect from a particular medication.

227

Other treatments: Omega-3 fatty acids. One study done on 30 women with borderline personality disorder showed that omega-3 fatty acids may help reduce symptoms of aggression and depression. The treatment seemed to be as well tolerated as commonly prescribed mood stabilizers and had few side effects. Fewer women who took omega-3 fatty acids dropped out of the study, compared to women who took a placebo (sugar pill).

With proper treatment, many people experience fewer or less severe symptoms. However, many factors affect the amount of time it takes for symptoms to improve, so it is important for people with borderline personality disorder to be patient and to receive appropriate support during treatment.

How can I help a friend or relative who has borderline personality disorder?

If you know someone who has borderline personality disorder, it affects you too. The first and most important thing you can do is help your friend or relative get the right diagnosis and treatment. You may need to make an appointment and go with your friend or relative to see the doctor. Encourage him or her to stay in treatment or to seek different treatment if symptoms do not appear to improve with the current treatment.

Never ignore comments about someone's intent or plan to harm himself or herself or someone else. Report such comments to the person's therapist or doctor. In urgent or potentially life-threatening situations, you may need to call the police.

How can I help myself if I have borderline personality disorder?

Taking that first step to help yourself may be hard. It is important to realize that, although it may take some time, you can get better with treatment.

- Talk to your doctor about treatment options and stick with treatment
- Try to maintain a stable schedule of meals and sleep times
- Engage in mild activity or exercise to help reduce stress
- Set realistic goals for yourself
- Break up large tasks into small ones, set some priorities, and do what you can, as you can

- Try to spend time with other people and confide in a trusted friend or family member

- Tell others about events or situations that may trigger symptoms

- Expect your symptoms to improve gradually, not immediately

- Identify and seek out comforting situations, places, and people

- Continue to educate yourself about this disorder.

What if I or someone I know is in crisis?

If you are thinking about harming yourself, or know someone who is call your doctor, call 911, or go to a hospital emergency room to get immediate help or ask a friend or family member to help you do these things.

Call the toll-free, 24-hour hotline of the National Suicide Prevention Lifeline at 800-273-TALK (800-273-8255) or TTY: 800-799-4TTY (4889) to talk to a trained counselor.

If you are in a crisis, make sure you are not left alone. If someone else is in a crisis, make sure he or she is not left alone.

Section 15.2

Other Personality Disorders

What is a personality disorder?

The word *personality* refers to the pattern of thoughts, feelings and behavior that makes each of us the individuals that we are. We don't always think, feel, and behave in exactly the same way. It depends on the situation we are in, the people with us, and many other things. But mostly we do tend to behave in fairly predictable ways, and can be described, accordingly, as shy, selfish, lively, and so on. We each have a set of these patterns, and this set makes up our personality.

Generally speaking, personality doesn't change very much, but it does develop as we go through different experiences in life, and as our circumstances change. We mature with time, and our thinking, feelings and behavior all change depending on our circumstances. We are usually flexible enough to learn from past experiences and to change our behavior to cope with life more effectively.

However, if you have a personality disorder, you are likely to find this more difficult. Your patterns of thinking, feeling and behaving are more difficult to change and you will have a more limited range of emotions, attitudes, and behaviors with which to cope with everyday life. This can lead to distress for you or for other people. If you have a personality disorder, you may find that your beliefs and attitudes are different from most other people's. They may find your behavior unusual, unexpected, and may find it difficult to spend time with you. This, of course, can make you feel very hurt and insecure; you may end up avoiding the company of others.

The diagnosis applies if you have personality difficulties which affect all aspects of your life, all the time, and make life difficult for you and for those around you. The diagnosis does not include personality changes caused by a life event such as a traumatic incident, or physical injury.

Personality disorders usually become noticeable in adolescence or early adulthood, but sometimes start in childhood. They can make it difficult for you to start and keep friendships or other relationships, and you may find it hard to work effectively with others. You may find other people very scary, and feel very alienated and alone.

However, with the right help you can learn to understand other people better, and cope better with social situations and relationships with other people. Working in groups of people with similar problems can be very helpful too.

What are the different types of personality disorder?

Personality disorder can show itself in different ways. Psychiatrists in the UK tend to use a system which identifies 10 different types of personality disorder, which can be grouped into three categories:

- **Suspicious:** Paranoid, schizoid, schizotypal, antisocial
- **Emotional and impulsive:** Borderline, histrionic, narcissistic
- **Anxious:** Avoidant, dependent, obsessive compulsive

Avoidant and dependent personality disorder are very similar, as are schizoid and schizotypal, and histrionic and narcissistic personality disorders.

One person may meet the criteria for several different disorders, while a wide range of people may fit different criteria for the same disorder, despite having very different personalities.

Paranoid personality disorder: You are likely to feel very wary of others, imagining they have hidden motives, will use you, or take advantage of you, if you don't stay vigilant. As a result, you will find it very difficult to trust other people. You will be suspicious and always on your guard, even with your friends, and you may feel that it's not safe to confide in them. You may watch others closely, looking for signs of betrayal or hostility, and you will read threats and menace—which others don't see—into everyday situations. Others may complain that you are far too mistrustful.

Schizoid personality disorder: Having a schizoid personality disorder means that you aren't really interested in forming close relationships with other people. You feel that relationships interfere with your freedom and tend to cause problems. You prefer to be solitary and inward looking, and choose to live your life without

231

interference from others. Other people will see you as a loner. Few things in life give you pleasure, and you may have little interest in sex or intimacy.

Schizotypal personality disorder: Making close relationships will be extremely difficult for you. People may describe you as eccentric, and you will find that you think differently to others. You might believe that you can read minds or that you have special powers, and you may feel anxious and tense with others who do not share these beliefs.

Borderline personality disorder (BPD): BPD may cause a number of problems in different areas of your life. You may feel that you don't have a strong sense of who you really are, and others may describe you as very changeable. You will suffer from mood swings, switching from one intense emotion to another very quickly, often with angry outbursts, and you may have brief psychotic episodes when you hear voices or see things that others can't. You may end up doing things on impulse, which you later regret. You may have episodes of harming yourself, and think about taking your own life. You will probably also have a history of stormy or broken relationships, and you will have a tendency to cling on to very damaging relationships, because you are terrified of being alone.

Histrionic personality disorder: Being ignored is probably very uncomfortable for you, and you feel much more at ease as the "life and soul of the party." But you may also feel that you have to entertain people and that you are dependent on their approval. You may flirt or behave provocatively to ensure that you remain the center of attention, or find that other people influence you too easily. You may earn a reputation for being dramatic and overemotional. Because you love excitement and don't tolerate boredom, you may behave recklessly or impulsively at times.

Narcissistic personality disorder: You may believe that there are special reasons that make you different, better, or more deserving than others, but because your self-esteem is rather fragile, you rely on others to recognize your worth and your needs. However, other people often ignore your special needs and don't give you what you feel you deserve, so that you then feel upset, and resent other people's successes. Because of this, you put your own needs above other people's, and demand they do too. People are likely to see you as selfish and "above yourself."

Antisocial personality disorder (ASPD): This is closely linked with adult criminal behavior, so if you are diagnosed with ASPD you are likely to have a criminal record. You may also be a heavy drinker or a drug-user. You are very easily bored and you may find it difficult to hold down a job for long or stay in a long-term relationship. You will tend to act impulsively and recklessly, often without considering the consequences for yourself or for other people. You may do things—even though they may hurt people—to get what you want, putting your needs above theirs. You believe that only the strongest survive and that you must do whatever it takes to lead a successful life, because if you don't grab opportunities, others will. You may be regarded as being selfish and hard. You will have had a diagnosis of conduct disorder before the age of 15.

Avoidant (or anxious) personality disorder: Feeling inadequate or inferior to other people, and avoiding work or other social activities, is one sign of avoidant personality disorder. You expect disapproval and criticism, and you worry constantly about being "found out" and rejected. You may be particularly worried about being ridiculed or shamed by others, so you avoid social relationships, friendships, and intimacy. However, you feel lonely and isolated, and long to have the very relationships you avoid. It's hard for others to understand the extent of your worries and not to believe you're exaggerating your fear of ordinary social situations. They will see you as a loner.

Dependent personality disorder: You are likely to feel needy, weak, and unable to make decisions or function properly without help or support. You allow others to assume responsibility for many areas of your life, finding it hard to say when you disagree with them because you fear losing their support. You could find yourself agreeing to things you feel are wrong, and put up with other people's unreasonable behavior to avoid being alone. Your self-confidence will be low, and you see other people as being much more capable than you are. Others may describe you as much too submissive and passive.

Obsessive-compulsive personality disorder (OCPD): If you are very concerned to keep everything in order and under control this can be a sign of OCPD. You are likely to set unrealistically high standards for yourself and others, and you generally think yours is the best way of making things happen, so you end up feeling responsible for everything. You worry when you or others make mistakes, and expect catastrophes if things aren't perfect.

OCPD is separate from obsessive compulsive disorder (OCD), which describes a form of behavior rather than a type of personality.

Are people with a personality disorder dangerous?

Despite the negative stories that often appear in the press, most people diagnosed with a personality disorder are not violent. If violence does occur, it tends to involve people diagnosed with ASPD. If you have a personality disorder, especially a borderline or paranoid personality disorder, you are much more likely to harm yourself than others.

What treatments are available?

For a long time it has been widely thought that personality disorders are difficult to treat because they involve such deeply rooted patterns of thoughts, feelings, and ways of relating to others. The type of treatment you are offered, and its success, may depend on where you are (at home, in hospital, or in prison) and on what is available locally.

If you have other conditions as well as a personality disorder, you should be offered treatment for these. This includes help with problems with misuse of alcohol or street drugs.

Personality disorders often improve as you get older, suggesting that as you gain life experience and mature you learn better ways of relating to others, gain better understanding of your responses and reactions to people and events, and learn to manage things better. Successful treatments aim to help you to make this happen by focusing on the way you think and behave, how to control your emotions, developing successful relationships, and getting more out of life.

Treatment plans need to include group and individual therapies, encouragement for you to continue with the program, education, and planning for crisis. You may receive treatment as an outpatient in a hospital or a day center, or as an inpatient.

Chapter 16

Eating and Body Image Disorders

Chapter Contents

Section 16.1

Anorexia Nervosa and Bulimia Nervosa

Excerpted from "Eating Disorders," National Institute of Mental Health
(www.nimh.nih.gov), September 16, 2011.

What are eating disorders?

An eating disorder is an illness that causes serious disturbances to your everyday diet, such as eating extremely small amounts of food or severely overeating. A person with an eating disorder may have started out just eating smaller or larger amounts of food, but at some point, the urge to eat less or more spiraled out of control. Severe distress or concern about body weight or shape may also characterize an eating disorder.

Eating disorders frequently appear during the teen years or young adulthood but may also develop during childhood or later in life. Common eating disorders include anorexia nervosa, bulimia nervosa, and binge-eating disorder.

Eating disorders affect both men and women. For the latest statistics on eating disorders, see the National Institute of Mental Health, (NIMH) website (www.nimh.nih.gov).

It is unknown how many adults and children suffer with other serious, significant eating disorders, including one category of eating disorders called eating disorders not otherwise specified (EDNOS). EDNOS includes eating disorders that do not meet the criteria for anorexia or bulimia nervosa. Binge-eating disorder is a type of eating disorder called EDNOS. EDNOS is the most common diagnosis among people who seek treatment.

Eating disorders are real, treatable medical illnesses. They frequently coexist with other illnesses such as depression, substance abuse, or anxiety disorders. Other symptoms, described below can become life-threatening if a person does not receive treatment. People with anorexia nervosa are 18 times more likely to die early compared with people of similar age in the general population.

What are the different types of eating disorders?

Anorexia nervosa: Anorexia nervosa typically is marked by these characteristics:

- Extreme thinness (emaciation)
- A relentless pursuit of thinness and unwillingness to maintain a normal or healthy weight
- Intense fear of gaining weight
- Distorted body image, a self-esteem that is heavily influenced by perceptions of body weight and shape, or a denial of the seriousness of low body weight
- Lack of menstruation among girls and women
- Extremely restricted eating.

Many people with anorexia nervosa see themselves as overweight, even when they are clearly underweight. Eating, food, and weight control become obsessions. People with anorexia nervosa typically weigh themselves repeatedly, portion food carefully, and eat very small quantities of only certain foods. Some people with anorexia nervosa may also engage in binge-eating followed by extreme dieting, excessive exercise, self-induced vomiting, and/or misuse of laxatives, diuretics, or enemas.

Some who have anorexia nervosa recover with treatment after only one episode. Others get well but have relapses. Still others have a more chronic, or long-lasting, form of anorexia nervosa, in which their health declines as they battle the illness.

Other symptoms may develop over time, including the following:

- Thinning of the bones (osteopenia or osteoporosis)
- Brittle hair and nails
- Dry and yellowish skin
- Growth of fine hair all over the body (lanugo)
- Mild anemia and muscle wasting and weakness
- Severe constipation
- Low blood pressure, slowed breathing and pulse
- Damage to the structure and function of the heart
- Brain damage
- Multiorgan failure
- Drop in internal body temperature, causing a person to feel cold all the time

- Lethargy, sluggishness, or feeling tired all the time
- Infertility

Bulimia nervosa: Bulimia nervosa is characterized by recurrent and frequent episodes of eating unusually large amounts of food and feeling a lack of control over these episodes. This binge-eating is followed by behavior that compensates for the overeating such as forced vomiting, excessive use of laxatives or diuretics, fasting, excessive exercise, or a combination of these behaviors.

Unlike anorexia nervosa, people with bulimia nervosa usually maintain what is considered a healthy or normal weight, while some are slightly overweight. But like people with anorexia nervosa, they often fear gaining weight, want desperately to lose weight, and are intensely unhappy with their body size and shape. Usually, bulimic behavior is done secretly because it is often accompanied by feelings of disgust or shame. The binge-eating and purging cycle happens anywhere from several times a week to many times a day.

Other symptoms include the following:

- Chronically inflamed and sore throat
- Swollen salivary glands in the neck and jaw area
- Worn tooth enamel, increasingly sensitive and decaying teeth as a result of exposure to stomach acid
- Acid reflux disorder and other gastrointestinal problems
- Intestinal distress and irritation from laxative abuse
- Severe dehydration from purging of fluids
- Electrolyte imbalance (too low or too high levels of sodium, calcium, potassium and other minerals) which can lead to heart attack

How are eating disorders treated?

Adequate nutrition, reducing excessive exercise, and stopping purging behaviors are the foundations of treatment. Specific forms of psychotherapy, or talk therapy, and medication are effective for many eating disorders. However, in more chronic cases, specific treatments have not yet been identified. Treatment plans often are tailored to individual needs and may include one or more of the following:

- Individual, group, and/or family psychotherapy
- Medical care and monitoring

- Nutritional counseling
- Medications

Some patients may also need to be hospitalized to treat problems caused by malnutrition or to ensure they eat enough if they are very underweight.

Treating anorexia nervosa: Treating anorexia nervosa involves three components:

- Restoring the person to a healthy weight
- Treating the psychological issues related to the eating disorder
- Reducing or eliminating behaviors or thoughts that lead to insufficient eating and preventing relapse.

Some research suggests that the use of medications, such as antidepressants, antipsychotics, or mood stabilizers, may be modestly effective in treating patients with anorexia nervosa. These medications may help resolve mood and anxiety symptoms that often occur along with anorexia nervosa. It is not clear whether antidepressants can prevent some weight-restored patients with anorexia nervosa from relapsing. Although research is still ongoing, no medication yet has shown to be effective in helping someone gain weight to reach a normal level.

Different forms of psychotherapy, including individual, group, and family-based, can help address the psychological reasons for the illness. In a therapy called the Maudsley approach, parents of adolescents with anorexia nervosa assume responsibility for feeding their child. This approach appears to be very effective in helping people gain weight and improve eating habits and moods. Shown to be effective in case studies and clinical trials, the Maudsley approach is discussed in some guidelines and studies for treating eating disorders in younger, nonchronic patients.

Other research has found that a combined approach of medical attention and supportive psychotherapy designed specifically for anorexia nervosa patients is more effective than psychotherapy alone. The effectiveness of a treatment depends on the person involved and his or her situation. Unfortunately, no specific psychotherapy appears to be consistently effective for treating adults with anorexia nervosa. However, research into new treatment and prevention approaches is showing some promise. One study suggests that an online intervention program may prevent some at-risk women from developing an eating disorder. Also, specialized treatment of anorexia nervosa may help reduce the risk of death.

Treating bulimia nervosa: As with anorexia nervosa, treatment for bulimia nervosa often involves a combination of options and depends upon the needs of the individual. To reduce or eliminate binge-eating and purging behaviors, a patient may undergo nutritional counseling and psychotherapy, especially cognitive behavioral therapy (CBT), or be prescribed medication. CBT helps a person focus on his or her current problems and how to solve them. The therapist helps the patient learn how to identify distorted or unhelpful thinking patterns, recognize, and change inaccurate beliefs, relate to others in more positive ways, and change behaviors accordingly.

CBT that is tailored to treat bulimia nervosa is effective in changing binge-eating and purging behaviors and eating attitudes. Therapy may be individual or group-based.

Some antidepressants, such as fluoxetine (Prozac), which is the only medication approved by the U.S. Food and Drug Administration (FDA) for treating bulimia nervosa, may help patients who also have depression or anxiety. Fluoxetine also appears to help reduce binge-eating and purging behaviors, reduce the chance of relapse, and improve eating attitudes.

How are males affected?

Like females who have eating disorders, males also have a distorted sense of body image. For some, their symptoms are similar to those seen in females. Others may have muscle dysmorphia, a type of disorder that is characterized by an extreme concern with becoming more muscular. Unlike girls with eating disorders, who mostly want to lose weight, some boys with muscle dysmorphia see themselves as smaller than they really are and want to gain weight or bulk up. Men and boys are more likely to use steroids or other dangerous drugs to increase muscle mass.

Although males with eating disorders exhibit the same signs and symptoms as females, they are less likely to be diagnosed with what is often considered a female disorder. More research is needed to understand the unique features of these disorders among males.

Section 16.2

Binge Eating Disorder

Excerpted from "Binge Eating Disorder," Weight-control Information Network, an information service of the National Institute of Diabetes and Digestive and Kidney Diseases (www.niddk.nih.gov), April 7, 2010.

How do I know if I have binge eating disorder?

Most of us overeat from time to time, and some of us often feel we have eaten more than we should have. Eating a lot of food does not necessarily mean that you have binge eating disorder. Experts generally agree that most people with serious binge eating problems often eat an unusually large amount of food and feel their eating is out of control. People with binge eating disorder also may have these experiences:

- Eat much more quickly than usual during binge episodes.

- Eat until they are uncomfortably full.

- Eat large amounts of food even when they are not really hungry.

- Eat alone because they are embarrassed about the amount of food they eat.

- Feel disgusted, depressed, or guilty after overeating.

Binge eating also occurs in another eating disorder called bulimia nervosa. Persons with bulimia nervosa, however, usually purge, fast, or do strenuous exercise after they binge eat. Purging means vomiting or using a lot of diuretics (water pills) or laxatives to keep from gaining weight. Fasting is not eating for at least 24 hours. Strenuous exercise, in this case, means exercising for more than an hour just to keep from gaining weight after binge eating. Purging, fasting, and overexercising are dangerous ways to try to control your weight.

How common is binge eating disorder, and who is at risk?

Binge eating disorder is the most common eating disorder. It affects about three percent of all adults in the United States. People of any age can have binge eating disorder, but it is seen more often in adults

241

age 46 to 55. Binge eating disorder is a little more common in women than in men; three women for every two men have it. The disorder affects Blacks as often as Whites, but it is not known how often it affects people in other ethnic groups.

Although most obese people do not have binge eating disorder, people with this problem are usually overweight or obese. The *Clinical Guidelines on the Identification, Evaluation, and Treatment of Overweight and Obesity in Adults*, published in 1998 by the National Heart, Lung, and Blood Institute, define overweight as a body mass index (BMI) of 25 to 29.9 and obesity as a BMI of 30 or more. BMI is calculated by dividing weight (in kilograms) by height (in meters) squared. Binge eating disorder is more common in people who are severely obese. Normal-weight people can also have the disorder.

People who are obese and have binge eating disorder often became overweight at a younger age than those without the disorder. They might also lose and gain weight more often, a process known as weight cycling (yo-yo dieting).

What causes binge eating disorder?

No one knows for sure what causes binge eating disorder. As many as half of all people with binge eating disorder are depressed or have been depressed in the past. Whether depression causes binge eating disorder, or whether binge eating disorder causes depression, is not known.

It is also unclear if dieting and binge eating are related, although some people binge eat after dieting. In these cases, dieting means skipping meals, not eating enough food each day, or avoiding certain kinds of food. These are unhealthy ways to try to change your body shape and weight.

Studies suggest that people with binge eating disorder may have trouble handling some of their emotions. Many people who are binge eaters say that being angry, sad, bored, worried, or stressed can cause them to binge eat.

Certain behaviors and emotional problems are more common in people with binge eating disorder. These include abusing alcohol, acting quickly without thinking (impulsive behavior), not feeling in charge of themselves, not feeling a part of their communities, and not noticing and talking about their feelings.

Researchers are looking into how brain chemicals and metabolism (the way the body uses calories) affect binge eating disorder. Other research suggests that genes may be involved in binge eating, since the disorder often occurs in several members of the same family. This research is still in the early stages.

What are the complications of binge eating disorder?

People with binge eating disorder are usually very upset by their binge eating and may become depressed. Research has shown that people with binge eating disorder report more health problems, stress, trouble sleeping, and suicidal thoughts than do people without an eating disorder. Other complications from binge eating disorder could include joint pain, digestive problems, headache, muscle pain, and menstrual problems.

People with binge eating disorder often feel bad about themselves and may miss work, school, or social activities to binge eat.

People with binge eating disorder may gain weight. Weight gain can lead to obesity, and obesity puts people at risk for many health problems, including type 2 diabetes, high blood pressure, high blood cholesterol levels, gallbladder disease, heart disease, and certain types of cancer.

Most people who binge eat, whether they are obese or not, feel ashamed and try to hide their problem. Often they become so good at hiding it that even close friends and family members do not know that their loved one binge eats.

How can people with binge eating disorder be helped?

People with binge eating disorder should get help from a health care professional such as a psychiatrist, psychologist, or clinical social worker. There are several different ways to treat binge eating disorder:

- Cognitive behavioral therapy teaches people how to keep track of their eating and change their unhealthy eating habits. It teaches them how to change the way they act in tough situations. It also helps them feel better about their body shape and weight.

- Interpersonal psychotherapy helps people look at their relationships with friends and family and make changes in problem areas.

- Drug therapy, such as antidepressants, may be helpful for some people.

The methods mentioned here seem to be equally helpful. Researchers are still trying to find the treatment that is the most helpful in controlling binge eating disorder. Combining drug and behavioral therapy has shown promising results for treating overweight and obese individuals with binge eating disorder. Drug therapy has been shown to benefit weight management and promote weight loss, while behavioral therapy has been shown to improve the psychological components of binge eating.

Other therapies being tried include dialectical behavior therapy, which helps people regulate their emotions; drug therapy with the anti-seizure medication topiramate; weight-loss surgery (bariatric surgery); exercise used alone or in combination with cognitive behavioral therapy; and self-help. Self-help books, videos, and groups have helped some people control their binge eating.

You are not alone: If you think you might have binge eating disorder, it is important to know that you are not alone. Most people who have the disorder have tried but failed to control it on their own. You may want to get professional help. Talk to your health care provider about the type of help that may be best for you. The good news is that most people do well in treatment and can overcome binge eating.

Section 16.3

Body Dysmorphic Disorder

"Body Dysmorphic Disorder," October 2010, reprinted with permission from www.kidshealth.org. This information was provided by KidsHealth®, one of the largest resources online for medically reviewed health information written for parents, kids, and teens. For more articles like this, visit www.KidsHealth.org or www.TeensHealth.org. Copyright © 1995-2012 The Nemours Foundation. All rights reserved.

Focusing on Appearance

Most of us spend time in front of the mirror checking our appearance. Some people spend more time than others, but taking care of our bodies and being interested in our appearance is natural.

How we feel about our appearance is part of our body image and self-image. Many people have some kind of dissatisfaction with their bodies. This can be especially true during the teen years when our bodies and appearance go through lots of changes.

Although many people feel dissatisfied with some aspect of their appearance, these concerns usually don't constantly occupy their thoughts or cause them to feel tormented. But for some people, concerns about appearance become quite extreme and upsetting.

Some people become so focused on imagined or minor imperfections in their looks that they can't seem to stop checking or obsessing about their appearance. Being constantly preoccupied and upset about body imperfections or appearance flaws is called body dysmorphic disorder.

What Is Body Dysmorphic Disorder?

Body dysmorphic disorder (BDD) is a condition that involves obsessions, which are distressing thoughts that repeatedly intrude into a person's awareness. With BDD, the distressing thoughts are about perceived appearance flaws.

People with BDD might focus on what they think is a facial flaw, but they can also worry about other body parts, such as short legs, breast size, or body shape. Just as people with eating disorders obsess about their weight, those with BDD become obsessed over an aspect of their appearance. They may worry their hair is thin, their face is scarred, their eyes aren't exactly the same size, their nose is too big, or their lips are too thin.

BDD has been called imagined ugliness because the appearance issues the person is obsessing about usually are so small that others don't even notice them. Or, if others do notice them, they consider them minor. But for someone with BDD, the concerns feel very real, because the obsessive thoughts distort and magnify any tiny imperfection.

Because of the distorted body image caused by BDD, a person might believe that he or she is too horribly ugly or disfigured to be seen.

Behaviors That Are Part of BDD

Besides obsessions, BDD also involves compulsions and avoidance behaviors.

A compulsion is something a person does to try to relieve the tension caused by the obsessive thoughts. For example, someone with obsessive thoughts that her nose is horribly ugly might check her appearance in the mirror, apply makeup, or ask someone many times a day whether her nose looks ugly. These types of checking, fixing, and asking are compulsions.

Somebody with obsessions usually feels a strong or irresistible urge to do compulsions because they can provide temporary relief from the terrible distress. The compulsions seem like the only way to escape bad feelings caused by bad thoughts. Compulsive actions often are repeated many times a day, taking up lots of time and energy.

Avoidance behaviors are also a part of BDD. A person might stay home or cover up to avoid being seen by others. Avoidance behaviors also include things like not participating in class or socializing, or avoiding mirrors.

With BDD, a pattern of obsessive thoughts, compulsive actions, and avoidance sets in. Even though the checking, fixing, asking, and avoiding seem to relieve terrible feelings, the relief is just temporary. In reality, the more someone performs compulsions or avoids things, the stronger the pattern of obsessions, compulsions, and avoidance becomes.

After a while, it takes more and more compulsions to relieve the distress caused by the bad thoughts. A person with BDD doesn't want to be preoccupied with these thoughts and behaviors, but with BDD it can seem impossible to break the pattern.

What Causes BDD?

Although the exact cause of BDD is still unclear, experts believe it is related to problems with serotonin, one of the brain's chemical neurotransmitters. Poor regulation of serotonin also plays a role in obsessive compulsive disorder (OCD) and other anxiety disorders, as well as depression.

Some people may be more prone to problems with serotonin balance, including those with family members who have problems with anxiety or depression. This may help explain why some people develop BDD but others don't.

Cultural messages can also play a role in BDD by reinforcing somebody's concerns about appearance. Critical messages or unkind teasing about appearance as someone is growing up may also contribute to a person's sensitivity to BDD. But while cultural messages, criticism, and teasing might harm someone's body image, these things alone usually do not result in BDD.

It's hard to know exactly how common BDD is because most people with BDD are unwilling to talk about their concerns or seek help. But compared with those who feel somewhat dissatisfied with their appearance, very few people have true BDD. BDD usually begins in the teen years, and if it's not treated, can continue into adulthood.

How BDD Can Affect a Person's Life

Sometimes people with BDD feel ashamed and keep their concerns secret. They may think that others will consider them vain or superficial.

Other people might become annoyed or irritated with somebody's obsessions and compulsions about appearance. They don't understand BDD or what the person is going through. As a result, those with BDD may feel misunderstood, unfairly judged, or alone. Because they avoid contact with others, they may have few friends or activities to enjoy.

It's extremely upsetting to be tormented by thoughts about appearance imperfections. These thoughts intrude into a person's awareness throughout the day and are hard to ignore. People with mild to moderate symptoms of BDD usually spend a great deal of time grooming themselves in the morning. Throughout the day, they may frequently check their appearance in mirrors or windows. In addition, they may repeatedly seek reassurance from people around them that they look OK.

Although people with mild BDD usually continue to go to school, the obsessions can interfere with their daily lives. For example, someone might measure or examine the "flawed" body part repeatedly or spend large sums of money and time on makeup to cover the problem.

Some people with BDD hide from others, and avoid going places because of fear of being seen. Spending so much time and energy on appearance concerns robs a person of pleasure and happiness, and of opportunities for fun and socializing.

People with severe symptoms may drop out of school, quit their jobs, or refuse to leave their homes. Many people with BDD also develop depression. Those with the most severe BDD might even consider or attempt suicide.

Many people with BDD seek the help of a dermatologist or cosmetic surgeon to try to correct appearance flaws. But dermatology treatments or plastic surgery don't change the BDD. Those who find cosmetic surgeons willing to perform surgery are often not satisfied with the results. They may find that even though their appearance has changes, the obsessive thinking is still present, and they begin to focus on some other imperfection.

Getting Help for BDD

If you or someone you know has BDD, the first step is recognizing what might be causing the distress. Many times, people with BDD are so focused on their appearance that they believe the answer lies in correcting how they look, not with their thoughts.

The real problem with BDD lies in the obsessions and compulsions, which distort body image, making someone feel ugly. Because people with BDD believe what they're perceiving is true and accurate, sometimes the most challenging part of overcoming the disorder is being open to new ideas about what might help.

BDD can be treated by an experienced mental health professional. Usually, the treatment involves a type of talk therapy called cognitive-behavioral therapy. This approach helps to correct the pattern that's causing the body image distortion and the extreme distress.

In cognitive behavioral therapy, a therapist helps a person to examine and change faulty beliefs, resist compulsive behaviors, and face stressful situations that trigger appearance concerns. Sometimes doctors prescribe medication along with the talk therapy.

Treatment for BDD takes time, hard work, and patience. It helps if a person has the support of a friend or loved one. If someone with BDD is also dealing with depression, anxiety, feeling isolated or alone, or other life situations, the therapy can address those issues, too.

Body dysmorphic disorder, like other obsessions, can interfere with a person's life, robbing it of pleasure and draining energy. An experienced psychologist or psychiatrist who is knowledgeable about BDD can help break the grip of the disorder so that a person can fully enjoy life.

Chapter 17

Addictions

Chapter Contents

Section 17.1

Alcoholism, Substance Abuse, and Addictive Behavior

From "Alcoholism, Substance Abuse, and Addictive Behavior," Office on Women's Health (www.womenshealth.gov), March 29, 2010.

Alcoholism

Alcohol abuse is a pattern of drinking that is harmful to the drinker or others. The following situations, occurring repeatedly in a 12-month period, would be indicators of alcohol abuse: missing work or skipping child care responsibilities because of drinking; drinking in situations that are dangerous, such as before or while driving; being arrested for driving under the influence of alcohol or for hurting someone while drunk; continuing to drink even though there are ongoing alcohol-related tensions with friends and family

Alcoholism is a disease. It is chronic, or lifelong, and it can get worse over time and be life-threatening. Alcoholism is based in the brain. These are some of the typical characteristics of alcoholism:

- **Craving:** A strong need to drink

- **Loss of control:** The inability to stop drinking

- **Physical dependence:** Withdrawal symptoms, such as nausea, sweating, shakiness, and anxiety, when alcohol use is stopped after a period of heavy drinking

- **Tolerance:** The need for increasing amounts of alcohol to get "high"

Know the Risks

Research suggests that people are more likely to drink too much if they have any of the following characteristics: parents and siblings (or other blood relatives) with alcohol problems; a partner who drinks too much; the ability to "hold their liquor" more than others; a history of depression; and a history of childhood physical or sexual abuse.

The presence of any of these factors is a good reason to be especially careful with drinking.

How Do You Know If You Have a Problem?

Answering the following four questions can help you find out if you or someone close to you has a drinking problem.

- Have you ever felt you should cut down on your drinking?
- Have people annoyed you by criticizing your drinking?
- Have you ever felt bad or guilty about your drinking?
- Have you ever had a drink first thing in the morning to steady your nerves or to get rid of a hangover?

One "yes" answer suggests a possible alcohol problem. If you responded "yes" to more than one question, it is very likely that you have a problem with alcohol. In either case, it is important that you see your health care provider right away to discuss your responses to these questions.

Even if you answered "no" to all of the above questions, if you are having drinking-related problems with your job, relationships, health, or with the law, you should still seek help.

Treatment for Alcohol Problems

Treatment for an alcohol problem depends on its severity. Routine doctor visits are an ideal time to discuss alcohol use and its potential problems. Health care professionals can help a person take a good hard look at what effect alcohol is having on his or her life and can give advice on ways to stop drinking or to cut down.

Alcoholism treatment works for many people. But like other chronic illnesses, such as diabetes, high blood pressure, and asthma, there are varying levels of success when it comes to treatment. Some people stop drinking and remain sober. Others have long periods of sobriety with bouts of relapse. And still others cannot stop drinking for any length of time. With treatment, one thing is clear, however: the longer a person stops drinking alcohol, the more likely he or she will be able to stay sober.

Substance Abuse

Many people do not understand why people become addicted to drugs. The truth is this: drugs change the brain and cause repeated drug abuse. Drug addiction is a brain disease. Drug use leads to changes in the structure and function of the brain. Although it is true that for most people

251

the initial decision to take drugs is voluntary, over time, the changes in the brain caused by repeated drug abuse can affect a person's self control and ability to make sound decisions. At the same time, drugs cause the brain to send intense impulses to take more drugs.

Treatment

Drug abuse is a treatable disease. There are many effective treatments for drug abuse. Some important points about substance abuse treatment include the following:

- Medical and behavioral therapy, alone or used together, are used to treat drug abuse.

- Sometimes treatment can be done on an outpatient basis.

- Severe drug abuse usually requires residential treatment, where the patient sleeps at the treatment center.

- Treatment can take place within the criminal justice systems, which can stop a convicted person from returning to criminal behavior.

- Studies show that treatment does not need to be voluntary to work.

Addictive behavior

Why do some people become addicted, while others do not?

Nothing can predict whether or not a person will become addicted to drugs. But there are some risk factors for drug addiction, including the following:

- **Biology:** Genes, gender, ethnicity, and the presence of other mental disorders may increase risk for drug abuse and addiction.

- **Environment:** Peer pressure, physical and sexual abuse, stress, and family relationships can influence the course of drug abuse and addiction in a person's life.

- **Development:** Although taking drugs at any age can lead to addiction, the earlier that drug use begins, the more likely it is to progress to more serious abuse.

Section 17.2

Comorbidity: Addiction and Other Mental Disorders

From "Comorbidity: Addiction and Other Mental Disorders," National
Institute on Drug Abuse (www.nida.nih.gov), March 2011.

What is comorbidity?

The term comorbidity describes two or more disorders or illnesses
occurring in the same person. They can occur at the same time or one
after the other. Comorbidity also implies interactions between the illnesses that can worsen the course of both.

Addiction changes the brain in fundamental ways, disturbing a person's
normal hierarchy of needs and desires and substituting new priorities
connected with procuring and using the drug. The resulting compulsive
behaviors that weaken the ability to control impulses, despite the negative
consequences, are similar to hallmarks of other mental illnesses.

Many people who are addicted to drugs are also diagnosed with
other mental disorders and vice versa. For example, compared with the
general population, people addicted to drugs are roughly twice as likely
to suffer from mood and anxiety disorders, with the reverse also true.

Why do these disorders often co-occur?

Although drug use disorders commonly occur with other mental illnesses, this does not mean that one caused the other, even if one appeared
first. In fact, establishing which came first or why can be difficult. Drug
abuse may bring about symptoms of another mental illness. Increased
risk of psychosis in vulnerable marijuana users suggests this possibility. Mental disorders can also lead to drug abuse, possibly as a means
of self-medication. Patients suffering from anxiety or depression may
rely on alcohol, tobacco, and other drugs to temporarily alleviate their
symptoms. These disorders could also be caused by shared risk factors.
Here are some possibilities:

- **Overlapping genetic vulnerabilities:** Predisposing genetic
  factors may make a person susceptible to both addiction and

other mental disorders or to having a greater risk of a second disorder once the first appears.

- **Overlapping environmental triggers:** Stress, trauma (such as physical or sexual abuse), and early exposure to drugs are common environmental factors that can lead to addiction and other mental illnesses.

- **Involvement of similar brain regions:** Brain systems that respond to reward and stress, for example, are affected by drugs of abuse and may show abnormalities in patients with certain mental disorders.

- **Drug use disorders and other mental illnesses are developmental disorders:** That means they often begin in the teen years or even younger—periods when the brain experiences dramatic developmental changes. Early exposure to drugs of abuse may change the brain in ways that increase the risk for mental disorders. Also, early symptoms of a mental disorder may indicate an increased risk for later drug use.

How are these comorbid conditions diagnosed and treated?

The high rate of comorbidity between drug use disorders and other mental illnesses calls for a comprehensive approach that identifies and evaluates both. Accordingly, anyone seeking help for either drug abuse/addiction or another mental disorder should be checked for both and treated accordingly.

Several behavioral therapies have shown promise for treating comorbid conditions. These approaches can be tailored to patients according to age, specific drug abused, and other factors. Some therapies have proven more effective for adolescents, while others have shown greater effectiveness for adults; some are designed for families and groups, others for individuals.

Effective medications exist for treating opioid, alcohol, and nicotine addiction and for alleviating the symptoms of many other mental disorders, yet most have not been well studied in comorbid populations. Some medications may benefit multiple problems. For example, evidence suggests that bupropion (trade names: Wellbutrin, Zyban), approved for treating depression and nicotine dependence, might also help reduce craving and use of the drug methamphetamine. More research is needed, however, to better understand how these medications work, particularly when combined in patients with comorbidities.

Chapter 18

Impulse Control Disorders

Chapter Contents

Section 18.1

What Are Impulse Control Disorders?

As humans, the ability to control our impulses—or urges—helps distinguish us from other species and marks our psychological maturity. Most of us take our ability to think before we act for granted. But this isn't easy for people who have problems controlling their impulses.

People with an impulse control disorder can't resist the urge to do something harmful to themselves or others. Impulse control disorders include addictions to alcohol or drugs, eating disorders, compulsive gambling, paraphilias (sexual fantasies), and behaviors involving non-human objects, suffering, humiliation or children, compulsive hair pulling, stealing, fire setting, and intermittent explosive attacks of rage.

Some of these disorders, such as intermittent explosive disorder, kleptomania, pyromania, compulsive gambling, and trichotillomania, are similar in terms of when they begin and how they progress. Usually, a person feels increasing tension or arousal before committing the act that characterizes the disorder. During the act, the person probably will feel pleasure, gratification, or relief. Afterward, the person may blame himself or feel regret or guilt.

People with these disorders may or may not plan the acts, but the acts generally fulfill their immediate, conscious wishes. Most people, however, find their disorders highly distressing and feel a loss of control over their lives.

How are they different from similar disorders?

While other disorders may involve difficulty controlling impulses, that is not their primary feature. For example, while people with attention-deficit/hyperactivity disorder (ADHD) or in a manic state of bipolar might have difficulty controlling their impulses, it is not their main problem.

Some health professionals consider impulse control disorders subgroups of other conditions, such as anxiety disorders or obsessive-compulsive

256

disorders. Some medications for treating depression and anxiety also have been successful in treating impulse disorders, particularly antidepressants known as serotonin reuptake inhibitors. This suggests the neurotransmitter serotonin plays a role in these disorders.

What causes impulse control disorders?

Scientists don't know what causes these disorders. But many things probably play a role, including physical or biological, psychological or emotional, and cultural or societal factors. Scientists do suspect that certain brain structures—including the limbic system, linked to emotions and memory functions, and the frontal lobe, the part of the brain's cortex linked to planning functions and controlling impulses—affect the disorder.

Hormones associated with violence and aggression, such as testosterone, also could play a role in the disorders. For example, researchers have suggested that women might be predisposed to less aggressive types of impulse control disorders such as kleptomania or trichotillomania, and men might be predisposed to more violent and aggressive types such as pyromania and intermittent explosive disorder.

Research also has shown connections between certain types of seizure disorders and violent impulsive behaviors. And studies have revealed that family members of people with impulse control disorders have a higher rate of addiction and mood disorders.

Section 18.2

Disruptive Behavior Disorders

What are disruptive behavior disorders?

Disruptive behavior disorders involve consistent patterns of behaviors that "break the rules." All young people break some rules, especially less important ones. More serious oppositional behavior is a normal part of childhood for children two and three years old and for young teenagers. At other times, when young people are routinely very, very oppositional and defiant of authority, a mental health disorder may be identified.

The main disruptive behavior disorders are oppositional defiant disorder and conduct disorder.

Oppositional defiant disorder: In oppositional defiant disorder, the rules broken are usually those in the family and the school. Oppositional defiant disorder may occur in children of any age and in adolescents. Sometimes oppositional defiant disorder leads to conduct disorder. Examples of oppositional defiant disorder behaviors are:

- Frequent defiance of the authority of parents, teachers and others

- Arguing and refusing to obey rules at home and school

- Failure to take responsibility for bad behavior or mistakes

- Resentment and looking for revenge

- Regular temper tantrums

Conduct disorder behaviors: In conduct disorder, the rules broken include the regulations and laws made by society. Conduct disorder usually occurs in older children and adolescents. Examples of conduct disorder behaviors are:

- Aggressive behaviors that threaten or harm people or animals

- Behaviors that destroy property such as fire setting, breaking windows, or graffiti

- Stealing, bullying, or lying to get something

- Serious violations of rules, including school truancy and running away from home

What causes disruptive behavior disorders?

Research has identified both biological and environmental causes for disruptive behavior disorders. Youngsters most at risk for oppositional defiant and conduct disorders are those who have low birth weight, neurological damage, or attention deficit hyperactivity disorder. Youngsters may also be at risk if they were rejected by their mothers as babies, separated from their parents and not given good foster care, physically or sexually abused, raised in homes with mothers who were abused, or living in poverty.

How can disruptive behavior disorders be treated?

Because so many of the factors that cause disruptive behavior disorders happen very early in a child's life, it is important to recognize the problems as early as possible and get treatment. The treatment that has shown the best results is a combination of:

- Specialized parent skills training

- Behavior therapies to teach young people how to control and express feelings in healthy ways

- Coordination of services with the young person's school and other involved agencies

- Parent training and therapy with the child or adolescent, most effective when done in the family home

No medications have been consistently useful in reducing the symptoms of oppositional defiant or conduct disorders. Medications may be helpful to some young people, but they tend to have side effects that must be monitored carefully.

Section 18.3

Self-Injury

Self-harm can be a way of coping with problems. It may help you express feelings you can't put into words, distract you from your life, or release emotional pain. If you want to stop but don't know how, remember this: you deserve to feel better, and you can get there without hurting yourself.

Understanding Cutting and Self-Harm

Self-harm is a way of expressing and dealing with deep distress and emotional pain. As counterintuitive as it may sound to those on the outside, hurting yourself makes you feel better. In fact, you may feel like you have no choice. Injuring yourself is the only way you know how to cope with feelings like sadness, self-loathing, emptiness, guilt, and rage.

The problem is that the relief that comes from self-harming doesn't last very long. It's like slapping on a Band-Aid when what you really need are stitches. It may temporarily stop the bleeding, but it doesn't fix the underlying injury. And it also creates its own problems.

If you're like most people who self-injure, you try to keep what you're doing secret. Maybe you feel ashamed or maybe you just think that no one would understand. But hiding who you are and what you feel is a heavy burden. Ultimately, the secrecy and guilt affects your relationships with your friends and family members and the way you feel about yourself. It can make you feel even more lonely, worthless, and trapped.

Myths and Facts about Cutting and Self-Harm

Because cutting and other means of self-harm tend to be taboo subjects, the people around you—and possibly even you—may harbor serious misconceptions about your motivations and state of mind. Don't let these myths get in the way of getting help or helping someone you care about.

Myth: People who cut and self-injure are trying to get attention.

Fact: The painful truth is that people who self-harm generally do so in secret. They aren't trying to manipulate others or draw attention to themselves. In fact, shame and fear can make it very difficult to come forward and ask for help.

Myth: People who self-injure are crazy and/or dangerous.

Fact: It is true that many people who self-harm suffer from anxiety, depression, or a previous trauma—just like millions of others in the general population. Self-injury is how they cope. Slapping them with a "crazy" or "dangerous" label isn't accurate or helpful.

Myth: People who self-injure want to die.

Fact: Self-injurers usually do not want to die. When they self-harm, they are not trying to kill themselves—they are trying to cope with their pain. In fact, self-injury may be a way of helping themselves go on living. However, in the long-term, people who self-injure have a much higher risk of suicide, which is why it's so important to seek help.

Myth: If the wounds aren't bad, it's not that serious.

Fact: The severity of a person's wounds has very little to do with how much he or she may be suffering. Don't assume that because the wounds or injuries are minor, there's nothing to worry about.

Signs and Symptoms of Cutting and Self-Harm

Self-harm includes anything you do to intentionally injure yourself. Some of the more common ways include:

- Cutting or severely scratching your skin;
- Burning or scalding yourself;
- Hitting yourself or banging your head;
- Punching things or throwing your body against walls and hard objects;
- Sticking objects into your skin;
- Intentionally preventing wounds from healing;
- Swallowing poisonous substances or inappropriate objects.

Self-harm can also include less obvious ways of hurting yourself or putting yourself in danger, such as driving recklessly, binge drinking, taking too many drugs, and having unsafe sex.

Warning Signs that a Family Member or Friend Is Cutting or Self-Injuring

Because clothing can hide physical injuries, and inner turmoil can be covered up by a seemingly calm disposition, self-injury can be hard to detect. However, there are red flags you can look for (but remember—you don't have to be sure that you know what's going on in order to reach out to someone you're worried about):

- Unexplained wounds or scars from cuts, bruises, or burns, usually on the wrists, arms, thighs, or chest.

- Blood stains on clothing, towels, or bedding; blood-soaked tissues.

- Sharp objects or cutting instruments, such as razors, knives, needles, glass shards, or bottle caps, in the person's belongings.

- Frequent "accidents." Someone who self-harms may claim to be clumsy or have many mishaps, in order to explain away injuries.

- Covering up. A person who self-injures may insist on wearing long sleeves or long pants, even in hot weather.

- Needing to be alone for long periods of time, especially in the bedroom or bathroom.

- Isolation and irritability.

How Does Cutting and Self-Harm Help?

It's important to acknowledge that self-harm helps you—otherwise you wouldn't do it. Some of the ways cutting and self-harming can help include:

- Expressing feelings you can't put into words;
- Releasing the pain and tension you feel inside;
- Helping you feel in control;
- Distracting you from overwhelming emotions or difficult life circumstances;
- Relieving guilt and punishing yourself;

- Making you feel alive, or simply feel something, instead of feeling numb.

In Your Own Words

- "It expresses emotional pain or feelings that I'm unable to put into words. It puts a punctuation mark on what I'm feeling on the inside!"

- "It's a way to have control over my body because I can't control anything else in my life."

- "I usually feel like I have a black hole in the pit of my stomach, at least if I feel pain it's better than feeling nothing."

- "I feel relieved and less anxious after I cut. The emotional pain slowly slips away into the physical pain."

Once you better understand why you self-harm, you can learn ways to stop self-harming, and find resources that can support you through this struggle.

If Self-Harm Helps, Why Stop?

- Although self-harm and cutting can give you temporary relief, it comes at a cost. In the long term, it causes far more problems than it solves.

- The relief is short lived, and is quickly followed by other feelings like shame and guilt. Meanwhile, it keeps you from learning more effective strategies for feeling better.

- Keeping the secret from friends and family members is difficult and lonely.

- You can hurt yourself badly, even if you don't mean to. It's easy to misjudge the depth of a cut or end up with an infected wound.

- If you don't learn other ways to deal with emotional pain, it puts you at risk for bigger problems down the line, including major depression, drug and alcohol addiction, and suicide.

- Self-harm can become addictive. It may start off as an impulse or something you do to feel more in control, but soon it feels like the cutting or self-harming is controlling you. It often turns into a compulsive behavior that seems impossible to stop.

The bottom line: Self-harm and cutting don't help you with the issues that made you want to hurt yourself in the first place.

Help for Cutting and Self-Harm Step 1: Confide in Someone

If you're ready to get help for cutting or self-harm, the first step is to confide in another person. It can be scary to talk about the very thing you have worked so hard to hide, but it can also be a huge relief to finally let go of your secret and share what you're going through.

Deciding whom you can trust with such personal information can be difficult. Choose someone who isn't going to gossip or try to take control of your recovery. Ask yourself who in your life makes you feel accepted and supported. It could be a friend, teacher, religious leader, counselor, or relative. But you don't necessarily have to choose someone you are close to.

Eventually, you'll want to open up to your inner circle of friends and family members, but sometimes it's easier to start by talking to an adult who you respect—such as a teacher, religious leader, or counselor—who has a little more distance from the situation and won't find it as difficult to be objective.

Need Help for Self-Harm?

If you're not sure where to turn, call the S.A.F.E. Alternatives information line in the U.S. at 800-366-8288 for referrals and support for cutting and self-harm. For helplines in other countries, see the Resources and References link available at http://www.helpguide.org/mental/self_injury.htm.

In the Middle of a Crisis?

If you're feeling suicidal and need help right now, call the National Suicide Prevention Lifeline in the U.S. at 800-273-8255. For a suicide helpline outside the U.S., visit Befrienders Worldwide at http://www.befrienders.org.

Tips for Talking about Cutting and Self-Injury

- Focus on your feelings. Instead of sharing sensational details of your self-harm behavior—what specifically you do to hurt yourself—focus on the feelings or situations that lead to it. This can help the person you're confiding in better understand where you're coming from. It also helps to let the person know why you're telling them. Do you want help or advice from them? Do you simply want another person to know so you can let go of the secret?

- Communicate in whatever way you feel most comfortable. If you're too nervous to talk in person, consider starting off the conversation with an e-mail or letter (although it's important to eventually follow-up with a face-to-face conversation). Don't feel pressured into sharing things you're not ready to talk about. You don't have to show the person your injuries or answer any questions you don't feel comfortable answering.

- Give the person time to process what you tell them. As difficult as it is for you to open up, it may also be difficult for the person you tell—especially if it's a close friend or family member. Sometimes, you may not like the way the person reacts. Try to remember that reactions such as shock, anger, and fear come out of concern for you. It may help to print out this article for the people you choose to tell. The better they understand self-harm, the better able they'll be to support you.

Talking about self-harm can be very stressful and bring up a lot of emotions. Don't be discouraged if the situation feels worse for a short time right after sharing your secret. It's uncomfortable to confront and change long-standing habits. But once you get past these initial challenges, you'll start to feel better.

Help for Cutting and Self-Harm Step 2: Figure Out Why You Cut

Learn to Manage Overwhelming Stress and Emotions

Understanding why you cut or self-harm is a vital first step toward your recovery. If you can figure out what function your self-injury serves, you can learn other ways to get those needs met—which in turn can reduce your desire to hurt yourself.

Identify Your Self-Harm Triggers

Remember, self-harm is most often a way of dealing with emotional pain. What feelings make you want to cut or hurt yourself? Sadness? Anger? Shame? Loneliness? Guilt? Emptiness?

Once you learn to recognize the feelings that trigger your need to self-injure, you can start developing healthier alternatives.

Get in Touch with Your Feelings

If you're having a hard time pinpointing the feelings that trigger your urge to cut, you may need to work on your emotional awareness. Emotional awareness means knowing what you are feeling and why. It's the ability to identify and express what you are feeling from moment to moment and to understand the connection between your feelings and your actions.

The idea of paying attention to your feelings—rather than numbing them or releasing them through self-harm—may sound frightening to you. You may be afraid that you'll get overwhelmed or be stuck with the pain. But the truth is that emotions quickly come and go if you let them. If you don't try to fight, judge, or beat yourself up over the feeling, you'll find that it soon fades, replaced by another emotion. It's only when you obsess over the feeling that it persists.

Help for Cutting and Self-Harm Step 3: Find New Coping Techniques

Self-harm is your way of dealing with feelings and difficult situations. So if you're going to stop, you need to have alternative ways of coping in place so you can respond differently when you start to feel like cutting or hurting yourself.

If You Cut to Express Pain and Intense Emotions

- Paint, draw, or scribble on a big piece of paper with red ink or paint
- Express your feelings in a journal
- Compose a poem or song to say what you feel
- Write down any negative feelings and then rip the paper up
- Listen to music that expresses what you're feeling

If You Cut to Calm and Soothe Yourself

- Take a bath or hot shower
- Pet or cuddle with a dog or cat
- Wrap yourself in a warm blanket

- Massage your neck, hands, and feet
- Listen to calming music

If You Cut Because You Feel Disconnected and Numb

- Call a friend (you don't have to talk about self-harm)
- Take a cold shower
- Hold an ice cube in the crook of your arm or leg
- Chew something with a very strong taste, like chili peppers, peppermint, or a grapefruit peel.
- Go online to a self-help website, chat room, or message board

If You Cut to Release Tension or Vent Anger

- Exercise vigorously—run, dance, jump rope, or hit a punching bag
- Punch a cushion or mattress or scream into your pillow
- Squeeze a stress ball or squish Play-Doh or clay
- Rip something up (sheets of paper, a magazine)
- Make some noise (play an instrument, bang on pots and pans)

Substitutes for the Cutting Sensation

- Use a red felt tip pen to mark where you might usually cut
- Rub ice across your skin where you might usually cut
- Put rubber bands on wrists, arms, or legs and snap them instead of cutting or hitting

Source: The Mental Health Foundation, UK

Professional Treatment for Cutting and Self-Harm

You may also need the help and support of a trained professional as you work to overcome the self-harm habit, so consider talking to a therapist. A therapist can help you develop new coping techniques and strategies to stop self-harming, while also helping you get to the root of why you cut or hurt yourself.

Remember, self-harm doesn't occur in a vacuum. It's an outward expression of inner pain—pain that often has its roots in early life. There is often a connection between self-harm and childhood trauma.

Self-harm may be your way of coping with feelings related to past abuse, flashbacks, negative feelings about your body, or other traumatic memories. This may be the case even if you're not consciously aware of the connection.

Finding the Right Therapist

Finding the right therapist may take some time. It's very important that the therapist you choose has experience treating both trauma and self-injury. But the quality of the relationship with your therapist is equally important. Trust your instincts. If you don't feel safe, respected, or understood, find another therapist.

There should be a sense of trust and warmth between you and your therapist. This therapist should be someone who accepts self-harm without condoning it, and who is willing to help you work toward stopping it at your own pace. You should feel at ease with him or her, even while talking through your most personal issues.

Helping a Friend or Family Member Who Cuts or Self-Injures

Perhaps you've noticed suspicious injuries on someone close to you, or that person has confided to you that he or she is cutting. Whatever the case may be, you may be feeling unsure of yourself. What should you say? How can you help?

- Deal with your own feelings. You may feel shocked, confused, or even disgusted by self-harming behaviors—and guilty about admitting these feelings. Acknowledging your feelings is an important first step toward helping your loved one.

- Learn about the problem. The best way to overcome any discomfort or distaste you feel about self-harm is by learning about it. Understanding why your friend or family member is self-injuring can help you see the world from his or her eyes.

- Don't judge. Avoid judgmental comments and criticism—they'll only make things worse. The first two tips will go a long way in helping you with this. Remember, the self-harming person already feels ashamed and alone.

- Offer support, not ultimatums. It's only natural to want to help, but threats, punishments, and ultimatums are counterproductive. Express your concern and let the person know that you're available whenever he or she wants to talk or needs support.

- Encourage communication. Encourage your loved one to express whatever he or she is feeling, even if it's something you might be uncomfortable with. If the person hasn't told you about the self-harm, bring up the subject in a caring, non-confrontational way: "I've noticed injuries on your body, and I want to understand what you're going through."

If the self-harmer is a family member, especially if it is your child, prepare yourself to address difficulties in the family. This is not about blame, but rather about learning ways of dealing with problems and communicating better that can help the whole family.

Section 18.4

Problem Gambling

"FAQ: Problem Gamblers," © 2009 National Council
on Problem Gambling (www.ncpgambling.org). All rights reserved.
Reprinted with permission.

What is problem gambling?

Problem gambling includes all gambling behavior patterns that compromise, disrupt, or damage personal, family, or vocational pursuits. The essential features are increasing preoccupation with gambling, a need to bet more money more frequently, restlessness or irritability when attempting to stop, "chasing" losses, and loss of control manifested by continuation of the gambling behavior in spite of mounting, serious, negative consequences. In extreme cases, problem gambling can result in financial ruin, legal problems, loss of career and family, or even suicide. For more information on criteria for gambling problems, see Problem Gambling Self Quiz available online at http://www.ncpgambling.org/i4a/survey/survey.cfm?id=6.

Isn't problem gambling just a financial problem?

No. Problem gambling is an emotional problem that has financial consequences. If you pay all of a problem gambler's debts, the person will still be a problem gambler. The real problem is that they have an uncontrollable obsession with gambling.

Isn't problem gambling really the result of irresponsible or weak-willed people?

No. Many people who develop problems have been viewed as responsible and strong by those who care about them. Precipitating factors often lead to a change in behavior, such as retirement or job related stress.

What kind of people become problem gamblers?

Anyone who gambles can develop problems if they are not aware of the risks and do not gamble responsibly. When gambling behavior interferes with finances, relationships, and the workplace, a serious problem already exists.

Do casinos, lotteries, and other types of gambling cause problem gambling?

The cause of a gambling problem is the individual's inability to control the gambling. This may be due in part to a person's genetic tendency to develop addiction, their ability to cope with normal life stress, and even their social upbringing and moral attitudes about gambling. The casino or lottery provides the opportunity for the person to gamble. It does not, in and of itself, create the problem any more than a liquor store would create an alcoholic.

What types of gambling cause the most problem gambling?

Again, the cause of a gambling problem is the individual's inability to control the gambling. Therefore, any type of gambling can become problematic, just as an alcoholic can get drunk on any type of alcohol. But some types of gambling have different characteristics that may exacerbate gambling problems. While these factors are still poorly understood, anecdotal reports indicate that one risk factor may be a fast speed of play. In other words, the faster the wager to response time with a game, the more likely players may be to develop problems with a particular game.

What is the responsibility of the gaming industry?

Everyone who provides gambling opportunities has a responsibility to develop policies and programs to address underage and problem gambling issues.

Can you be a problem gambler if you don't gamble every day?

The frequency of a person's gambling does not determine whether or not they have a gambling problem. Even though the problem gambler may only go on periodic gambling binges, the emotional and financial consequences will still be evident in the gambler's life, including the effects on the family.

How much money do you have to lose before gambling becomes a problem?

The amount of money lost or won does not determine when gambling becomes a problem. Gambling becomes a problem when it causes a negative impact on any area of the individual's life.

How can a person be addicted to something that isn't a substance?

Although no substance is ingested, the problem gambler gets the same effect from gambling as someone else might get from taking a tranquilizer or having a drink. The gambling alters the person's mood and the gambler keeps repeating the behavior attempting to achieve that same effect. But just as tolerance develops to drugs or alcohol, the gambler finds that it takes more and more of the gambling experience to achieve the same emotional effect as before. This creates an increased craving for the activity and the gambler finds they have less and less ability to resist as the craving grows in intensity and frequency.

Are problem gamblers usually addicted to other things too?

It is generally accepted that people with one addiction are more at risk to develop another. Some problem gamblers also find they have a problem with alcohol or drugs. This does not, however, mean that if you have a gambling problem you are guaranteed to become addicted to other things. Some problem gamblers never experience any other addiction because no other substance or activity gives them the same feeling as the gambling does. There also appears to be evidence of family patterns regarding dependency as many problem gamblers report one or both parents had a drinking and or gambling problem.

How widespread is problem gambling in the U.S.?

Two million (1%) of U.S. adults are estimated to meet criteria for pathological gambling in a given year. Another 4–6 million (2–3%)

would be considered problem gamblers; that is, they do not meet the full diagnostic criteria for pathological gambling, but meet one of more of the criteria and are experiencing problems due to their gambling behavior. Research also indicates that most adults who choose to gamble are able to do responsibly.

How widespread is gambling in the U.S.?

Approximately 85% of U.S. adults have gambled at least once in their lives; 60% in the past year. Some form of legalized gambling is available in 48 states plus the District of Columbia. The two without legalized gambling are Hawaii and Utah.

Can children or teenagers develop gambling problems?

A number of states allow children under 18 to gamble, and youth also participate in illegal forms of gambling, such as gambling on the internet or betting on sports. Therefore, it is not surprising that research shows that a vast majority of kids have gambled before their 18th birthday, and that children may be more likely to develop problems related to gambling than adults. While debate continues on this issue, there appears to be a number of factors influencing this finding. Parental attitudes and behavior play a role. Age of exposure plays a part, in that adults who seek treatment for problem gambling report having started gambling at an early age. A number of adolescents reported a preoccupation with everything related to gambling prior to developing problems.

Section 18.5

Paraphilias

Paraphilias are frequent, intense, sexually arousing fantasies or behaviors that involve inanimate objects, children or nonconsenting adults, or suffering or humiliation of oneself or the partner.

Sexual arousal may depend on one of the above. Once these arousal patterns are established, usually in late childhood or near puberty, they are often lifelong.

Some degree of variety in sexual activity is very common in healthy adult sexual relationships and fantasies. When people mutually agree to engage in them, noninjurious sexual behaviors of an unusual nature may be part of a loving and caring relationship. When taken to the extreme, however, such sexual behaviors are paraphilias—psychosexual disorders that seriously impair the capacity for affectionate, reciprocal sexual activity. Partners of people with a paraphilia may feel like an object or as if they are unimportant or unnecessary in the sexual relationship. Paraphilias cause significant distress and interfere with functioning. Distress may result from other people's reactions or from guilt about doing something socially unacceptable.

The most common paraphilias are transvestic fetishism, pedophilia, exhibitionism, and voyeurism. Others include sexual masochism and sadism. Most people with paraphilias are men, and many have more than one type of paraphilia. Some of them also have a severe personality disorder, such as an antisocial or narcissistic personality. Some paraphilias are against the law.

Fetishism

Fetishism is use of a physical object (the fetish) as the preferred way to produce sexual arousal.

People with fetishes may become sexually stimulated and gratified by wearing another person's undergarments, wearing rubber or leather, or holding, rubbing, or smelling objects, such as high-heeled shoes. People with this disorder may not be able to function sexually without their fetish. The fetish may replace typical sexual activity with a partner or may be integrated into sexual activity with a willing partner.

Transvestic fetishism: In transvestic fetishism (cross-dressing), men prefer to wear women's clothing, or, far less commonly, women prefer to wear men's clothing. However, they do not wish to change their sex, as transsexuals do. Cross-dressing may not hurt a couple's sexual relationship, although if a partner is not cooperative, transvestites may feel anxious, depressed, and guilty and ashamed about their desire.

Transvestic fetishism is considered a mental health disorder only if it causes distress, interferes with functioning, or involves daredevil behavior likely to lead to injury, loss of a job, or imprisonment. Transvestites also cross-dress for reasons other than sexual stimulation—for example, to reduce anxiety, to relax, or, in the case of male transvestites, to experiment with the feminine side of their otherwise male personalities. Some men who appear to be transvestites only in their teens and twenties develop gender identity disorder later in life and may seek to change their body through hormones and genital surgery.

Only a few transvestites seek medical care. They may be motivated by an unhappy spouse or by worry about how the cross-dressing is affecting their social life and work. Some seek medical care for other problems, such as substance abuse or depression. Treatment involves psychotherapy to help them accept themselves and control behaviors that could cause problems.

Pedophilia

Pedophilia is a preference for sexual activity with young children.

In Western societies, pedophilia is defined as sexual fantasy about or sexual relations with a prepubertal child younger than 13 by a person 16 or older. Some pedophiles are attracted only to children, often of a specific age range or developmental stage. Others are attracted to both children and adults. Pedophiles may be attracted to young boys, young girls, or both, but most pedophiles prefer children of the opposite sex. Usually, the adult is known to the child and may be a family member, stepparent, or a person with authority (such as a teacher). Looking or general touching seems more common than touching the genitals or having sexual intercourse.

Although state laws vary in the United States, the law generally considers a person older than 18 to be committing statutory rape if the victim is 16 or younger. Statutory rape cases often do not meet the definition of pedophilia, highlighting the somewhat arbitrary nature of selecting a specific age cutoff point in a medical or legal definition. In many other countries and cultures, children as young as 12 can legally marry, further complicating the definition of pedophilia and statutory rape.

Pedophilia is much more common among men than among women. Both boys and girls can be victims, although more reported cases involve girls. Pedophiles may focus only on children within their families (incest), or they may prey on children in the community. Force or coercion may be used to engage children sexually, and threats (for example, to harm the child or the child's pets) may be invoked to prevent the child from telling anyone.

Many pedophiles have or develop substance abuse or dependence and depression. They often come from dysfunctional families, and marital conflict is common.

Treatment

Pedophilia can be treated with long-term psychotherapy and drugs that alter the sex drive and reduce testosterone levels. Results vary. Outcome is best when participation is voluntary and the person receives training in social skills and treatment of other problems, such as drug abuse or depression. Treatment that is sought only after criminal apprehension and legal action may be less effective. Simple incarceration, even long-term, does not change pedophilic desires or fantasies. However, some incarcerated pedophiles who are committed to long-term, monitored treatment (usually including drugs) can refrain from pedophilic activity and be reintegrated into society.

For drug treatment, doctors in the United States usually use the drug medroxyprogesterone acetate (a trade name is Provera), which is injected into a muscle. This drug (a progestin) is similar to the female hormone progesterone (some trade names are Crinone and Endometrin). Alternatives are drugs such as leuprolide (Lupron) and goserelin (Zoladex) that stop the pituitary gland from signaling the testicles to produce testosterone. It is not clear how useful these drugs are in women who are pedophiles.

Exhibitionism

Exhibitionism involves exposing the genitals in order to become sexually excited or having a strong desire to be observed by other people during sexual activity.

Exhibitionists (usually males) expose their genitals, usually to unsuspecting strangers, and become sexually excited when doing so. They may be aware of their need to surprise, shock, or impress the unwilling observer. The victim is almost always a woman or a child of either sex. Actual sexual contact is almost never sought, so exhibitionists rarely commit rape. Exhibitionism usually starts when people are in their mid 20s. Most exhibitionists are married, but the marriage is often troubled.

About 30% of male sex offenders who are arrested are exhibitionists. They tend to persist in their behavior. About 20 to 50% are re-arrested.

Exposure of genitals to unsuspecting strangers for sexual excitement is rare among women. Women have other venues to expose themselves: dressing provocatively (which is increasingly accepted as normal) and appearing in various media and entertainment venues. Participation in these venues may not constitute a mental health disorder.

For some people, exhibitionism is expressed as a strong desire to have other people watch their sexual acts. Such people want to be seen by a consenting audience, rather than to surprise people. People with this form of exhibitionism may make pornographic films or become adult entertainers. They are rarely troubled by their desire and thus may not have a mental health disorder.

Treatment

Treatment usually begins after exhibitionists are arrested. It includes psychotherapy, support groups, and antidepressants called selective serotonin reuptake inhibitors (SSRIs). If these drugs are ineffective, drugs that alter the sex drive and reduce testosterone levels may be used. People must give their informed consent to the use of these drugs, and doctors periodically do blood tests to monitor the drug's effects on liver function and serum testosterone levels.

Voyeurism

Voyeurism involves becoming sexually aroused by watching someone who is disrobing, naked, or engaged in sexual activity.

In voyeurism, it is the act of observing (peeping) that is arousing, not sexual activity with the observed person. Voyeurs do not seek sexual contact with the people being observed. When voyeurs observe unsuspecting people, they may have problems with the law.

Voyeurism usually begins during adolescence or early adulthood. Some degree of voyeurism is common, more among boys and men but increasingly among women. Society often regards mild forms of this behavior as normal when involving consenting adults. Viewing sexually explicit pictures and shows, now widely available in private on the internet, is not considered voyeurism because it lacks the element of secret observation, which is the hallmark of voyeurism.

As a disorder, voyeurism is much more common among men. When voyeurism is a disorder, voyeurs spend a lot of time seeking out viewing opportunities. It may become the preferred method of sexual activity and consume countless hours of watching.

Treatment

When voyeurs are arrested, treatment usually begins. It includes therapy, support groups, and antidepressants called selective serotonin reuptake inhibitors (SSRIs). If these drugs are ineffective, drugs that alter the sex drive and reduce testosterone levels may be used. People must give their informed consent to the use of these drugs, and doctors periodically do blood tests to monitor the drug's effects on liver function and serum testosterone levels.

Sexual Masochism and Sadism

Sexual masochism involves acts in which a person experiences sexual excitement from being humiliated, beaten, bound, or otherwise abused. Sexual sadism involves acts in which a person experiences sexual excitement from inflicting physical or psychologic suffering on another person.

Some amount of sadism and masochism is commonly play-acted in healthy sexual relationships, and mutually compatible partners often seek one another out. For example, the use of silk handkerchiefs for simulated bondage and mild spanking during sexual activity are common practices between consenting partners and are not considered sadomasochistic.

Most sadists interact with a consenting partner (who may have sexual masochism). In these relationships, the humiliation and beating are simply acted out, with participants knowing that it is a game and carefully avoiding actual humiliation or injury. Fantasies of total control and dominance are often important, and sadists may bind and gag their partner in elaborate ways.

In contrast, the disorder of sexual masochism or of sexual sadism takes these acts to an extreme or involves nonconsenting victims (and thus constitutes a crime). Some acts result in severe bodily or psychologic harm and even death. For example, masochistic sexual activity may involve asphyxiophilia, in which the person is partially choked or strangled (by a partner or by self-application of a noose around the neck). A temporary decrease in oxygen to the brain at the point of orgasm is sought as an enhancement to sexual release, but the practice may accidentally result in death.

Treatment of masochism and sadism is usually ineffective.

Chapter 19

Tourette Syndrome

What is Tourette syndrome?

Tourette syndrome (TS) is a neurological disorder characterized by repetitive, stereotyped, involuntary movements and vocalizations called tics. The disorder is named for Dr. Georges Gilles de la Tourette, the pioneering French neurologist who in 1885 first described the condition in an 86-year-old French noblewoman.

The early symptoms of TS are typically noticed first in childhood, with the average onset between the ages of three and nine years. TS occurs in people from all ethnic groups; males are affected about three to four times more often than females. It is estimated that 200,000 Americans have the most severe form of TS, and as many as one in 100 exhibit milder and less complex symptoms such as chronic motor or vocal tics. Although TS can be a chronic condition with symptoms lasting a lifetime, most people with the condition experience their worst tic symptoms in their early teens, with improvement occurring in the late teens and continuing into adulthood.

What are the symptoms?

Tics are classified as either simple or complex. Simple motor tics are sudden, brief, repetitive movements that involve a limited number of muscle groups. Some of the more common simple tics include eye

"Tourette Syndrome Fact Sheet," National Institute of Neurological Disorders and Stroke (www.ninds.nih.gov), November 16, 2011.

blinking and other eye movements, facial grimacing, shoulder shrugging, and head or shoulder jerking. Simple vocalizations might include repetitive throat-clearing, sniffing, or grunting sounds. Complex tics are distinct, coordinated patterns of movements involving several muscle groups. Complex motor tics might include facial grimacing combined with a head twist and a shoulder shrug. Other complex motor tics may actually appear purposeful, including sniffing or touching objects, hopping, jumping, bending, or twisting. Simple vocal tics may include throat-clearing, sniffing/snorting, grunting, or barking. More complex vocal tics include words or phrases. Perhaps the most dramatic and disabling tics include motor movements that result in self-harm such as punching oneself in the face or vocal tics including coprolalia (uttering socially inappropriate words such as swearing) or echolalia (repeating the words or phrases of others). However, coprolalia is only present in a small number (10 to 15 percent) of individuals with TS. Some tics are preceded by an urge or sensation in the affected muscle group, commonly called a premonitory urge. Some with TS will describe a need to complete a tic in a certain way or a certain number of times in order to relieve the urge or decrease the sensation.

Tics are often worse with excitement or anxiety and better during calm, focused activities. Certain physical experiences can trigger or worsen tics, for example tight collars may trigger neck tics, or hearing another person sniff or throat-clear may trigger similar sounds. Tics do not go away during sleep but are often significantly diminished.

What is the course of TS?

Tics come and go over time, varying in type, frequency, location, and severity. The first symptoms usually occur in the head and neck area and may progress to include muscles of the trunk and extremities. Motor tics generally precede the development of vocal tics and simple tics often precede complex tics. Most patients experience peak tic severity before the mid-teen years with improvement for the majority of patients in the late teen years and early adulthood. Approximately 10–15 percent of those affected have a progressive or disabling course that lasts into adulthood.

Can people with TS control their tics?

Although the symptoms of TS are involuntary, some people can sometimes suppress, camouflage, or otherwise manage their tics in an effort to minimize their impact on functioning. However, people with TS often report a substantial buildup in tension when suppressing their tics to the point where they feel that the tic must be expressed (against their will). Tics in response to an environmental trigger can appear to be voluntary or purposeful but are not.

What causes TS?

Although the cause of TS is unknown, current research points to abnormalities in certain brain regions (including the basal ganglia, frontal lobes, and cortex), the circuits that interconnect these regions, and the neurotransmitters (dopamine, serotonin, and norepinephrine) responsible for communication among nerve cells. Given the often complex presentation of TS, the cause of the disorder is likely to be equally complex.

What disorders are associated with TS?

Many individuals with TS experience additional neurobehavioral problems that often cause more impairment than the tics themselves. These include inattention, hyperactivity and impulsivity (attention deficit hyperactivity disorder—ADHD); problems with reading, writing, and arithmetic; and obsessive-compulsive symptoms such as intrusive thoughts/worries and repetitive behaviors. For example, worries about dirt and germs may be associated with repetitive hand-washing, and concerns about bad things happening may be associated with ritualistic behaviors such as counting, repeating, or ordering and arranging. People with TS have also reported problems with depression or anxiety disorders, as well as other difficulties with living, that may or may not be directly related to TS. In addition, although most individuals with TS experience a significant decline in motor and vocal tics in late adolescence and early adulthood, the associated neurobehavioral conditions may persist. Given the range of potential complications, people with TS are best served by receiving medical care that provides a comprehensive treatment plan.

How is TS diagnosed?

TS is a diagnosis that doctors make after verifying that the patient has had both motor and vocal tics for at least one year. The existence of other neurological or psychiatric conditions can also help doctors arrive at a diagnosis. Common tics are not often misdiagnosed by knowledgeable clinicians. However, atypical symptoms or atypical presentations (for example, onset of symptoms in adulthood) may require specific specialty expertise for diagnosis. There are no blood, laboratory, or imaging tests needed for diagnosis. In rare cases, neuroimaging studies, such as magnetic resonance imaging (MRI) or computerized tomography (CT), electroencephalogram (EEG) studies, or certain blood tests may be used to rule out other conditions that might be confused with TS when the history or clinical examination is atypical.

It is not uncommon for patients to obtain a formal diagnosis of TS only after symptoms have been present for some time. The reasons for this are many. For families and physicians unfamiliar with TS, mild and even moderate tic symptoms may be considered inconsequential, part of a developmental phase, or the result of another condition. For example, parents may think that eye blinking is related to vision problems or that sniffing is related to seasonal allergies. Many patients are self-diagnosed after they, their parents, other relatives, or friends read or hear about TS from others.

How is TS treated?

Because tic symptoms often do not cause impairment, the majority of people with TS require no medication for tic suppression. However, effective medications are available for those whose symptoms interfere with functioning. Neuroleptics (drugs that may be used to treat psychotic and non-psychotic disorders) are the most consistently useful medications for tic suppression; a number are available but some are more effective than others (for example, haloperidol and pimozide).

Unfortunately, there is no one medication that is helpful to all people with TS, nor does any medication completely eliminate symptoms. In addition, all medications have side effects. Many neuroleptic side effects can be managed by initiating treatment slowly and reducing the dose when side effects occur. The most common side effects of neuroleptics include sedation, weight gain, and cognitive dulling. Neurological side effects such as tremor, dystonic reactions (twisting movements or postures), parkinsonian-like symptoms, and other dyskinetic (involuntary) movements are less common and are readily managed with dose reduction.

Discontinuing neuroleptics after long-term use must be done slowly to avoid rebound increases in tics and withdrawal dyskinesias. One form of dyskinesia called tardive dyskinesia is a movement disorder distinct from TS that may result from the chronic use of neuroleptics. The risk of this side effect can be reduced by using lower doses of neuroleptics for shorter periods of time.

Other medications may also be useful for reducing tic severity, but most have not been as extensively studied or shown to be as consistently useful as neuroleptics. Additional medications with demonstrated efficacy include alpha-adrenergic agonists such as clonidine and guanfacine. These medications are used primarily for hypertension but are also used in the treatment of tics. The most common side effect from these medications that precludes their use is sedation. However, given the lower side effect risk associated with these medications, they are often used as first-line agents before proceeding to treatment with neuroleptics.

Effective medications are also available to treat some of the associated neurobehavioral disorders that can occur in patients with TS. Recent research shows that stimulant medications such as methylphenidate and dextroamphetamine can lessen ADHD symptoms in people with TS without causing tics to become more severe. However, the product labeling for stimulants currently contraindicates the use of these drugs in children with tics/TS and those with a family history of tics. Scientists hope that future studies will include a thorough discussion of the risks and benefits of stimulants in those with TS or a family history of TS and will clarify this issue. For obsessive-compulsive symptoms that significantly disrupt daily functioning, the serotonin reuptake inhibitors (clomipramine, fluoxetine, fluvoxamine, paroxetine, and sertraline) have been proven effective in some patients.

Behavioral treatments such as awareness training and competing response training can also be used to reduce tics. A recent multi-center randomized control trial funded by the National Institutes of Health (NIH), called Cognitive Behavioral Intervention for Tics, or CBIT, showed that training to voluntarily move in response to a premonitory urge can reduce tic symptoms. Other behavioral therapies, such as biofeedback or supportive therapy, have not been shown to reduce tic symptoms. However, supportive therapy can help a person with TS better cope with the disorder and deal with the secondary social and emotional problems that sometimes occur.

Is TS inherited?

Evidence from twin and family studies suggests that TS is an inherited disorder. Although early family studies suggested an autosomal dominant mode of inheritance (an autosomal dominant disorder is one in which only one copy of the defective gene, inherited from one parent, is necessary to produce the disorder), more recent studies suggest that the pattern of inheritance is much more complex. Although there may be a few genes with substantial effects, it is also possible that many genes with smaller effects and environmental factors may play a role in the development of TS.

Genetic studies also suggest that some forms of ADHD and OCD (obsessive-compulsive disorder) are genetically related to TS, but there is less evidence for a genetic relationship between TS and other neurobehavioral problems that commonly co-occur with TS. It is important for families to understand that genetic predisposition may not necessarily result in full-blown TS; instead, it may express itself as a milder tic disorder or as obsessive-compulsive behaviors. It is also possible that the gene-carrying offspring will not develop any TS symptoms.

The gender of the person also plays an important role in TS gene expression. At-risk males are more likely to have tics and at-risk females are more likely to have obsessive-compulsive symptoms.

Genetic counseling of individuals with TS should include a full review of all potentially hereditary conditions in the family.

What is the prognosis?

Although there is no cure for TS, the condition in many individuals improves in the late teens and early 20s. As a result, some may actually become symptom-free or no longer need medication for tic suppression. Although the disorder is generally lifelong and chronic, it is not a degenerative condition. Individuals with TS have a normal life expectancy. TS does not impair intelligence. Although tic symptoms tend to decrease with age, it is possible that neurobehavioral disorders such as ADHD, OCD, depression, generalized anxiety, panic attacks, and mood swings can persist and cause impairment in adult life.

What is the best educational setting for children with TS?

Although students with TS often function well in the regular classroom, ADHD, learning disabilities, obsessive-compulsive symptoms, and frequent tics can greatly interfere with academic performance or social adjustment. After a comprehensive assessment, students should be placed in an educational setting that meets their individual needs. Students may require tutoring, smaller or special classes, and in some cases special schools.

All students with TS need a tolerant and compassionate setting that both encourages them to work to their full potential and is flexible enough to accommodate their special needs. This setting may include a private study area, exams outside the regular classroom, or even oral exams when the child's symptoms interfere with his or her ability to write. Untimed testing reduces stress for students with TS.

What research is being done?

Within the federal government, the National Institute of Neurological Disorders and Stroke (NINDS), a part of the National Institutes of Health (NIH), is responsible for supporting and conducting research on the brain and nervous system. The NINDS and other NIH components, such as the National Institute of Mental Health, the Eunice Kennedy Shriver National Institute of Child Health and Human Development, the National Institute on Drug Abuse, and the National Institute on Deafness and Other Communication Disorders, support research of relevance to TS, either at NIH laboratories or through grants to major research institutions across the country. Another component of the Department of Health and Human Services, the Centers for Disease Control and Prevention, funds professional education programs as well as TS research.

Knowledge about TS comes from studies across a number of medical and scientific disciplines, including genetics, neuroimaging, neuropathology, clinical trials (medication and non-medication), epidemiology, neurophysiology, neuroimmunology, and descriptive/diagnostic clinical science.

Genetic studies: Currently, NIH-funded investigators are conducting a variety of large-scale genetic studies. Rapid advances in the technology of gene discovery will allow for genome-wide screening approaches in TS, and finding a gene or genes for TS would be a major step toward understanding genetic risk factors. In addition, understanding the genetics of TS genes may strengthen clinical diagnosis, improve genetic counseling, lead to the clarification of pathophysiology, and provide clues for more effective therapies.

Neuroimaging studies: Advances in imaging technology and an increase in trained investigators have led to an increasing use of novel and powerful techniques to identify brain regions, circuitry, and neurochemical factors important in TS and related conditions.

Neuropathology: There has been an increase in the number and quality of donated postmortem brains from TS patients available for research purposes. This increase, coupled with advances in neuropathological techniques, has led to initial findings with implications for neuroimaging studies and animal models of TS.

Clinical trials: A number of clinical trials in TS have recently been completed or are currently underway. These include studies of stimulant treatment of ADHD in TS and behavioral treatments for reducing tic severity in children and adults. Smaller trials of novel approaches to treatment such as dopamine agonists and glutamatergic medications also show promise.

Epidemiology and clinical science: Careful epidemiological studies now estimate the prevalence of TS to be substantially higher than previously thought with a wider range of clinical severity. Furthermore, clinical studies are providing new findings regarding TS and co-existing conditions. These include subtyping studies of TS and OCD, an examination of the link between ADHD and learning problems in children with TS, a new appreciation of sensory tics, and the role of co-existing disorders in rage attacks. One of the most important and controversial areas of TS science involves the relationship between TS and autoimmune brain injury associated with group A beta-hemolytic streptococcal infections or other infectious processes. There are a number of epidemiological and clinical investigations currently underway in this intriguing area.

Part Three

Mental Health Treatments

Chapter 20

Recognizing a Mental Health Emergency

Recognizing a Mental Health Crisis

For a variety of reasons, mental health issues can be difficult to recognize and address. When people live with chronic, low to moderate levels of depression or anxiety, a new "baseline" emotional state gets established and can actually start to feel normal. Many continue to function superficially well despite their mental health problems because of various mechanisms such as: emotional numbness and denial; compensatory overwork and/or extreme perfectionism; self-medication with caffeine, nicotine and/or alcohol—if not (illegal or misused prescription) drugs; and of course, the "enabling" behavior of family, friends and work associates.

Even when more severe psychiatric symptoms manifest, people might delay seeking help because of impaired thinking/judgment, poor insight, or fear of being stigmatized. And some who do recognize the need for treatment receive confusing messages from friends and relatives, who might assume that mental illness can be overcome by simply adjusting one's attitude or "trying harder."

People who are in denial about a mental health problem or their need for professional help might only begin to take responsibility when allowed to experience natural consequences. But often, well-intended others enable with the assumption that the person will get better if everyone is more "supportive", i.e., does not hold him/her accountable for the effects of the untreated psychiatric problem or addiction. For example, if a depressed employee is allowed to come late to work or leave early most days, he/she might have no incentive to get help. And a relative who continues being invited to family events despite becoming drunk and obnoxious each time can remain oblivious to the impact of this destructive behavior.

Whereas some people might respond to direct expressions of concern by seeking help, others will continue to deny until the situation gets out of control. Often, the most effective approach for concerned others is to develop "healthy detachment" (i.e., focus on taking care of yourself, and don't protect the troubled person from consequences—including more distance in your relationship, if necessary). However, in a crisis which seems to present a direct threat to anyone's health and safety, a more immediate response might be required. Below are some guidelines to help you differentiate a problem from a crisis.

Signs of a Problem Include

- Declining educational/vocational or social functioning
- Apparent depression—sad mood, low energy, sleep/appetite problems
- Stress-related symptoms—physical, emotional, or behavioral
- Pervasive worry or anxiety; mild-moderate panic symptoms
- Indications of alcohol or drug abuse, and related health or legal problems
- Compulsive behavior (e.g., "workaholism", eating disorder symptoms, overspending)
- Possible domestic violence (with adult victim who is not actively seeking help); someone suffering the effects of any past or recent trauma.

Signs of a Crisis Include

- Any mention or threat of suicide, up to and including "gestures" or attempts
- Any threat or motion to harm another person
- Observed violent or reckless behavior, including property destruction
- Extreme agitation, anxiety, panic
- Person seems immobilized by depression, unable to care for self

- Person seems extremely irrational, confused, illogical (possibly paranoid)

- Alcohol or drug intoxication/withdrawal that could present an immediate health threat.

How to Respond When Someone Is in Crisis

If there has been any violence or aggression (or threat thereof), get to a safe place and call the police. In addition to protecting yourself and others, this can also create another avenue by which the troubled person might get help. If you feel threatened but the situation does no seem to warrant calling 911, you can still contact the police for help with revising a safety plan that could include:

1. A restraining order;

2. A psychiatric detention, wherein a magistrate orders that the troubled person be held and evaluated in a secure hospital unit for a specified time period. Many police departments have a victim assistance unit which provides information and support services, even if no criminal charges are being brought.

If the aggressive behavior has been ongoing (or episodic) and directed against a spouse/romantic partner or a child, there are specialized services available for victims of domestic violence and child abuse. Again, depending on how immediate the threat, you can call 911; a non-emergency police number; a mental health crisis center or hotline; child protective services; or a local victim assistance program.

If there has been any type of suicide attempt or gesture, take the person to a hospital emergency room or call for an ambulance—even assured that he/she is "fine." (If it seems possible that someone might jump from a moving car, don't transport the person yourself.)

If someone is making direct or indirect comments about suicide, or showing behavioral indications such as giving away their possessions, try to convince the troubled person to:

1. Contact his/her therapist or psychiatrist if already in treatment, or perhaps allow you to talk with the professional;

2. Call an emergency hotline or crisis center; or

3. Go to the nearest hospital emergency room.

If you are afraid to leave someone alone, this means that you probably need to make sure some type of intervention is made (vs. trying to keep your own "suicide watch" or continually worrying about the person while you're away).

If there is any question of someone being suicidal or potentially violent, try to ensure that there are no guns available. Ask if the troubled person will let you take any weapons and put them in a secure, locked place. If he/she will not relinquish a gun, or if you're aware of another easy means of suicide such as stockpiled medication, you should bring this to the attention of whatever (mental health or law enforcement) professionals end up getting involved. Also make sure the professional knows of any previous suicide attempts.

Finally, never leave a child in the care of someone who might be suicidal, violent/aggressive or suffering from any serious, untreated mental illness or substance abuse problem.

Other Response Options

- If your company has an Employee Assistance Program, this can be a good place to get (free, confidential) consultation on how to help someone in crisis. Many EAP's have 24- hour telephone counseling/referral services available.

- Call your local mental health crisis center for advice. If there is only a hotline staffed by volunteers, don't hesitate to ask for the supervising professional to make sure you get the most helpful guidance. Some centers have a "mobile crisis unit", providing on-site assessment/intervention for psychiatrically impaired persons who refuse to go for help.

- In crisis situations which involve the police, ask if they can dispatch a team that includes a mental health professional to help address any relevant psychiatric issues.

- If someone seems severely impaired or unable to care for him- or herself because of mental illness, talk with a primary care physician about treatment options including psychiatric referrals and hospitalization. If a mentally ill person is willing to see an MD but not a psychiatrist, sometimes the doctor can do the initial prescribing and case management—and work towards getting the patient into formal treatment.

- If there is a child who might be affected by a parent's mental illness or addiction, consider letting his/her school counselor know of the situation. This will help the counselor be alert to signs that the child is suffering emotionally or is at any type of risk, so that appropriate support services can be made available.

Chapter 21

Mental Health Care Services

Chapter Contents

Section 21.1

Types of Mental Health Professionals

Reprinted with permission from "Mental Health Professionals:
Who They Are and How to Find One," © 2012 NAMI, the National
Alliance on Mental Illness, www.nami.org.

Mental health services are provided by several different professions, each of which has its own training and areas of expertise. Finding the right professional(s) for you or a loved one can be a critical ingredient in the process of diagnosis, treatment, and recovery when faced with serious mental illness.

Types of Mental Health Professionals

Psychiatrist: A psychiatrist is a physician with a doctor of medicine (M.D.) degree or osteopathic (D.O.) degree, with at least four more years of specialized study and training in psychiatry. Psychiatrists are licensed as physicians to practice medicine by individual states. "Board certified" psychiatrists have passed the national examination administered by the American Board of Psychiatry and Neurology. Psychiatrists provide medical and psychiatric evaluations, treat psychiatric disorders, provide psychotherapy, and prescribe and monitor medications.

Psychologist: Some psychologists have a master's degree (M.A. or M.S.) in psychology while others have a doctoral degree (Ph.D., Psy.D., or Ed.D.) in clinical, educational, counseling, or research psychology. Most states license psychologists to practice psychology. They can provide psychological testing, evaluations, treat emotional and behavioral problems and mental disorders, and provide psychotherapy.

Social worker: Social workers have either a bachelor's degree (B.A., B.S., or B.S.W.), a master's degree (M.A., M.S., M.S.W., or M.S.S.W), or doctoral degree (D.S.W. or Ph.D.). In most states, social workers take an examination to be licensed to practice social work (L.C.S.W. or L.I.C.S.W.), and the type of license depends on their level of education and practice experience. Social workers provide various services including assessment and treatment of psychiatric illnesses, case management, hospital discharge planning, and psychotherapy.

Psychiatric/mental health nurse: Psychiatric/mental health nurses may have various degrees ranging from associate's to bachelor's (B.S.N.) to master's (M.S.N. or A.P.R.N) to doctoral (D.N.Sc., Ph.D.). Depending on their level of education and licensing, they provide a broad range of psychiatric and medical services, including the assessment and treatment of psychiatric illnesses, case management, and psychotherapy. In some states, some psychiatric nurses may prescribe and monitor medication.

Licensed professional counselors: Licensed Professional Counselors have a master's degree (M.A.) in psychology, counseling or a similar discipline and typically have two years of post-graduate experience. They may provide services that include diagnosis and counseling (individual, family/group or both). They have a license issued in their state and may be certified by the National Academy of Certified Clinical Mental Health Counselors.

Resources for Locating a Mental Health Professional

The following sources may help you locate a mental health professional or treatment facility to meet your needs:

- **NAMI local affiliates and support groups:** Speaking with NAMI members (consumers and family members) can be a good way to exchange information about mental health professionals in your local community.

- **Primary care physician (PCP):** If you are part of an HMO or other managed care insurance plan, your primary physician can refer you to a specialist or therapist.

- **Your insurance provider:** Contact your insurance company or "behavioral health care organization" for a list of mental health care providers included in your insurance plan.

- **District branch of the American Psychiatric Association:** The APA can give you names of APA members in your area. Find your district branch online or consult your local phone book under the headings "district branch" or "psychiatric society."

- **Psychiatry department** at local teaching hospital or medical school.

- **National Association of Social Workers (NASW)** has an online directory of clinical social workers. Visit www.socialworkers. org and click on Resources.

- **American Psychological Association** can refer to local psychologists by calling 800-964-2000.

- **The Substance Abuse and Mental Health Services Administration's (SAMHSA) Center for Mental Health Services** has an online database of mental health services and facilities in each state. Visit www.mentalhealth.org and click on Services Locator.

Section 21.2

Types of Psychotherapies

"Psychotherapies," National Institute of Mental Health
(www.nimh.nih.gov), August 16, 2010.

Psychotherapy

Psychotherapy, or "talk therapy," is a way to treat people with a mental disorder by helping them understand their illness. It teaches people strategies and gives them tools to deal with stress and unhealthy thoughts and behaviors. Psychotherapy helps patients manage their symptoms better and function at their best in everyday life.

Sometimes psychotherapy alone may be the best treatment for a person, depending on the illness and its severity. Other times, psychotherapy is combined with medications. Therapists work with an individual or families to devise an appropriate treatment plan.

Types of Psychotherapy

Many kinds of psychotherapy exist. There is no "one-size-fits-all" approach. In addition, some therapies have been scientifically tested more than others. Some people may have a treatment plan that includes only one type of psychotherapy. Others receive treatment that includes elements of several different types. The kind of psychotherapy a person receives depends on his or her needs.

This section explains several of the most commonly used psychotherapies. However, it does not cover every detail about psychotherapy. Patients should talk to their doctor or a psychotherapist about planning treatment that meets their needs.

Cognitive Behavioral Therapy

Cognitive behavioral therapy (CBT) is a blend of two therapies: cognitive therapy (CT) and behavioral therapy. CT was developed by psychotherapist, Aaron Beck, M.D., in the 1960s. CT focuses on a person's thoughts and beliefs, and how they influence a person's mood and actions, and it aims to change a person's thinking to be more adaptive and healthy. Behavioral therapy focuses on a person's actions and aims to change unhealthy behavior patterns.

CBT helps a person focus on his or her current problems and how to solve them. Both patient and therapist need to be actively involved in this process. The therapist helps the patient learn how to identify distorted or unhelpful thinking patterns, recognize and change inaccurate beliefs, relate to others in more positive ways, and change behaviors accordingly. CBT can be applied and adapted to treat many specific mental disorders.

CBT for depression: Many studies have shown that CBT is a particularly effective treatment for depression, especially minor or moderate depression. Some people with depression may be successfully treated with CBT only. Others may need both CBT and medication. CBT helps people with depression restructure negative thought patterns. Doing so helps people interpret their environment and interactions with others in a positive and realistic way. It may also help a person recognize things that may be contributing to the depression and help him or her change behaviors that may be making the depression worse.

CBT for anxiety disorders: CBT for anxiety disorders aims to help a person develop a more adaptive response to a fear. A CBT therapist may use "exposure" therapy to treat certain anxiety disorders, such as a specific phobia, post traumatic stress disorder, or obsessive compulsive disorder. Exposure therapy has been found to be effective in treating anxiety-related disorders. It works by helping a person confront a specific fear or memory while in a safe and supportive environment. The main goals of exposure therapy are to help the patient learn that anxiety can lessen over time and give him or her the tools to cope with fear or traumatic memories. A recent study sponsored by the Centers for Disease Control and Prevention concluded that CBT is effective in treating trauma-related disorders in children and teens.

CBT for bipolar disorder: People with bipolar disorder usually need to take medication, such as a mood stabilizer. But CBT is often used as an added treatment. The medication can help stabilize a person's mood so that he or she is receptive to psychotherapy and can get the most out of it. CBT can help a person cope with bipolar symptoms and learn to recognize when a mood shift is about to occur. CBT also helps a person with bipolar disorder stick with a treatment plan to reduce the chances of relapse (when symptoms return).

CBT for eating disorders: Eating disorders can be very difficult to treat. However, some small studies have found that CBT can help reduce the risk of relapse in adults with anorexia who have restored their weight. CBT may also reduce some symptoms of bulimia, and it may also help some people reduce binge-eating behavior.

CBT for schizophrenia: Treating schizophrenia with CBT is challenging. The disorder usually requires medication first. But research has shown that CBT, as an add-on to medication, can help a patient cope with schizophrenia. CBT helps patients learn more adaptive and realistic interpretations of events. Patients are also taught various coping techniques for dealing with "voices" or other hallucinations. They learn how to identify what triggers episodes of the illness, which can prevent or reduce the chances of relapse.

CBT for schizophrenia also stresses skill-oriented therapies. Patients learn skills to cope with life's challenges. The therapist teaches social, daily functioning, and problem-solving skills. This can help patients with schizophrenia minimize the types of stress that can lead to outbursts and hospitalizations.

Dialectical Behavior Therapy

Dialectical behavior therapy (DBT), a form of CBT, was developed by Marsha Linehan, Ph.D. At first, it was developed to treat people with suicidal thoughts and actions. It is now also used to treat people with borderline personality disorder (BPD). BPD is an illness in which suicidal thinking and actions are more common.

The term *dialectical* refers to a philosophic exercise in which two opposing views are discussed until a logical blending or balance of the two extremes—the middle way—is found. In keeping with that philosophy, the therapist assures the patient that the patient's behavior and feelings are valid and understandable. At the same time, the therapist coaches the patient to understand that it is his or her personal responsibility to change unhealthy or disruptive behavior.

DBT emphasizes the value of a strong and equal relationship between patient and therapist. The therapist consistently reminds the patient when his or her behavior is unhealthy or disruptive—when boundaries are overstepped—and then teaches the skills needed to better deal with future similar situations. DBT involves both individual and group therapy. Individual sessions are used to teach new skills, while group sessions provide the opportunity to practice these skills.

Research suggests that DBT is an effective treatment for people with BPD. A recent study funded by the National Institute of Mental Health (NIMH) funded study found that DBT reduced suicide attempts by half compared to other types of treatment for patients with BPD.

Interpersonal Therapy

Interpersonal therapy (IPT) is most often used on a one-on-one basis to treat depression or dysthymia (a more persistent but less severe form of depression). The current manual-based form of IPT used today was developed in the 1980s by Gerald Klerman, M.D., and Myrna Weissman, M.D.

IPT is based on the idea that improving communication patterns and the ways people relate to others will effectively treat depression. IPT helps identify how a person interacts with other people. When a behavior is causing problems, IPT guides the person to change the behavior. IPT explores major issues that may add to a person's depression, such as grief, or times of upheaval or transition. Sometimes IPT is used along with antidepressant medications.

IPT varies depending on the needs of the patient and the relationship between the therapist and patient. Basically, a therapist using IPT helps the patient identify troubling emotions and their triggers. The therapist helps the patient learn to express appropriate emotions in a healthy way. The patient may also examine relationships in his or her past that may have been affected by distorted mood and behavior. Doing so can help the patient learn to be more objective about current relationships.

Studies vary as to the effectiveness of IPT. It may depend on the patient, the disorder, the severity of the disorder, and other variables. In general, however, IPT is found to be effective in treating depression.

A variation of IPT called interpersonal and social rhythm therapy (IPSRT) was developed to treat bipolar disorder. IPSRT combines the basic principles of IPT with behavioral psychoeducation designed to help patients adopt regular daily routines and sleep/wake cycles, stick with medication treatment, and improve relationships. Research has found that when IPSRT is combined with medication, it is an effective treatment for bipolar disorder. IPSRT is as effective as other types of psychotherapy combined with medication in helping to prevent a relapse of bipolar symptoms.

Family-Focused Therapy

Family-focused therapy (FFT) was developed by David Miklowitz, Ph.D., and Michael Goldstein, Ph.D., for treating bipolar disorder. It was designed with the assumption that a patient's relationship with his or her family is vital to the success of managing the illness. FFT includes family members in therapy sessions to improve family relationships, which may support better treatment results.

Therapists trained in FFT work to identify difficulties and conflicts among family members that may be worsening the patient's illness. Therapy is meant to help members find more effective ways to resolve those difficulties. The therapist educates family members about their loved one's disorder, its symptoms and course, and how to help their relative manage it more effectively. When families learn about the disorder, they may be able to spot early signs of a relapse and create an action plan that involves all family members. During therapy, the therapist will help family members recognize when they express unhelpful criticism or hostility toward their relative with bipolar disorder. The therapist will teach family members how to communicate negative emotions in a better way. Several studies have found FFT to be effective in helping a patient become stabilized and preventing relapses.

FFT also focuses on the stress family members feel when they care for a relative with bipolar disorder. The therapy aims to prevent family members from "burning out" or disengaging from the effort. The therapist helps the family accept how bipolar disorder can limit their relative. At the same time, the therapist holds the patient responsible for his or her own well being and actions to a level that is appropriate for the person's age.

Generally, the family and patient attend sessions together. The needs of each patient and family are different, and those needs determine the exact course of treatment. However, the main components of a structured FFT usually include family education on bipolar disorder, building communication skills to better deal with stress, and solving problems together as a family.

It is important to acknowledge and address the needs of family members. Research has shown that primary caregivers of people with bipolar disorder are at increased risk for illness themselves. For example, a 2007 study based on results from the NIMH-funded Systematic Treatment Enhancement Program for Bipolar Disorder (STEP-BD) trial found that primary caregivers of participants were at high risk for developing sleep problems and chronic conditions, such as high blood pressure. However, the caregivers were less likely to see a doctor for their own health issues. In addition, a 2005 study found that 33 percent of caregivers of bipolar patients had clinically significant levels of depression.

Psychotherapies for Children and Adolescents

Psychotherapies can be adapted to the needs of children and adolescents, depending on the mental disorder. For example, the NIMH-funded Treatment of Adolescents with Depression Study (TADS) found that CBT, when combined with antidepressant medication, was the most effective treatment over the short term for teens with major depression. CBT by itself was also an effective treatment, especially over the long term. Studies have found that individual and group-based CBT are effective treatments for child and adolescent anxiety disorders. Other studies have found that IPT is an effective treatment for child and adolescent depression.

Psychosocial treatments that involve a child's parents and family also have been shown to be effective, especially for disruptive disorders such as conduct disorder or oppositional defiant disorder. Some effective treatments are designed to reduce the child's problem behaviors and improve parent-child interactions. Focusing on behavioral parent management training, parents are taught the skills they need to encourage and reward positive behaviors in their children. Similar training helps parents manage their child's attention deficit/hyperactivity disorder (ADHD). This approach, which has been shown to be effective, can be combined with approaches directed at children to help them learn problem-solving, anger management and social interaction skills.

Family-based therapy may also be used to treat adolescents with eating disorders. One type is called the Maudsley approach, named after the Maudsley Hospital in London, where the approach was developed. This type of outpatient family therapy is used to treat anorexia nervosa in adolescents. It considers the active participation of parents to be essential in the recovery of their teen. The Maudsley approach proceeds through three phases:

- **Weight restoration:** Parents become fully responsible for ensuring that their teen eats. A therapist helps parents better understand their teen's disease. Parents learn how to avoid criticizing their teen, but they also learn to make sure that their teen eats.

- **Returning control over eating to the teen:** Once the teen accepts the control parents have over his or her eating habits, parents may begin giving up that control. Parents are encouraged to help their teen take more control over eating again.

- **Establishing healthy adolescent identity:** When the teen has reached and maintained a healthy weight, the therapist helps him or her begin developing a healthy sense of identity and autonomy.

Several studies have found the Maudsley approach to be successful in treating teens with anorexia. Currently a large-scale, NIMH-funded study on the approach is under way.

Other Types of Therapies

In addition to the therapies listed above, many more approaches exist. Some types have been scientifically tested more than others. Also, some of these therapies are constantly evolving. They are often combined with more established psychotherapies. A few examples of other therapies are described here.

Psychodynamic Therapy

Historically, psychodynamic therapy was tied to the principles of psychoanalytic theory, which asserts that a person's behavior is affected by his or her unconscious mind and past experiences. Now therapists who use psychodynamic therapy rarely include psychoanalytic methods. Rather, psychodynamic therapy helps people gain greater self-awareness and understanding about their own actions. It helps patients identify and explore how their nonconscious emotions and motivations can influence their behavior. Sometimes ideas from psychodynamic therapy are interwoven with other types of therapy, like CBT or IPT, to treat various types of mental disorders. Research on psychodynamic therapy is mixed. However, a review of 23 clinical trials involving psychodynamic therapy found it to be as effective as other established psychotherapies.

Light Therapy

Light therapy is used to treat seasonal affective disorder (SAD), a form of depression that usually occurs during the autumn and winter months, when the amount of natural sunlight decreases. Scientists think SAD occurs in some people when their bodies' daily rhythms are upset by short days and long nights. Research has found that the hormone melatonin is affected by this seasonal change. Melatonin normally works to regulate the body's rhythms and responses to light and dark. During light therapy, a person sits in front of a "light box" for periods of time, usually in the morning. The box emits a full spectrum light, and sitting in front of it appears to help reset the body's daily rhythms. Also, some research indicates that a low dose of melatonin, taken at specific times of the day, can also help treat SAD.

Additional Therapies

Other types of therapies sometimes used in conjunction with the more established therapies include:

Expressive or creative arts therapy: Expressive or creative arts therapy is based on the idea that people can help heal themselves through art, music, dance, writing, or other expressive acts. One study has found that expressive writing can reduce depression symptoms among women who were victims of domestic violence. It also helps college students at risk for depression.

Animal-assisted therapy: Working with animals, such as horses, dogs, or cats, may help some people cope with trauma, develop empathy, and encourage better communication. Companion animals are sometimes introduced in hospitals, psychiatric wards, nursing homes, and other places where they may bring comfort and have a mild therapeutic effect. Animal-assisted therapy has also been used as an added therapy for children with mental disorders. Research on the approach is limited, but a recent study found it to be moderately effective in easing behavioral problems and promoting emotional well-being.

Play therapy: This therapy is used with children. It involves the use of toys and games to help a child identify and talk about his or her feelings, as well as establish communication with a therapist. A therapist can sometimes better understand a child's problems by watching how he or she plays. Research in play therapy is minimal.

Section 21.3

Assertive Community Treatment

"ACT Model," © Assertive Community Treatment Association
(www.actassociation.org), reviewed 2012. Reprinted with permission.

Assertive Community Treatment (ACT) is a team treatment approach designed to provide comprehensive, community-based psychiatric treatment, rehabilitation, and support to persons with serious and persistent mental illness such as schizophrenia.

The ACT model of care evolved out of the work of Arnold Marx, M.D., Leonard Stein, and Mary Ann Test, Ph.D., in the late 1960s. ACT has been widely implemented in the United States, Canada, and England. The Department of Veterans Affairs has also implemented ACT across the United States.

A team of professionals whose backgrounds and training include social work, rehabilitation, counseling, nursing, and psychiatry provide Assertive Community Treatment services. Among the services ACT teams provide are: case management, initial and ongoing assessments; psychiatric services; employment and housing assistance; family support and education; substance abuse services; and other services and supports critical to an individual's ability to live successfully in the community. ACT services are available 24 hours per day, 365 days per year.

An evidence based practice, ACT has been extensively researched and evaluated and has proven clinical and cost effectiveness. The Schizophrenia Patient Outcomes Research Team (PORT) has identified ACT as an effective and underutilized treatment modality for persons with serious mental illness.

Persons Served by ACT

Clients served by ACT are individuals with serious and persistent mental illness or personality disorders, with severe functional impairments, who have avoided or not responded well to traditional outpatient mental health care and psychiatric rehabilitation services. Persons served by ACT often have co-existing problems such as homelessness, substance abuse problems, or involvement with the judicial system.

Principles of ACT

Assertive Community Treatment services adhere to certain essential standards and the following basic principles:

- **Primary provider of services:** The multidisciplinary make-up of each team (psychiatrist, nurses, social workers, rehabilitation, etc.) and the small client to staff ratio, helps the team provide most services with minimal referrals to other mental health programs or providers. The ACT team members share offices and their roles are interchangeable when providing services to ensure that services are not disrupted due to staff absence or turnover.

- **Services are provided out of office:** Services are provided within community settings, such as a person's own home and neighborhood, local restaurants, parks and nearby stores.

- **Highly individualized services:** Treatment plans, developed with the client, are based on individual strengths and needs, hopes and desires. The plans are modified as needed through an ongoing assessment and goal setting process.

- **Assertive approach:** ACT team members are pro-active with clients, assisting them to participate in and continue treatment, live independently, and recover from disability.

- **Long-term services:** ACT services are intended to be long-term due to the severe impairments often associated with serious and persistent mental illness. The process of recovery often takes many years.

- **Emphasis on vocational expectations:** The team encourages all clients to participate in community employment and provides many vocational rehabilitation services directly.

- **Substance abuse services:** The team coordinates and provides substance abuse services.

- **Psychoeducational services:** Staff work with clients and their family members to become collaborative partners in the treatment process. Clients are taught about mental illness and the skills needed to better manage their illnesses and their lives.

- **Family support and education:** With the active involvement of the client, ACT staff work to include the client's natural support systems (family, significant others) in treatment, educating them and including them as part of the ACT services. It is often necessary to help improve family relationships in order to reduce conflicts and increase client autonomy.

* **Community integration:** ACT staff help clients become less socially isolated and more integrated into the community by encouraging participation in community activities and membership in organizations of their choice.

* **Attention to health care needs:** The ACT team provides health education, access, and coordination of health care services.

Chapter 22

Mental Health Medications

Introduction

Medications are used to treat the symptoms of mental disorders such as schizophrenia, depression, bipolar disorder (sometimes called manic-depressive illness), anxiety disorders, and attention deficit-hyperactivity disorder (ADHD). Sometimes medications are used with other treatments such as psychotherapy. This chapter describes the types of medications used to treat mental disorders and their side effects. Information about medications is frequently updated. Check the FDA website (www.fda.gov) for the latest information on warnings, patient medication guides, or newly approved medications. Throughout this chapter, except in the alphabetical lists of trade names at the end, you will see two names for medications—the generic name and in parenthesis, the trade name. An example is fluoxetine (Prozac).

Psychiatric Medications

Psychiatric medications treat mental disorders. Sometimes called psychotropic or psychotherapeutic medications, they have changed the lives of people with mental disorders for the better. Many people with mental disorders live fulfilling lives with the help of these medications. Without them, people with mental disorders might suffer serious and disabling symptoms.

Excerpted from "Medications," National Institute of Mental Health (www .nimh.nih.gov), April 25, 2011.

Medications Used to Treat Mental Disorders

Medications treat the symptoms of mental disorders. They cannot cure the disorder, but they make people feel better so they can function.

Medications work differently for different people. Some people get great results from medications and only need them for a short time. For example, a person with depression may feel much better after taking a medication for a few months and may never need it again. People with disorders like schizophrenia or bipolar disorder or people who have long-term or severe depression or anxiety may need to take medication for a much longer time.

Some people get side effects from medications and other people don't. Doses can be small or large, depending on the medication and the person. The following are examples of factors that can affect how medications work in people:

- Type of mental disorder, such as depression, anxiety, bipolar disorder, and schizophrenia
- Age, sex, and body size
- Physical illnesses
- Habits like smoking and drinking
- Liver and kidney function
- Genetics
- Other medications and herbal/vitamin supplements
- Diet
- Whether medications are taken as prescribed.

Medications Used to Treat Schizophrenia

Antipsychotic medications are used to treat schizophrenia and schizophrenia-related disorders. Some of these medications have been available since the mid-1950s. They are also called conventional, *typical*, antipsychotics. Some of the more commonly used medications include the chlorpromazine (Thorazine), haloperidol (Haldol), perphenazine (generic only), and fluphenazine (generic only).

In the 1990s, new antipsychotic medications were developed. These new medications are called second generation, or *atypical* antipsychotics.

One of these medications was clozapine (Clozaril). It is a very effective medication that treats psychotic symptoms, hallucinations, and breaks with reality, such as when a person believes he or she is the president. But clozapine can sometimes cause a serious problem called agranulocytosis, which is a loss of the white blood cells that help a person fight infection. Therefore, people who take clozapine must get their white blood cell counts checked every week or two. This problem and the cost of blood tests make treatment with clozapine difficult for many people. Still, clozapine is potentially helpful for people who do not respond to other antipsychotic medications.

Other atypical antipsychotics were developed. All of them are effective, and none cause agranulocytosis. These include risperidone (Risperdal), olanzapine (Zyprexa), quetiapine (Seroquel), ziprasidone (Geodon), aripiprazole (Abilify), and paliperidone (Invega).

The antipsychotics listed here are some of the medications used to treat symptoms of schizophrenia. Additional antipsychotics and other medications used for schizophrenia are listed at the end of this chapter.

Note: The FDA issued a Public Health Advisory for atypical antipsychotic medications. The FDA determined that death rates are higher for elderly people with dementia when taking this medication. A review of data has found a risk with conventional antipsychotics as well. Antipsychotic medications are not FDA-approved for the treatment of behavioral disorders in patients with dementia.

What are the side effects?

Some people have side effects when they start taking these medications. Most side effects go away after a few days and often can be managed successfully. People who are taking antipsychotics should not drive until they adjust to their new medication. Side effects of many antipsychotics include drowsiness, dizziness when changing positions, blurred vision, rapid heartbeat, sensitivity to the sun, skin rashes, and for women, menstrual problems.

Atypical antipsychotic medications can cause major weight gain and changes in a person's metabolism. This may increase a person's risk of getting diabetes and high cholesterol. A person's weight, glucose levels, and lipid levels should be monitored regularly by a doctor while taking an atypical antipsychotic medication.

Typical antipsychotic medications can cause side effects related to physical movement. Some examples include rigidity, persistent muscle spasms, tremors, and restlessness.

Long-term use of typical antipsychotic medications may lead to a condition called tardive dyskinesia (TD). TD causes muscle movements a person can't control. The movements commonly happen around the mouth. TD can range from mild to severe, and in some people the problem cannot be cured. Sometimes people with TD recover partially or fully after they stop taking the medication.

Every year, an estimated five percent of people taking typical antipsychotics get TD. The condition happens to fewer people who take the new, atypical antipsychotics, but some people may still get TD. People who think that they might have TD should check with their doctor before stopping their medication.

How are antipsychotics taken and how do people respond to them?

Antipsychotics are usually pills that people swallow, or liquid they can drink. Some antipsychotics are shots that are given once or twice a month.

Symptoms of schizophrenia, such as feeling agitated and having hallucinations, usually go away within days. Symptoms like delusions usually go away within a few weeks. After about six weeks, many people will see a lot of improvement.

However, people respond in different ways to antipsychotic medications, and no one can tell beforehand how a person will respond. Sometimes a person needs to try several medications before finding the right one. Doctors and patients can work together to find the best medication or medication combination, and dose.

Some people may have a relapse—their symptoms come back or get worse. Usually, relapses happen when people stop taking their medication, or when they only take it sometimes. Some people stop taking the medication because they feel better or they may feel they don't need it anymore. But no one should stop taking an antipsychotic medication without talking to his or her doctor. When a doctor says it is okay to stop taking a medication, it should be gradually tapered off, never stopped suddenly.

How do antipsychotics interact with other medications?

Antipsychotics can produce unpleasant or dangerous side effects when taken with certain medications. For this reason, all doctors treating a patient need to be aware of all the medications that person is taking. Doctors need to know about prescription and over-the-counter medicine, vitamins, minerals, and herbal supplements. People also need to discuss any alcohol or other drug use with their doctor.

To find out more about how antipsychotics work, the National Institute of Mental Health (NIMH) funded a study called CATIE (Clinical

Antipsychotic Trials of Intervention Effectiveness). This study compared the effectiveness and side effects of five antipsychotics used to treat people with schizophrenia. In general, the study found that the older medication perphenazine worked as well as the newer, atypical medications. But because people respond differently to different medications, it is important that treatments be designed carefully for each person.

Medications Used to Treat Depression

Depression is commonly treated with antidepressant medications. Antidepressants work to balance some of the natural chemicals in our brains. These chemicals are called neurotransmitters, and they affect our mood and emotional responses. Antidepressants work on neurotransmitters such as serotonin, norepinephrine, and dopamine.

The most popular types of antidepressants are called selective serotonin reuptake inhibitors (SSRIs). These include fluoxetine (Prozac), citalopram (Celexa), sertraline (Zoloft), paroxetine (Paxil), and escitalopram (Lexapro). Other types of antidepressants are serotonin and norepinephrine reuptake inhibitors (SNRIs). SNRIs are similar to SSRIs and include venlafaxine (Effexor) and duloxetine (Cymbalta). Another antidepressant that is commonly used is bupropion (Wellbutrin). Bupropion, which works on the neurotransmitter dopamine, is unique in that it does not fit into any specific drug type.

SSRIs and SNRIs are popular because they do not cause as many side effects as older classes of antidepressants. Older antidepressant medications include tricyclics, tetracyclics, and monoamine oxidase inhibitors (MAOIs). Tricyclics, tetracyclics, or MAOIs may be the best medications for some people.

What are the side effects?

Antidepressants may cause mild side effects that usually do not last long. Any unusual reactions or side effects should be reported to a doctor immediately.

The most common side effects associated with SSRIs and SNRIs include the following:

- Headache, which usually goes away within a few days

- Nausea (feeling sick to your stomach), which usually goes away within a few days

- Sleeplessness or drowsiness, which may happen during the first few weeks but then goes away (Sometimes the medication dose

311

needs to be reduced or the time of day it is taken needs to be adjusted to help lessen these side effects.)

- Agitation (feeling jittery)

- Sexual problems, which can affect both men and women and may include reduced sex drive, and problems having and enjoying sex

Tricyclic antidepressants can cause side effects such as these:

- Dry mouth

- Constipation

- Bladder problems. It may be hard to empty the bladder, or the urine stream may not be as strong as usual. Older men with enlarged prostate conditions may be more affected.

- Sexual problems, which can affect both men and women and may include reduced sex drive, and problems having and enjoying sex

- Blurred vision, which usually goes away quickly

- Drowsiness. Usually, antidepressants that make you drowsy are taken at bedtime.

People taking MAOIs need to be careful about the foods they eat and the medicines they take. Foods and medicines that contain high levels of a chemical called tyramine are dangerous for people taking MAOIs. Tyramine is found in some cheeses, wines, and pickles. The chemical is also in some medications, including decongestants and over-the-counter cold medicine.

Mixing MAOIs and tyramine can cause a sharp increase in blood pressure, which can lead to stroke. People taking MAOIs should ask their doctors for a complete list of foods, medicines, and other substances to avoid. An MAOI skin patch has recently been developed and may help reduce some of these risks. A doctor can help a person figure out if a patch or a pill will work for him or her.

How should antidepressants be taken?

People taking antidepressants need to follow their doctors' directions. The medication should be taken in the right dose for the right amount of time. It can take three or four weeks until the medicine takes effect. Some people take the medications for a short time, and some people take them for much longer periods. People with long-term or severe depression may need to take medication for a long time.

Once a person is taking antidepressants, it is important not to stop taking them without the help of a doctor. Sometimes people taking antidepressants feel better and stop taking the medication too soon, and the depression may return. When it is time to stop the medication, the doctor will help the person slowly and safely decrease the dose. It's important to give the body time to adjust to the change. People don't get addicted, or "hooked," on the medications, but stopping them abruptly can cause withdrawal symptoms.

If a medication does not work, it is helpful to be open to trying another one. A study funded by NIMH found that if a person with difficult-to-treat depression did not get better with a first medication, chances of getting better increased when the person tried a new one or added a second medication to his or her treatment. The study was called STAR*D (Sequenced Treatment Alternatives to Relieve Depression).

Are herbal medicines used to treat depression?

The herbal medicine St. John's wort has been used for centuries in many folk and herbal remedies. Today in Europe, it is used widely to treat mild-to-moderate depression. In the United States, it is one of the top-selling botanical products.

The National Institutes of Health conducted a clinical trial to determine the effectiveness of treating adults who have major depression with St. John's wort. The study included 340 people diagnosed with major depression. One-third of the people took the herbal medicine, one-third took an SSRI, and one-third took a placebo ("sugar pill"). The people did not know what they were taking. The study found that St. John's wort was no more effective than the placebo in treating major depression. A study currently in progress is looking at the effectiveness of St. John's wort for treating mild or minor depression.

Other research has shown that St. John's wort can dangerously interact with other medications, including those used to control HIV. On February 10, 2000, the FDA issued a Public Health Advisory letter stating that the herb appears to interfere with certain medications used to treat heart disease, depression, seizures, certain cancers, and organ transplant rejection. Also, St. Johns wort may interfere with oral contraceptives.

Because St. John's wort may not mix well with other medications, people should always talk with their doctors before taking it or any herbal supplement.

FDA Warning on Antidepressants

Antidepressants are safe and popular, but some studies have suggested that they may have unintentional effects, especially in young people. In 2004, the FDA looked at published and unpublished data on trials of antidepressants that involved nearly 4,400 children and adolescents. They found that four percent of those taking antidepressants thought about or tried suicide (although no suicides occurred) compared to two percent of those receiving placebos.

In 2005, the FDA decided to adopt a black box warning label—the most serious type of warning—on all antidepressant medications. The warning says there is an increased risk of suicidal thinking or attempts in children and adolescents taking antidepressants. In 2007, the FDA proposed that makers of all antidepressant medications extend the warning to include young adults up through age 24.

The warning also says that patients of all ages taking antidepressants should be watched closely, especially during the first few weeks of treatment. Possible side effects to look for are depression that gets worse, suicidal thinking or behavior, or any unusual changes in behavior such as trouble sleeping, agitation, or withdrawal from normal social situations. Families and caregivers should report any changes to the doctor. To find the latest information visit the FDA website.

Results of a comprehensive review of pediatric trials conducted between 1988 and 2006 suggested that the benefits of antidepressant medications likely outweigh their risks to children and adolescents with major depression and anxiety disorders. The study was funded in part by NIMH.

Finally, the FDA has warned that combining the newer SSRI or SNRI antidepressants with one of the commonly used triptan medications used to treat migraine headaches could cause a life-threatening illness called serotonin syndrome. A person with serotonin syndrome may be agitated, have hallucinations (see or hear things that are not real), have a high temperature, or have unusual blood pressure changes. Serotonin syndrome is usually associated with the older antidepressants called MAOIs, but it can happen with the newer antidepressants as well if they are mixed with the wrong medications.

Medications Used to Treat Bipolar Disorder

Bipolar disorder, also called manic-depressive illness, is commonly treated with mood stabilizers. Sometimes, antipsychotics and antidepressants are used along with a mood stabilizer.

Mood stabilizers: People with bipolar disorder usually try mood stabilizers first. In general, people continue treatment with mood stabilizers for years. Lithium is a very effective mood stabilizer. It was the first mood stabilizer approved by the FDA in the 1970s for treating both manic and depressive episodes.

Anticonvulsant medications also are used as mood stabilizers. They were originally developed to treat seizures, but they were found to help control moods as well. One anticonvulsant commonly used as a mood stabilizer is valproic acid, also called divalproex sodium (Depakote). For some people, it may work better than lithium. Other anticonvulsants used as mood stabilizers are carbamazepine (Tegretol), lamotrigine (Lamictal) and oxcarbazepine (Trileptal).

Atypical antipsychotics: Atypical antipsychotic medications are sometimes used to treat symptoms of bipolar disorder. Often, antipsychotics are used along with other medications.

Antipsychotics used to treat people with bipolar disorder include the following:

- Olanzapine (Zyprexa), which helps people with severe or psychotic depression, which often is accompanied by a break with reality, hallucinations, or delusions

- Aripiprazole (Abilify), which can be taken as a pill or as a shot

- Risperidone (Risperdal)

- Ziprasidone (Geodon)

- Clozapine (Clozaril), which is often used for people who do not respond to lithium or anticonvulsants.

Antidepressants: Antidepressants are sometimes used to treat symptoms of depression in bipolar disorder. Fluoxetine (Prozac), paroxetine (Paxil), or sertraline (Zoloft) are a few that are used. However, people with bipolar disorder should not take an antidepressant on its own. Doing so can cause the person to rapidly switch from depression to mania, which can be dangerous. To prevent this problem, doctors give patients a mood stabilizer or an antipsychotic along with an antidepressant.

Research on whether antidepressants help people with bipolar depression is mixed. An NIMH-funded study called STEP-BD (Systematic Treatment Enhancement Program for Bipolar Disorder) found that antidepressants were no more effective than a placebo to help treat depression in people with bipolar disorder. The people were taking mood stabilizers along with the antidepressants.

What are the side effects?

Treatments for bipolar disorder have improved over the last 10 years. But everyone responds differently to medications. If you have any side effects, tell your doctor right away. He or she may change the dose or prescribe a different medication.

Different medications for treating bipolar disorder may cause different side effects. Some medications used for treating bipolar disorder have been linked to unique and serious symptoms, which are described below.

Lithium can cause several side effects, and some of them may become serious. Lithium's side effects include loss of coordination, excessive thirst, frequent urination, blackouts, seizures, slurred speech, fast, slow, irregular, or pounding heartbeat, hallucinations (seeing things or hearing voices that do not exist), changes in vision, itching, rash, and swelling of the eyes, face, lips, tongue, throat, hands, feet, ankles, or lower legs.

If a person with bipolar disorder is being treated with lithium, he or she should visit the doctor regularly to check the levels of lithium in the blood, and make sure the kidneys and the thyroid are working normally.

Some possible side effects linked with valproic acid/divalproex sodium include changes in weight, nausea, stomach pain, vomiting, anorexia, and loss of appetite. Valproic acid may also cause damage to the liver or pancreas, so people taking it should see their doctors regularly.

Valproic acid may affect young girls and women in unique ways. Sometimes, valproic acid may increase testosterone (a male hormone) levels in teenage girls and lead to a condition called polycystic ovarian syndrome (PCOS). PCOS is a disease that can affect fertility and make the menstrual cycle become irregular, but symptoms tend to go away after valproic acid is stopped. It also may cause birth defects in women who are pregnant.

Lamotrigine can cause a rare but serious skin rash that needs to be treated in a hospital. In some cases, this rash can cause permanent disability or be life-threatening.

In addition, valproic acid, lamotrigine, carbamazepine, oxcarbazepine and other anticonvulsant medications (listed at the end of this chapter) have an FDA warning. The warning states that their use may increase the risk of suicidal thoughts and behaviors. People taking anticonvulsant medications for bipolar or other illnesses should be closely monitored for new or worsening symptoms of depression, suicidal thoughts or behavior, or any unusual changes in mood or behavior.

People taking these medications should not make any changes without talking to their health care professional.

Other medications for bipolar disorder may also be linked with rare but serious side effects. Always talk with the doctor or pharmacist about any potential side effects before taking the medication. For more information on side effects of antipsychotics, see the section on medications for treating schizophrenia. For more information on side effects and FDA warnings of antidepressants, see the section on medications for treating depression.

How should medications for bipolar disorder be taken?

Medications should be taken as directed by a doctor. Sometimes a person's treatment plan needs to be changed. When changes in medicine are needed, the doctor will guide the change. A person should never stop taking a medication without asking a doctor for help.

There is no cure for bipolar disorder, but treatment works for many people. Treatment works best when it is continuous, rather than on and off. However, mood changes can happen even when there are no breaks in treatment. Patients should be open with their doctors about treatment. Talking about how treatment is working can help it be more effective.

It may be helpful for people or their family members to keep a daily chart of mood symptoms, treatments, sleep patterns, and life events. This chart can help patients and doctors track the illness. Doctors can use the chart to treat the illness most effectively.

Because medications for bipolar disorder can have serious side effects, it is important for anyone taking them to see the doctor regularly to check for possibly dangerous changes in the body.

Medications Used to Treat Anxiety Disorders

Antidepressants, anti-anxiety medications, and beta-blockers are the most common medications used for anxiety disorders. Obsessive compulsive disorder (OCD), post-traumatic stress disorder (PTSD), generalized anxiety disorder (GAD), panic disorder, and social phobia are examples of anxiety disorders.

Antidepressants: Antidepressants were developed to treat depression, but they also help people with anxiety disorders. SSRIs such as fluoxetine (Prozac), sertraline (Zoloft), escitalopram (Lexapro), paroxetine (Paxil), and citalopram (Celexa) are commonly prescribed for panic disorder, OCD, PTSD, and social phobia. The SNRI venlafaxine (Effexor) is commonly used to treat GAD. The antidepressant bupropion (Wellbutrin) is also sometimes used. When treating anxiety disorders, antidepressants generally are started at low doses and increased over time.

Some tricyclic antidepressants work well for anxiety. For example, imipramine (Tofranil) is prescribed for panic disorder and GAD. Clomipramine (Anafranil) is used to treat OCD. Tricyclics are also started at low doses and increased over time.

MAOIs are also used for anxiety disorders. Doctors sometimes prescribe phenelzine (Nardil), tranylcypromine (Parnate), and isocarboxazid (Marplan). People who take MAOIs must avoid certain food and medicines that can interact with their medicine and cause dangerous increases in blood pressure. For more information, see the section on medications used to treat depression.

Benzodiazepines (anti-anxiety medications): The anti-anxiety medications called benzodiazepines can start working more quickly than antidepressants. The ones used to treat anxiety disorders include clonazepam (Klonopin), which is used for social phobia and GAD; lorazepam (Ativan), which is used for panic disorder; and alprazolam (Xanax), which is used for panic disorder and GAD. Buspirone (BuSpar) is an anti-anxiety medication used to treat GAD. Unlike benzodiazepines, however, it takes at least two weeks for buspirone to begin working. Clonazepam is an anticonvulsant medication. See FDA warning on anticonvulsants under the bipolar disorder section.

Beta-blockers: Beta-blockers control some of the physical symptoms of anxiety, such as trembling and sweating. Propranolol (Inderal) is a beta-blocker usually used to treat heart conditions and high blood pressure. The medicine also helps people who have physical problems related to anxiety. For example, when a person with social phobia must face a stressful situation, such as giving a speech, or attending an important meeting, a doctor may prescribe a beta-blocker. Taking the medicine for a short period of time can help the person keep physical symptoms under control.

What are the side effects?

See the section on antidepressants for a discussion on side effects. The most common side effects for benzodiazepines are drowsiness and dizziness. Other possible side effects include upset stomach, blurred vision, headache, confusion, grogginess, and nightmares.

Buspirone (BuSpar) may cause side effects such as dizziness, headaches, nausea, nervousness, lightheadedness, excitement, and trouble sleeping.

Common side effects from beta-blockers include fatigue, cold hands, dizziness, and weakness. In addition, beta-blockers generally are not recommended for people with asthma or diabetes because they may worsen symptoms.

How should medications for anxiety disorders be taken?

People can build a tolerance to benzodiazepines if they are taken over a long period of time and may need higher and higher doses to get the same effect. Some people may become dependent on them. To avoid these problems, doctors usually prescribe the medication for short periods, a practice that is especially helpful for people who have substance abuse problems or who become dependent on medication easily. If people suddenly stop taking benzodiazepines, they may get withdrawal symptoms, or their anxiety may return. Therefore, they should be tapered off slowly.

Buspirone and beta-blockers are similar. They are usually taken on a short-term basis for anxiety. Both should be tapered off slowly. Talk to the doctor before stopping any anti-anxiety medication.

Medications Used to Treat ADHD

Attention deficit/hyperactivity disorder (ADHD) occurs in both children and adults. ADHD is commonly treated with stimulants, such as methylphenidate (Ritalin, Metadate, Concerta, Daytrana), amphetamine (Adderall), and dextroamphetamine (Dexedrine, Dextrostat).

In 2002, the FDA approved the nonstimulant medication atomoxetine (Strattera) for use as a treatment for ADHD. In February 2007, the FDA approved the use of the stimulant lisdexamfetamine dimesylate (Vyvanse) for the treatment of ADHD in children ages 6 to 12 years.

What are the side effects?

Most side effects are minor and disappear when dosage levels are lowered. The most common side effects include the following:

- **Decreased appetite:** Children seem to be less hungry during the middle of the day, but they are often hungry by dinnertime as the medication wears off.

- **Sleep problems:** If a child cannot fall asleep, the doctor may prescribe a lower dose. The doctor might also suggest that parents give the medication to their child earlier in the day, or stop the afternoon or evening dose. To help ease sleeping problems, a doctor may add a prescription for a low dose of an antidepressant or a medication called clonidine.

- **Stomachaches and headaches**

- **Less common side effects:** A few children develop sudden, repetitive movements or sounds called tics. These tics may or may not be noticeable. Changing the medication dosage may make tics go away. Some children also may appear to have a personality change, such as appearing "flat" or without emotion. Talk with your child's doctor if you see any of these side effects.

How are ADHD medications taken?

Stimulant medications can be short-acting or long-acting, and can be taken in different forms such as a pill, patch, or powder. Long-acting, sustained, and extended release forms allow children to take the medication just once a day before school. Parents and doctors should decide together which medication is best for the child and whether the child needs medication only for school hours or for evenings and weekends too.

ADHD medications help many children and adults who are hyperactive and impulsive. They help people focus, work, and learn. Stimulant medication also may improve physical coordination. However, different people respond differently to medications, so children taking ADHD medications should be watched closely.

Are ADHD medications safe?

Stimulant medications are safe when given under a doctor's supervision. Some children taking them may feel slightly different or "funny." Some parents worry that stimulant medications may lead to drug abuse or dependence, but there is little evidence of this. Research shows that teens with ADHD who took stimulant medications were less likely to abuse drugs than those who did not take stimulant medications.

FDA Warning on Possible Rare Side Effects

In 2007, the FDA required that all makers of ADHD medications develop Patient Medication Guides. The guides must alert patients to possible heart and psychiatric problems related to ADHD medicine. The FDA required the Patient Medication Guides because a review of data found that ADHD patients with heart conditions had a slightly higher risk of strokes, heart attacks, and sudden death when taking the medications. The review also found a slightly higher risk (about 1 in 1,000) for medication-related psychiatric problems, such as hearing voices, having hallucinations, becoming suspicious for no reason, or becoming manic. This happened to patients who had no history of psychiatric problems.

The FDA recommends that any treatment plan for ADHD include an initial health and family history examination. This exam should look for existing heart and psychiatric problems.

The non-stimulant ADHD medication called atomoxetine (Strattera) carries another warning. Studies show that children and teenagers with ADHD who take atomoxetine are more likely to have suicidal thoughts than children and teenagers with ADHD who do not take atomoxetine. If your child is taking atomoxetine, watch his or her behavior carefully. A child may develop serious symptoms suddenly, so it is important to pay attention to your child's behavior every day. Ask other people who spend a lot of time with your child, such as brothers, sisters, and teachers, to tell you if they notice changes in your child's behavior. Call a doctor right away if your child shows any of the following symptoms: acting more subdued or withdrawn than usual; feeling helpless, hopeless, or worthless; new or worsening depression; thinking or talking about hurting himself or herself; extreme worry; agitation; panic attacks; trouble sleeping; irritability; aggressive or violent behavior; acting without thinking; extreme increase in activity or talking; frenzied, abnormal excitement; or any sudden or unusual changes in behavior.

While taking atomoxetine, your child should see a doctor often, especially at the beginning of treatment. Be sure that your child keeps all appointments with his or her doctor.

Groups That Have Special Needs When Taking Psychiatric Medications

Psychiatric medications are taken by all types of people, but some groups have special needs, especially children and adolescents, older adults, and women who are pregnant or may become pregnant.

Children and Adolescents

Most medications used to treat young people with mental illness are safe and effective. However, many medications have not been studied or approved for use with children. Researchers are not sure how these medications affect a child's growing body. Still, a doctor can give a young person an FDA-approved medication on an *off-label* basis. This means that the doctor prescribes the medication to help the patient even though the medicine is not approved for the specific mental disorder or age.

For these reasons, it is important to watch young people who take these medications. Young people may have different reactions and side effects than adults. Also, some medications, including antidepressants and ADHD medications, carry FDA warnings about potentially dangerous side effects for young people. See the sections on antidepressants and ADHD medications for more information about these warnings.

More research is needed on how these medications affect children and adolescents. NIMH has funded studies on this topic. For example, NIMH funded the Preschoolers with ADHD Treatment Study (PATS), which involved 300 preschoolers (three to five years old) diagnosed with ADHD. The study found that low doses of the stimulant methylphenidate are safe and effective for preschoolers. However, children of this age are more sensitive to the side effects of the medication, including slower growth rates. Children taking methylphenidate should be watched closely.

In addition to medications, other treatments for young people with mental disorders should be considered. Psychotherapy, family therapy, educational courses, and behavior management techniques can help everyone involved cope with the disorder.

Older Adults

Because older people often have more medical problems than other groups, they tend to take more medications than younger people, including prescribed, over-the-counter, and herbal medications. As a result, older people have a higher risk for experiencing bad drug interactions, missing doses, or overdosing.

Older people also tend to be more sensitive to medications. Even healthy older people react to medications differently than younger people because their bodies process it more slowly. Therefore, lower or less frequent doses may be needed.

Sometimes memory problems affect older people who take medications for mental disorders. An older adult may forget his or her regular dose and take too much or not enough. A good way to keep track of medicine is to use a seven-day pill box, which can be bought at any pharmacy. At the beginning of each week, older adults and their caregivers fill the box so that it is easy to remember what medicine to take. Many pharmacies also have pillboxes with sections for medications that must be taken more than once a day.

Women Who Are Pregnant or May Become Pregnant

The research on the use of psychiatric medications during pregnancy is limited. The risks are different depending on what medication is taken, and at what point during the pregnancy the medication is taken. Research has shown that antidepressants, especially SSRIs, are safe during pregnancy. Birth defects or other problems are possible, but they are very rare.

However, antidepressant medications do cross the placental barrier and may reach the fetus. Some research suggests the use of SSRIs during pregnancy is associated with miscarriage or birth defects, but other studies do not support this. Studies have also found that fetuses exposed to SSRIs during the third trimester may be born with withdrawal symptoms such as breathing problems, jitteriness, irritability, trouble feeding, or hypoglycemia (low blood sugar).

Most studies have found that these symptoms in babies are generally mild and short-lived, and no deaths have been reported. On the flip side, women who stop taking their antidepressant medication during pregnancy may get depression again and may put both themselves and their infant at risk.

In 2004, the FDA issued a warning against the use of certain antidepressants in the late third trimester. The warning said that doctors may want to gradually taper pregnant women off antidepressants in the third trimester so that the baby is not affected. After a woman delivers, she should consult with her doctor to decide whether to return to a full dose during the period when she is most vulnerable to postpartum depression.

Some medications should not be taken during pregnancy. Benzodiazepines may cause birth defects or other infant problems, especially if taken during the first trimester. Mood stabilizers are known to cause birth defects. Benzodiazepines and lithium have been shown to cause floppy baby syndrome, which is when a baby is drowsy and limp and cannot breathe or feed well.

Research suggests that taking antipsychotic medications during pregnancy can lead to birth defects, especially if they are taken during the first trimester. But results vary widely depending on the type of antipsychotic. The conventional antipsychotic haloperidol has been studied more than others, and has been found not to cause birth defects.

After the baby is born, women and their doctors should watch for postpartum depression, especially if they stopped taking their medication during pregnancy. In addition, women who nurse while taking psychiatric medications should know that a small amount of the medication passes into the breast milk. However, the medication may or may not affect the baby. It depends on the medication and when it is taken. Women taking psychiatric medications and who intend to breastfeed should discuss the potential risks and benefits with their doctors.

Decisions on medication should be based on each woman's needs and circumstances. Medications should be selected based on available scientific research, and they should be taken at the lowest possible dose. Pregnant women should be watched closely throughout their pregnancy and after delivery.

What to Ask Your Doctor about Psychiatric Medications

You and your family can help your doctor find the right medications for you. The doctor needs to know your medical history; family history; information about allergies; other medications, supplements or herbal remedies you take; and other details about your overall health. You or a family member should ask the following questions when a medication is prescribed:

- What is the name of the medication?
- What is the medication supposed to do?
- How and when should I take it?
- How much should I take?
- What should I do if I miss a dose?
- When and how should I stop taking it?
- Will it interact with other medications I take?
- Do I need to avoid any types of food or drink while taking the medication? What should I avoid?
- Should it be taken with or without food?
- Is it safe to drink alcohol while taking this medication?
- What are the side effects? What should I do if I experience them?
- Is the Patient Package Insert for the medication available?

After taking the medication for a short time, tell your doctor how you feel, if you are having side effects, and any concerns you have about the medicine.

Alphabetical List of Medications

This section identifies antipsychotic medications, antidepressant medications, mood stabilizers, anticonvulsant medications, anti-anxiety medications, and ADHD medications. Some medications are marketed under trade names, not all of which can be listed here. The first section lists the medications by trade name; the second section lists the medications by generic name. If your medication does not appear in this section, refer to the FDA website (www.fda.gov). Also, ask your doctor or pharmacist for more information about any medication.

Medications Organized by Trade Name

Combination Antipsychotic and Antidepressant Medication

- Symbyax [Prozac & Zyprexa] (fluoxetine and olanzapine): FDA approved age 18 and older

Antipsychotic Medications

- Abilify (aripiprazole): FDA approved age 10 and older for bipolar disorder, manic or mixed episodes; 13 to 17 for schizophrenia and bipolar;
- Clozaril (clozapine): FDA approved age 18 and older
- Fanapt (iloperidone): FDA approved age 18 and older
- Fluphenazine (generic only): FDA approved age 18 and older
- Geodon (ziprasidone): FDA approved age 18 and older
- Haldol (haloperidol): FDA approved age 3 and older
- Invega (paliperidone): FDA approved age 18 and older
- Loxitane (loxapine): FDA approved age 18 and older
- Moban (molindone): FDA approved age 18 and older
- Navane (thiothixene): FDA approved age 18 and older
- Orap [for Tourette's syndrome] (pimozide): FDA approved age 12 and older
- Perphenazine (generic only): FDA approved age 18 and older
- Risperdal (risperidone): FDA approved age 13 and older for schizophrenia; 10 and older for bipolar mania and mixed episodes; 5 to 16 for irritability associated with autism
- Seroquel (quetiapine): FDA approved age 13 and older for schizophrenia; 18 and older for bipolar disorder; 10-17 for treatment of manic and mixed episodes of bipolar disorder.
- Stelazine (trifluoperazine): FDA approved age 18 and older
- Thioridazine (generic only): FDA approved age 2 and older
- Thorazine (chlorpromazine): FDA approved age 18 and older

- Zyprexa (olanzapine): FDA approved age 18 and older; ages 13–17 as second line treatment for manic or mixed episodes of bipolar disorder and schizophrenia.

Antidepressant Medications (also used for anxiety disorders)

- Anafranil [tricyclic] (clomipramine): FDA approved age 10 and older [for OCD only]
- Asendin (amoxapine): FDA approved age 18 and older
- Aventyl [tricyclic] (nortriptyline): FDA approved age 18 and older
- Celexa [SSRI] (citalopram): FDA approved age 18 and older
- Cymbalta [SNRI] (duloxetine): FDA approved age 18 and older
- Desyrel (trazodone): FDA approved age 18 and older
- Effexor [SNRI] (venlafaxine): FDA approved age 18 and older
- Elavil [tricyclic] (amitriptyline): FDA approved age 18 and older
- Emsam (selegiline): FDA approved age 18 and older
- Lexapro [SSRI] (escitalopram): FDA approved age 18 and older; 12–17 (for major depressive disorder)
- Ludiomil [tricyclic] (maprotiline): FDA approved age 18 and older
- Luvox [SSRI] (fluvoxamine): FDA approved age 8 and older (for OCD only)
- Marplan [MAOI] (isocarboxazid): FDA approved age 18 and older
- Nardil [MAOI] (phenelzine): FDA approved age 18 and older
- Norpramin [tricyclic] (desipramine): FDA approved age 18 and older
- Pamelor [tricyclic] (nortriptyline): FDA approved age 18 and older
- Parnate [MAOI] (tranylcypromine): FDA approved age 18 and older
- Paxil [SSRI] (paroxetine): FDA approved age 18 and older
- Pexeva [SSRI] (paroxetine-mesylate): FDA approved age 18 and older
- Pristiq (desvenlafaxine [SNRI]): FDA approved age 18 and older
- Prozac [SSRI] (fluoxetine): FDA approved age 8 and older
- Remeron (mirtazapine): FDA approved age 18 and older

- Sarafem [SSRI] (fluoxetine): FDA approved age 18 and older for premenstrual dysphoric disorder (PMDD)

- Sinequan[tricyclic] (doxepin): FDA approved age 12 and older

- Surmontil[tricyclic] (trimipramine): FDA approved age 18 and older

- Tofranil[tricyclic] (imipramine): FDA approved age 6 and older (for bedwetting)

- Tofranil-PM[tricyclic] (imipramine pamoate): FDA approved age 18 and older

- Vivactil[tricyclic] (protriptyline): FDA approved age 18 and older

- Wellbutrin (bupropion): FDA approved age 18 and older

- Zoloft [SSRI] (sertraline): FDA approved age 6 and older (for OCD only)

Mood Stabilizing and Anticonvulsant Medications

- Depakote (divalproex sodium [valproic acid]): FDA approved age 2 and older (for seizures)

- Eskalith (lithium carbonate): FDA approved age 12 and older

- Lamictal (lamotrigine): FDA approved age 18 and older

- Lithium citrate (generic only): FDA approved age 12 and older

- Lithobid (lithium carbonate): FDA approved age 12 and older

- Neurontin (gabapentin): FDA approved age 18 and older

- Tegretol (carbamazepine): FDA approved age any age (for seizures)

- Topamax (topiramate): FDA approved age 18 and older

- Trileptal (oxcarbazepine): FDA approved age 4 and older

Anti-Anxiety Medications

All of these anti-anxiety medications are benzodiazepines, except BuSpar.

- Ativan (lorazepam): FDA approved age 18 and older

- BuSpar (buspirone): FDA approved age 18 and older

- Klonopin (clonazepam): FDA approved age 18 and older

- Librium (chlordiazepoxide): FDA approved age 18 and older
- Oxazepam (generic only): FDA approved age 18 and older
- Tranxene (clorazepate): FDA approved age 18 and older
- Valium (diazepam): FDA approved age 18 and older
- Xanax (alprazolam): FDA approved age 18 and older

ADHD Medications

All of these ADHD medications are stimulants, except Intuniv and Strattera.

- Adderall (amphetamine): FDA approved age 3 and older
- Adderall XR (amphetamine [extended release]): FDA approved age 6 and older
- Concerta (methylphenidate [long acting]): FDA approved age 6 and older
- Daytrana (methylphenidate patch): FDA approved age 6 and older
- Desoxyn (methamphetamine): FDA approved age 6 and older
- Dexedrine (dextroamphetamine): FDA approved age 3 and older
- Dextrostat (dextroamphetamine): FDA approved age 3 and older
- Focalin (dexmethylphenidate): FDA approved age 6 and older
- Focalin XR (dexmethylphenidate [extended release]): FDA approved age 6 and older
- Intuniv (guanfacine): FDA approved age 6 and older
- Metadate ER (methylphenidate [extended release]): FDA approved age 6 and older
- Metadate CD (methylphenidate [extended release]): FDA approved age 6 and older
- Methylin (methylphenidate [oral solution and chewable tablets]): FDA approved age 6 and older
- Ritalin (methylphenidate): FDA approved age 6 and older
- Ritalin SR (methylphenidate [extended release]): FDA approved age 6 and older
- Ritalin LA (methylphenidate [long-acting]): FDA approved age 6 and older

- Strattera (atomoxetine): FDA approved age 6 and older
- Vyvanse (lisdexamfetamine dimesylate): FDA approved age 6 and older

Medications Organized by Generic Name

Combination Antipsychotic and Antidepressant Medication

- fluoxetine and olanzapine (Symbyax [Prozac and Zyprexa]): FDA approved age 18 and older

Antipsychotic Medications

- aripiprazole (Abilify): FDA approved age 10 and older for bipolar disorder, manic or mixed episodes; 13 to 17 for schizophrenia and bipolar disorder
- chlorpromazine (Thorazine): FDA approved age 18 and older
- clozapine (Clozaril): FDA approved age 18 and older
- fluphenazine (generic only): FDA approved age 18 and older
- haloperidol (Haldol): FDA approved age 3 and older
- iloperidone (Fanapt): FDA approved age 18 and older
- loxapine (Loxitane): FDA approved age 18 and older
- molindone (Moban): FDA approved age 18 and older
- olanzapine (Zyprexa): FDA approved age 18 and older; ages 13–17 as second line treatment for manic or mixed episodes of bipolar disorder and schizophrenia
- paliperidone (Invega): FDA approved age 18 and older
- perphenazine (generic only): FDA approved age 18 and older
- pimozide [for Tourette's syndrome] (Orap): FDA approved age 12 and older
- quetiapine (Seroquel): FDA approved age 13 and older for schizophrenia;18 and older for bipolar disorder; 10–17 for treatment of manic and mixed episodes of bipolar disorder
- risperidone (Risperdal): FDA approved age 13 and older for schizophrenia;10 and older for bipolar mania and mixed episodes; 5 to 16 for irritability associated with autism
- thioridazine (generic only): FDA approved age 2 and older

- thiothixene (Navane): FDA approved age 18 and older

- trifluoperazine (Stelazine): FDA approved age 18 and older

- ziprasidone (Geodon): FDA approved age 18 and older

Antidepressant Medications (also used for anxiety disorders)

- amitriptyline [tricyclic] (Elavil): FDA approved age 18 and older

- amoxapine (Asendin): FDA approved age 18 and older

- bupropion (Wellbutrin): FDA approved age 18 and older

- citalopram [SSRI] (Celexa): FDA approved age 18 and older

- clomipramine [tricyclic] (Anafranil): FDA approved age 10 and older (for OCD only)

- desipramine [tricyclic] (Norpramin): FDA approved age 18 and older

- desvenlafaxine [SNRI] (Pristiq): FDA approved age 18 and older

- doxepin [tricyclic] (Sinequan): FDA approved age 12 and older

- duloxetine [SNRI] (Cymbalta): FDA approved age 18 and older

- escitalopram [SSRI] (Lexapro): FDA approved age 18 and older; 12–17 (for major depressive disorder)

- fluoxetine [SSRI] (Prozac): FDA approved age 8 and older

- fluoxetine [SSRI] (Sarafem): FDA approved age 18 and older for premenstrual dysphoric disorder (PMDD)

- fluvoxamine [SSRI] (Luvox): FDA approved age 8 and older (for OCD only)

- imipramine [tricyclic] (Tofranil): FDA approved age 6 and older (for bedwetting)

- imipramine pamoate [tricyclic] (Tofranil-PM): FDA approved age 18 and older

- isocarboxazid [MAOI] (Marplan): FDA approved age 18 and older

- maprotiline [tricyclic] (Ludiomil): FDA approved age 18 and older

- mirtazapine (Remeron): FDA approved age 18 and older

- nortriptyline [tricyclic] (Aventyl, Pamelor): FDA approved age 18 and older

- paroxetine [SSRI] (Paxil): FDA approved age 18 and older

- paroxetine mesylate [SSRI] (Pexeva): FDA approved age 18 and older
- phenelzine [MAOI] (Nardil): FDA approved age 18 and older
- protriptyline [tricyclic] (Vivactil): FDA approved age 18 and older
- selegiline (Emsam): FDA approved age 18 and older
- sertraline [SSRI] (Zoloft): FDA approved age 6 and older (for OCD only)
- tranylcypromine [MAOI] (Parnate): FDA approved age 18 and older
- trazodone (Desyrel): FDA approved age 18 and older
- trimipramine [tricyclic] (Surmontil): FDA approved age 18 and older
- venlafaxine [SNRI] (Effexor): FDA approved age 18 and older

Mood Stabilizing and Anticonvulsant Medications

- carbamazepine (Tegretol): FDA approved age any age (for seizures)
- divalproex sodium [valproic acid] (Depakote): FDA approved age 2 and older (for seizures)
- gabapentin (Neurontin): FDA approved age 18 and older
- lamotrigine (Lamictal): FDA approved age 18 and older
- lithium carbonate (Eskalith, Lithobid): FDA approved age 12 and older
- lithium citrate (generic only): FDA approved age 12 and older
- oxcarbazepine (Trileptal): FDA approved age 4 and older
- topiramate (Topamax): FDA approved age 18 and older

Anti-Anxiety Medications

All of these anti-anxiety medications are benzodiazepines, except buspirone.

- alprazolam (Xanax): FDA approved age 18 and older
- buspirone (BuSpar): FDA approved age 18 and older
- chlordiazepoxide (Librium): FDA approved age 18 and older
- clonazepam (Klonopin): FDA approved age 18 and older
- clorazepate (Tranxene): FDA approved age 18 and older

- diazepam (Valium): FDA approved age 18 and older

- lorazepam (Ativan): FDA approved age 18 and older

- oxazepam (generic only): FDA approved age 18 and older

ADHD Medications

All of these ADHD medications are stimulants, except atomoxetine and guanfacine.

- amphetamine (Adderall): FDA approved age 3 and older

- amphetamine [extended release] (Adderall XR): FDA approved age 6 and older

- atomoxetine (Strattera): FDA approved age 6 and older

- dexmethylphenidate (Focalin): FDA approved age 6 and older

- dexmethylphenidate [extended release] (Focalin XR): FDA approved age 6 and older

- dextroamphetamine (Dexedrine, Dextrostat): FDA approved age 3 and older

- guanfacine (Intuniv): FDA approved age 6 and older

- lisdexamfetamine dimesylate (Vyvanse): FDA approved age 6 and older

- methamphetamine (Desoxyn): FDA approved age 6 and older

- methylphenidate (Ritalin): FDA approved age 6 and older

- methylphenidate [extended release] (Metadate CD, Metadate ER, Ritalin SR): FDA approved age 6 and older

- methylphenidate [long-acting] (Ritalin LA, Concerta): FDA approved age 6 and older

- methylphenidate patch (Daytrana): FDA approved age 6 and older

- methylphenidate [oral solution and chewable tablets] (Methylin): FDA approved age 6 and older

Chapter 23

Tardive Dyskinesia: A Side Effect of Some Psychiatric Drugs

What is tardive dyskinesia?

Tardive dyskinesia, or TD, is one of the muscular side effects of antipsychotic drugs, especially the older generation like haloperidol. TD does not occur until after many months or years of taking antipsychotic drugs, unlike akathisia (restlessness), dystonia (sudden and painful muscle stiffness), and Parkinsonism (tremors and slowing down of all body muscles), which can occur within hours to days of taking an antipsychotic drug. TD is primarily characterized by random movements in the tongue, lips, or jaw as well as facial grimacing, movements of arms, legs, fingers and toes, or even swaying movements of the trunk or hips. TD can be quite embarrassing to the affected patient when in public. The movements disappear during sleep. They can be mild, moderate, or severe.

How does an individual get TD?

Essentially, prolonged exposure to antipsychotic treatment (which is necessary for many persons who have chronic schizophrenia) is the major reason that TD occurs in an individual. Some persons get it sooner than others. The risk factors that increase the chances of developing TD are A) duration of exposure to antipsychotics (especially

Reprinted with permission from "Tardive Dyskinesia," © 2003 NAMI, the National Alliance on Mental Illness, www.nami.org. Reviewed by David A. Cooke, MD, FACP, June 16, 2012.

the older generation), B) older age, D) postmenopausal females, D) alcoholism and substance abuse, E) mental retardation and F) experiencing a lot of extrapyramidal symptoms (EPS) in the acute stage of antipsychotic therapy.

The mechanism of TD is still unknown despite extensive research. However, it is generally believed that long-term blocking of dopamine D2 receptors (which is what all antipsychotics on the market do) causes an increase in the number of D2 receptors in the striated region of the brain (which controls muscle coordination). This up-regulation of D2 receptors may cause spontaneous and random muscle contractions or movements throughout the body, but particularly in the perioral and facial muscles.

How many individuals currently have TD?

It is not known how many individuals currently have TD. No large scale epidemiological prevalence survey has been done. It would also change because TD can be transient or persistent, and it can be more common in some persons with risk factors than others.

However, there have been several follow-up studies of individuals who start taking antipsychotics in order to measure the annual occurrence (incidence) of TD. Eight studies in young individuals (average age 29 years) receiving the older antipsychotics showed practically the same rate of 5% of those persons develop TD every year, year after year, until eventually almost 50–60% develop TD over their lifetime. The incidence of TD is higher in older individuals (average age 65 years) where our studies have shown that TD occurs in 26% after only one year of exposure to haloperidol, which increases to 52% after two years and up to 60% after three years.

Do the newer generation atypical antipsychotics pose a lower risk of TD?

Yes, the newer atypical antipsychotics are much safer than the older generation when it comes to TD. The first year incidence of TD with risperidone, olanzapine, quetiapine, and ziprasidone in young persons about 0.5%, which is ten-fold lower than with haloperidol. Similarly, the incidence of TD with atypical antipsychotics in the first year in geriatric patients is 2.5%, which is also ten-fold lower than with haloperidol. There is also growing evidence that the incidence is even lower in subsequent years of exposure to atypicals. The problem of TD has been significantly reduced with the advent and wide-spread use of atypical antipsychotics.

What are the symptoms of TD and is TD reversible?

As described above, the main symptoms of TD are continuous and random muscular movements in the tongue, mouth, and face, but sometimes the limbs and trunks are affected as well. Rarely, the respiration muscles may be affected resulting in grunts and even breathing difficulties. Sometimes, the legs can be so severely affected that walking becomes difficult.

It must be noted that there are many other conditions that resemble TD and must be ruled out before a diagnosis of TD is made. For example, several neurodegenerative brain diseases may cause movement disorders. Very old persons may also develop mouth and facial movements with age that may be mistaken for TD. Blepharospasm is another condition that may be mistaken for TD. It should be emphasized that a history of several months or years of antipsychotic intake must be documented before TD is even considered.

TD is often mild and reversible. The percentage of patients who develop severe or irreversible TD is quite low as a proportion of those receiving long-term antipsychotic therapy.

What should you do if you notice symptoms of TD in yourself or in a family member?

Consult a psychiatrist with an established experience in using antipsychotic drugs or a neurologist who specializes in movement disorders. That physician will take a detailed history and conduct an examination and decide whether you have TD or something else, and will recommend the appropriate management.

The pattern and severity of TD is usually measured on a rating scale called The Abnormal Involuntary Movement Scale, (AIMS for short). Psychiatrists generally assess patients receiving long-term antipsychotic medication for TD symptoms at least annually using the AIMS.

Are there effective treatments for TD?

There has never been a definitive, validated, and widely accepted treatment for TD. Dozens of drugs have been tested over the past 30 years with mixed results at best. The atypical antipsychotic clozapine has been reported to reverse persistent TD after 6–12 months, possibly through gradual down-regulation of supersensitive dopamine D2 receptors. Some preliminary reports suggest that other atypical antipsychotics may also help reverse TD.

However, given that a large majority of persons who need antipsychotic treatment are now receiving the new atypicals and given the drastically lower incidence of TD with atypical antipsychotics, the issue of developing a treatment for TD may have become a moot one. Preventing the occurrence of TD is much more preferable to treating TD.

Chapter 24

Brain Stimulation Therapies

What Are Brain Stimulation Therapies?

Brain stimulation therapies involve activating or touching the brain directly with electricity, magnets, or implants to treat depression and other disorders. Electroconvulsive therapy is the most researched stimulation therapy and has the longest history of use. Other stimulation therapies discussed here—vagus nerve stimulation, repetitive transcranial magnetic stimulation, magnetic seizure therapy, and deep brain stimulation—are newer, more experimental methods.

Electroconvulsive Therapy

First developed in 1938, electroconvulsive therapy (ECT) for years had a poor reputation with many negative depictions in popular culture. However, the procedure has improved significantly since its initial use and is safe and effective. People who undergo ECT do not feel any pain or discomfort during the procedure.

ECT is usually considered only after a patient's illness has not improved after other treatment options, such as antidepressant medication or psychotherapy, are tried. It is most often used to treat severe, treatment-resistant depression, but occasionally it is used to treat other mental disorders, such as bipolar disorder or schizophrenia. It also may be used in life-threatening circumstances, such as when a

---

"Brain Stimulation Therapies," National Institute of Mental Health (www.nimh .nih.gov), November 19, 2009.

patient is unable to move or respond to the outside world (for example, catatonia), is suicidal, or is malnourished as a result of severe depression. One study, the Consortium for Research in ECT study, found an 86 percent remission rate for those with severe major depression. The same study found it to be effective in reducing chances of relapse when the patients underwent follow-up treatments.

How does it work?

Before ECT is administered, a person is sedated with general anesthesia and given a medication called a muscle relaxant to prevent movement during the procedure. An anesthesiologist monitors breathing, heart rate, and blood pressure during the entire procedure, which is conducted by a trained physician. Electrodes are placed at precise locations on the head. Through the electrodes, an electric current passes through the brain, causing a seizure that lasts generally less than one minute.

Scientists are unsure how the treatment works to relieve depression, but it appears to produce many changes in the chemistry and functioning of the brain. Because the patient is under anesthesia and has taken a muscle relaxant, the patient's body shows no signs of seizure, nor does he or she feel any pain, other than the discomfort associated with inserting an IV.

Five to ten minutes after the procedure ends, the patient awakens. He or she may feel groggy at first as the anesthesia wears off. But after about an hour, the patient usually is alert and can resume normal activities.

A typical course of ECT is administered about three times a week until the patient's depression lifts (usually within six to twelve treatments). After that, maintenance ECT treatment is sometimes needed to reduce the chance that symptoms will return. ECT maintenance treatment varies depending on the needs of the individual, and may range from one session per week to one session every few months. Frequently, a person who underwent ECT will take antidepressant medication or a mood stabilizing medication as well.

What are the side effects?

The most common side effects associated with ECT are headache, upset stomach, and muscle aches. Some people may experience memory problems, especially of memories around the time of the treatment. People may also have trouble remembering information learned shortly after the procedure, but this difficulty usually disappears over the days and weeks following the end of an ECT course. It is possible that a person may have gaps in memory over the weeks during which he or she receives treatment.

Research has found that memory problems seem to be more associated with the traditional type of ECT called bilateral ECT, in which the electrodes are placed on both sides of the head. Unilateral ECT, in which the electrodes are placed on just one side of the head—typically the right side because it is opposite the brain's learning and memory areas—appears less likely to cause memory problems and therefore is preferred by many doctors. In the past, a sine wave was used to administer electricity in a constant, high dose. However, studies have found that a brief pulse of electricity administered in several short bursts is less likely to cause memory loss, and therefore is most commonly used today.

Vagus Nerve Stimulation

Vagus nerve stimulation (VNS) works through a device implanted under the skin that sends electrical pulses through the left vagus nerve, half of a prominent pair of nerves that run from the brainstem through the neck and down to each side of the chest and abdomen. The vagus nerves carry messages from the brain to the body's major organs like the heart, lungs and intestines, and to areas of the brain that control mood, sleep, and other functions.

VNS was originally developed as a treatment for epilepsy. However, it became evident that it also had effects on mood, especially depressive symptoms. Using brain scans, scientists found that the device affected areas of the brain that are also involved in mood regulation. The pulses also appeared to alter certain neurotransmitters (brain chemicals) associated with mood, including serotonin, norepinephrine, GABA, and glutamate.

In 2005, the U.S. Food and Drug Administration (FDA) approved VNS for use in treating major depression in certain circumstances—if the illness has lasted two years or more, if it is severe or recurrent, and if the depression has not eased after trying at least four other treatments. Despite FDA approval, VNS remains a controversial treatment for depression because results of studies testing its effectiveness in treating major depression have been mixed.

How does it work?

A device called a pulse generator, about the size of a stopwatch, is surgically implanted in the upper left side of the chest. Connected to the pulse generator is a lead wire, which is guided under the skin up to the neck, where it is attached to the left-side vagus nerve.

Typically, electrical pulses that last about 30 seconds are sent about every five minutes from the generator to the vagus nerve. The duration and frequency of the pulses may vary depending on how the generator is programmed. The vagus nerve, in turn, delivers those signals to the brain. The pulse generator, which operates continuously, is powered by a battery that lasts around ten years, after which it must be replaced. Normally, a person does not feel any sensation in the body as the device works, but it may cause coughing or the voice may become hoarse while the nerve is being stimulated.

The device also can be temporarily deactivated by placing a magnet over the chest where the pulse generator is implanted. A person may want to deactivate it if side effects become intolerable, or before engaging in strenuous activity or exercise because it may interfere with breathing. The device reactivates when the magnet is removed.

What are the side effects?

VNS is not without risk. There may be complications such as infection from the implant surgery, or the device may come loose, move around or malfunction, which may require additional surgery to correct. Long-term side effects are unknown.

Other potential side effects include the following:

- Voice changes or hoarseness

- Cough or sore throat

- Neck pain

- Discomfort or tingling in the area where the device is implanted

- Breathing problems, especially during exercise

- Difficulty swallowing

Repetitive Transcranial Magnetic Stimulation

Repetitive transcranial magnetic stimulation (rTMS) uses a magnet instead of an electrical current to activate the brain. First developed in 1985, rTMS has been studied as a possible treatment for depression, psychosis, and other disorders since the mid-1990s.

Clinical trials studying the effectiveness of rTMS reveal mixed results. When compared to a placebo or inactive (sham) treatment, some studies have found that rTMS is more effective in treating patients with major depression. But other studies have found no difference in response compared to inactive treatment.

In October 2008, rTMS was approved for use by the FDA as a treatment for major depression for patients who have not responded to at least one antidepressant medication. It is also used in countries such as in Canada and Israel as a treatment for depression for patients who have not responded to medications and who might otherwise be considered for ECT.

How does it work?

Unlike ECT, in which electrical stimulation is more generalized, rTMS can be targeted to a specific site in the brain. Scientists believe that focusing on a specific spot in the brain reduces the chance for the type of side effects that are associated with ECT. But opinions vary as to what spot is best.

A typical rTMS session lasts 30 to 60 minutes and does not require anesthesia. An electromagnetic coil is held against the forehead near an area of the brain that is thought to be involved in mood regulation. Then, short electromagnetic pulses are administered through the coil. The magnetic pulse easily passes through the skull, and causes small electrical currents that stimulate nerve cells in the targeted brain region. And because this type of pulse generally does not reach further than two inches into the brain, scientists can select which parts of the brain will be affected and which will not be. The magnetic field is about the same strength as that of a magnetic resonance imaging (MRI) scan. Generally, the person will feel a slight knocking or tapping on the head as the pulses are administered.

Not all scientists agree on the best way to position the magnet on the patient's head or give the electromagnetic pulses. They also do not yet know if rTMS works best when given as a single treatment or combined with medication. More research, including a large trial funded by the National Institute of Mental Health (NIMH), is underway to determine the safest and most effective use of rTMS.

What are the side effects?

Sometimes a person may have discomfort at the site on the head where the magnet is placed. The muscles of the scalp, jaw or face may contract or tingle during the procedure. Mild headache or brief lightheadedness may result. It is also possible that the procedure could cause a seizure, although documented incidences of this are uncommon. A recent large-scale study on the safety of rTMS found that most side effects, such as headaches or scalp discomfort, were mild or moderate, and no seizures occurred. Because the treatment is new, however, long-term side effects are unknown.

Magnetic Seizure Therapy

Magnetic seizure therapy (MST) borrows certain aspects from both ECT and rTMS. Like rTMS, it uses a magnetic pulse instead of electricity to stimulate a precise target in the brain. However, unlike rTMS, MST aims to induce a seizure like ECT. So the pulse is given at a higher frequency than that used in rTMS. Therefore, like ECT, the patient must be anesthetized and given a muscle relaxant to prevent movement. The goal of MST is to retain the effectiveness of ECT while reducing the cognitive side effects usually associated with it.

MST is currently in the early stages of testing, but initial results are promising. Studies on both animals and humans have found that MST produces fewer memory side effects, shorter seizures, and allows for a shorter recovery time than ECT. However, its effect on treatment-resistant depression is not yet established. Studies are underway to determine its antidepressant effects.

Deep Brain Stimulation

Deep brain stimulation (DBS) was first developed as a treatment for Parkinson disease to reduce tremor, stiffness, walking problems, and uncontrollable movements. In DBS, a pair of electrodes is implanted in the brain and controlled by a generator that is implanted in the chest. Stimulation is continuous and its frequency and level is customized to the individual.

DBS has only recently been studied as a treatment for depression or obsessive compulsive disorder (OCD). Currently, it is available on an experimental basis only. So far, very little research has been conducted to test DBS for depression treatment, but the few studies that have been conducted show that the treatment may be promising. One small trial involving people with severe, treatment-resistant depression found that four out of six participants showed marked improvement in their symptoms either immediately after the procedure, or soon after. Another study involving ten people with OCD found continued improvement among the majority three years after the surgery.

How does it work?

DBS requires brain surgery. The head is shaved and then attached with screws to a sturdy frame that prevents the head from moving during the surgery. Scans of the head and brain using MRI are taken. The surgeon uses these images as guides during the surgery. Patients are awake during the procedure to provide the surgeon with feedback, but they feel no pain because the head is numbed with a local anesthetic.

Once ready for surgery, two holes are drilled into the head. From there, the surgeon threads a slender tube down into the brain to place electrodes on each side of a specific part of the brain. In the case of depression, the part of the brain targeted is called Area 25. This area has been found to be overactive in depression and other mood disorders. In the case of OCD, the electrodes are placed in a different part of the brain believed to be associated with the disorder.

After the electrodes are implanted and the patient provides feedback about the placement of the electrodes, the patient is put under general anesthesia. The electrodes are then attached to wires that are run inside the body from the head down to the chest, where a pair of battery-operated generators are implanted. From here, electrical pulses are continuously delivered over the wires to the electrodes in the brain. Although it is unclear exactly how the device works to reduce depression or OCD, scientists believe that the pulses help to "reset" the area of the brain that is malfunctioning so that it works normally again.

What are the side effects?

DBS carries risks associated with any type of brain surgery. For example, the procedure may lead to conditions such as the following:

- Bleeding in the brain or stroke
- Infection
- Disorientation or confusion
- Unwanted mood changes
- Movement disorders
- Lightheadedness
- Trouble sleeping

Because the procedure is still experimental, other side effects that are not yet identified may be possible. Long-term benefits and side effects are unknown.

Research Is Underway on Brain Stimulation Therapies

Brain stimulation therapies hold promise for treating certain mental disorders that do not respond to more conventional treatments. Therefore, they are of high interest and are the subject of many studies. For example, researchers continue to look for ways to reduce the side effects of ECT while retaining the benefits. Studies on rTMS are ongoing and include a trial in which the procedure is being tested for safety and effectiveness for the treatment of major depression in 240 participants. Similar studies are being conducted using MST.

Other researchers are studying how the brain responds to VNS by using imaging techniques such as positron emission tomography (PET) scans. Finally, although DBS as a depression treatment is still very new, researchers are beginning to conduct studies with people to determine its effectiveness and safety in treating depression, OCD and other mental disorders.

Chapter 25

Complementary and Alternative Medicine for Mental Health Care

Chapter Contents

Section 25.1

Herbal Remedies and Supplements for Mental Health

What Are Complementary and Alternative Medicines (CAMs)?

They are ways of treating illness that have developed outside the mainstream of modern medicine. Many are traditional remedies that have developed in different cultures over the centuries. They include:

- herbal medicines

- foods

- nutritional supplements, such as vitamins and minerals

All these treatments can be used on their own, or with conventional medicine.

CAMs and Mental Health Problems

Many CAMs have been used for mental health problems, but there is little good evidence to support their use. Some of these treatments may work, but most have not been thoroughly tested. The studies have often been too small to give a clear answer. We know most about the treatments for depression, anxiety, and insomnia.

Despite the lack of evidence, people all over the world take CAMs, and many report that they find them helpful. Ultimately, whether taking CAMs is a good idea depends on individual circumstances. We recommend that you talk to your health care provider or mental health team first.

If you are considering taking CAMs, you should seek specialist advice if:

- you are pregnant or breastfeeding

- you want to give CAMs to children

- you are competing in sports to make sure that the CAM you are considering taking is not in breach of doping regulations.

How to Use CAMs Safely?

Do

- Choose a qualified practitioner who is a member of a recognized society.

- Ask about their qualification and experience.

- Ask about side-effects.

- If in doubt, ask your doctor, nurse or pharmacist.

- Tell the professionals involved in your care, including your CAM practitioner, about all your treatments and medications.

- Tell them if you are pregnant, plan to become pregnant or breast-feed.

- Tell them about your physical health and allergies.

- Discuss your concerns about treatment.

- Seek medical advice if you experience unusual symptoms.

- Make special time for your treatment sessions.

- Find a reliable source for your information about therapies.

Don't

- Stop conventional medicines without telling your doctor.

- Believe claims for "wonder cures."

- Take high doses of supplements unless confirmed with an experienced health professional.

- Combine many different remedies.

- Take complementary medicines without knowing what they are for.

- Take somebody else's complementary medicines.

- Give remedies to children without seeking specialist advice.

- Take remedies from an unreliable source—this includes the internet.

- Eat or drink raw plant material, such as flowers, fruits, leaves, seeds, or the root unless you are sure it is absolutely safe (many plants are poisonous and need to be processed before they can be used safely).

- Prepare your own teas and extracts unless you are sure it is safe.

- Smoke raw plant material.

- Pay large sums of money up front.

- Practice acupuncture or any other physical treatment on yourself unless you have been trained.

- Blame yourself if a treatment does not work.

Herbal Remedies and Supplements

Herbal remedies come from plants. If possible, choose a remedy which has been standardized, that is, the contents are approximately the same in each bottle or tablet you buy. Plant remedies are not always safer than ordinary medicines. All of them can have side-effects and interact with other medicines.

Supplements include vitamins, minerals, and animal and plant products, such as cod liver oil. They can also have side-effects and interact with other medicines. Some people take supplements, like vitamin C in high doses, but this can damage the liver or kidneys. Many supplements have a recommended daily intake (RDI), or allowance (RDA). Do not go beyond this dose without talking to an experienced health professional.

Brain Function and Dementia

These are called cognitive enhancers and can improve concentration. They include:

- Ginkgo (*Ginkgo biloba*)

- Ginseng (*Panax ginseng*)

- Hydergine (Ergot) (*Claviceps purpurea*)

- Sage (*Salvia officinalis, Salvia lavandulaefolia*)

- Vitamin E (alpha-tocopheril)

Ginkgo

Ginkgo is a tree originating in China. Extracts of its seeds and leaves are used to improve thinking in healthy people, as well as people with dementia.

How does it work?

We don't know. It may:

- Act as an antioxidant to prevent cell damage
- Increase the blood flow in the brain or increase chemical transmitters in the brain

How good is it?

Research shows that ginkgo may help in dementia. The same is true of its use in healthy adults. However, more recently its effectiveness has been put in doubt.

Side-effects

It may rarely cause bleeding into the brain and into the eye or prolong bleeding time during surgery. About twenty such cases have been reported, and patients undergoing surgery may consider avoiding gingko. Gingko should not be taken together with blood thinning medications, such as aspirin and ibuprofen. There is an increased risk of fits and lower fertility in both men and women.

Drug interactions with

- Blood thinning drugs such as aspirin, ibuprofen, warfarin (increases bleeding time)
- Trazodone (one case of coma has been reported)
- Antidepressants (increase the risk of going high—mania)
- Anticonvulsants (reduces their effectiveness)

Ginseng

Ginseng grows in many parts of the world. *Panax ginseng* or Korean ginseng are most commonly used.

How does it work?

We don't know. It may:

- Thin the blood
- Prevent cell damage through antioxidant activity

How good is it?

It might improve cognitive performance, but there is no evidence that it delays ageing.

Side-effects

- Agitation and mania; sleep problems; blood pressure changes; changes in bleeding time so people with bleeding disorders such as stroke and blood clots (thrombosis) should avoid it. It may possibly stimulate breast cancers.

Drug interactions with

- Drugs used in diabetes (lower blood sugar)
- Blood thinning agents such as aspirin, ibuprofen and warfarin (changes in bleeding time)
- MAOI antidepressants (for example, Phenelzine), may lead to agitation and sleep problems

Hydergine

This comes from a fungus which lives on rye. For hundreds of years it has caused epidemics of poisoning (ergotism). This is caused by eating bread made from infected rye flour.

How does it work?

It may affect the activity of brain transmitters.

How good is it?

It may improve memory in dementia.

Side-effects

It can cause fits, confusion, hallucinations, and psychosis. Severe poisoning can cause gangrene.

Drug interactions with

- Antidepressants and some pain killers
- Drugs for dementia
- Drugs for migraine

Sage

Sage produces oils which are used in aromatherapy. It is used to improve concentration and memory and has been suggested as a treatment of depression and anxiety.

How does it work?

It may:

- Increase some brain transmitters
- Have antioxidant, anti-inflammatory and oestrogen effects

How good is it?

There is some evidence for improved memory in volunteers. One study found that it improved mood, alertness, calmness and contentedness. It may help concentration in people with dementia.

Side-effects

- Although safe when used in amounts commonly found in foods, some types when taken orally can cause convulsions. Sage may also lower blood sugar. It should not be used in pregnancy or when breastfeeding.

Drug interactions with

- Drugs for diabetes
- Drugs for epilepsy
- Sedatives

Vitamin E (Alpha-Tocopherol)

Vitamin E is found in plant oils, nuts, vegetables, and, to a lesser degree, in meat and dairy products.

How does it work?

Antioxidant properties may prevent cell damage.

How good is it?

It may improve behavior in dementia, but there is no good evidence that it improves memory or slows the progress of the disease.

Side-effects

A recent study found that a daily intake of more than 400IU (270 mg of alpha-tocopherol) resulted in an increase of death from all causes, and an increased risk of bleeding and stroke.

Drug interactions with

- Drugs to thin the blood
- Anesthetics and cocaine
- Drugs to lower cholesterol and some cancer treatments

Anxiety and Sleep Problems

Most of these treatments seem to work on gamma-amino-butyric acid (GABA), a chemical in the brain linked to anxiety. We do not know if these drugs cause addiction. They are less powerful than conventional sedatives or sleeping tablets.

Note

- Kava (*Piper methysticum*) has been withdrawn in the UK due to concerns that it might cause liver damage. It should not be used.
- Combinations of extracts may be less safe. There have been concerns about liver damage from combinations of valerian and other herbs.

Remedies Include

- Valerian (valeriana officinalis)
- Passion flower (passiflora incarnata)
- German chamomile (matricaria recutita)
- Hops (humulus lupulus)

- Oats (avena sativa)
- Starflower / borage (borago officinalis)
- Lemon balm (melissa officinalis)
- Lavender (lavendula angustifolia)
- Bach flower remedies
- Melatonin (N-acetyl-S-metoxy tryptamine)
- Aminoacids
- Roseroot
- Vitamins, trace elements and supplements

Valerian

Valeriana officinalis is thought to be safe and is available as a standard extract in the UK. Some other species may cause liver problems

How does it work?

- It probably acts on GABA.
- It may also counteract the effects of caffeine.

How good is it?

This remains unclear at the moment, but some studies have shown that people report sleeping better having taken Valerian.

Side-effects

- Drowsiness or excitability. It may slow down reactions, so you should not drive or operate dangerous machinery after taking it. It may cause liver damage, but this seems to be confined to some formulations. You should not take it in pregnancy.

Drug interactions with

- Sedatives
- Alcohol
- The pill
- HIV medicines

- Cancer treatments
- Epilepsy and anti-fungal treatments
- Blood thinning medicines

Passion Flower

Passion flower is used to treat anxiety. It has also been suggested as a treatment in alcohol craving and opiate withdrawal.

How does it work?

It probably acts on GABA.

How good is it?

Very few studies have been conducted, One trial found it to be as good as conventional tranquillizers.

Side-effects

- Isolated reports of severe toxicity even at normal doses. It can cause dizziness, confusion, heart problems, and inflammation of blood vessels. Some species may contain cyanides, so toxicity may depend on the preparation.

Drug interactions with

- Warfarin, a blood thinner

German Chamomile

Chamomile is a mild sedative. It is also used to treat stomach upsets and mucosal irritations. Traditionally the flowers are prepared as a tea.

How does it work?

It acts on GABA.

How good is it?

We know very little, but one recent study has shown that it may make people less anxious, as long as the anxiety is not too bad.

Side-effects

- It may increase bleeding time and may stimulate breast cancer cell growth in estrogen sensitive cancers.

Drug interactions with

- Blood thinning drugs
- Oral contraception (the pill)

Hops

Dried hops have been used to treat anxiety and sleep problems.

How does it work?

We don't know.

How good is it?

One study showed that a valerian-hops combination helped sleep.

Side effects

- None reported

Drug interactions with

- Increases sedation when used with:
  - Sedatives
  - Sleeping tablets
  - Other herbs
  - Alcohol

Oats

People use this to lower cholesterol and for stomach upsets, such as irritable bowel syndrome. It has also been used to treat anxiety and tiredness. It has even been suggested for use in alcohol and nicotine addiction.

How does it work?

We don't know.

How good is it?

We don't know.

Side-effects

- None known

Drug interactions with

- None known

Starflower (Borage)

Starflower oil is used for rheumatoid arthritis, premenstrual syndrome (PMS), and sedation.

How does it work?

We do not know.

How good is it?

We do not know.

Side-effects

- Some extracts can cause liver problems or possibly cancer. It should not be used in pregnancy, and it may increase epileptic fits.

Drug interactions with

- Blood thinning drugs such as: aspirin, ibuprofen, warfarin.

Lemon Balm

Lemon balm is a herb of the mint family. It is used for anxiety, sleep problems, heavy periods, and period pain. It is also used to treat agitation in dementia. Lemon balm is used as tea or extract. The oil is also used in aromatherapy.

How does it work?

It may work on brain transmitters.

How good is it?

Some evidence of calming in dementia. No research on its use in anxiety and insomnia. In combination with valerian and hops, it can improve sleep.

Side-effects

- Very few

Drug interactions with

- Increases sedation when used with:
  - Sedatives
  - Herbs
  - Alcohol

Lavender

Lavender is also a member of the mint family. Drops of lavender oil or seeds put onto pillows have been used to help sleep. It is used in aromatherapy, and as an extract or tea.

How does it work?

We don't know.

How good is it?

May act as a mild sedative when used in aromatherapy.

Side-effects

- Skin irritation

Drug interactions with

- Increased sedation when used with:
  - Sedatives
  - Herbs
  - Alcohol

Bach Flower Remedies

This is an extract from a combination of flowers which is used to treat anxiety, panic and trauma.

How does it work?

We don't know.

How good is it?

No good evidence.

Side-effects

We don't know.

Drug interactions with

We don't know.

Melatonin

Melatonin is a hormone made by the pineal gland in the base of the brain. It controls our body clock. If you are over 55, your doctor can prescribe melatonin for you. The prescribed brand is called Circadin.

How does it work?

By regulating the body clock.

How good is it?

It may improve sleep quality in older adults.

Side-effects

• Sleepiness and low mood

Drug interactions with

• Blood thinning drugs
• Increases sedation when used with:
  • Sedatives
  • Herbs

Aminoacids

A mixture of two amino acids—L-Arginine and L-Lysine—has been used to try to reduce stress and anxiety.

How does it work?

By modifying hormones which are released under stress.

How good is it?

Only a few studies exist so we don't know.

Side-effects

- L-Lysine: one case of severe kidney problems has been reported.

- L-Arginine: drugs which lower blood pressure and nitrates. A few deaths have occurred in people who had a recent heart attack. If in doubt, avoid or seek an opinion from a heart specialist first.

Drug interactions with

- L-Lysine: calcium supplements.

- L-Arginine: drugs which lower blood pressure and nitrates. Avoid such combinations because they may make your blood pressure fall too much. Even combinations with medicines, such as Viagra, may make your blood pressure go too low.

Roseroot

Roseroot is also known as artic root or rhodolia. It is also a so called adaptogen which should help the body cope better with stress, anxiety and tiredness. Roseroot has also been used as an energy booster, for instance to enhance athletic performance.

How does it work?

We don't know. Some components of roseroot may modify hormones which are released under stress, others may be mildly stimulating.
It also has antioxidant activity.

How good is it?

We don't know at present. More studies are needed to confirm the effects.

Side-effects

No serious effects reported. It may cause dizziness or dry mouth.

Drug interactions with

- None reported

Vitamins, Trace Elements, and Supplements

It has been suggested that certain vitamins, trace elements, and supplements may help anxiety. However, there are very few studies to rely on at present. One problem is that studies tend to test combinations rather than individual substances, so that it's difficult to tell which ingredient does what.

The Food Standards Agency has produced a website (http://www.food.gov.uk) which explains all about vitamins, trace elements, and supplements.

Depression and Bipolar Disorder

Remedies include:

- St John's wort (*Hypericum perforatum*)
- S-adenosyl-methionine
- Folic acid (folate)
- Selenium
- Omega-3 fatty acids

In bipolar disorder (manic depression), adding omega-3 fatty acids may reduce the chance of becoming ill again. Some people buy natural lithium, but we do not recommend this because the doses offered in the tablets are much lower than in prescription preparations. Also, lithium at any dose should be closely monitored.

Most treatments for depression are supplements, which are building blocks in the production of serotonin. This is a chemical in the brain that seems to be involved in depression. L-tryptophan, is one of these building blocks, but it has not yet been cleared as safe.

St John's Wort

St John's wort gets its name from St John's day on June 24. This is when the plant starts to flower. For a long time it was thought that the red dye, hypericin, which is produced when the plant is crushed, was responsible for its action. Research now suggests that another ingredient, hyperforin, may produce the antidepressant effect. St John's wort has also been suggested as a treatment of anxiety, addiction, and premenstrual stress.

How does it work?

- Increases serotonin in the brain.

How good is it?

It has been shown to be effective in many trials.

Side-effects

- People taking St John's wort may burn more easily in the sun; if in doubt use sun screen. It may cause mania in people with bipolar disorder.

Drug interactions with

- Antidepressants
- Strong painkillers
- Oral contraceptives (the pill), reduces its effectiveness
- Some cancer drugs.

Can also reduce the effect of:
- Some epilepsy drugs, such as carbamazepine
- Digoxin
- Warfarin
- HIV drugs
- Some cancer drugs

There is also a risk of organ rejection in people taking St John's wort who undergo transplant surgery.

S-Adenosyl-Methionine

S-adenosyl-methionine (SAMe) is another building block of serotonin. It is not often used in the UK, but is popular in Europe and the U.S. It is also popular with HIV sufferers because it has few side-effects. It is often given as an injection. However, oral preparations are available, but some do not work. SAMe can be expensive.

How does it work?

It helps to produce serotonin and other neurotransmitters.

How good is it?

Two trials show that SAMe has a good antidepressant effect.

Side-effects

- May cause mania in people with bipolar disorder.

Drug interactions with

- Antidepressants
- Strong painkillers

Folic Acid

Folic acid is used by women who want to become pregnant or are pregnant to prevent spina bifida, a malformation of the baby's spine. In some countries, folic acid is added to the flour.

How does it work?

It is another building block of serotonin and other neurotransmitters.

How good is it?

It may increase the effect of some antidepressants.

Side-effects

It may make it more difficult to diagnose pernicious anaemia which can occur in people who do not have enough Vitamin B12. Large doses can cause agitation, sleep problems, confusion, and fits.

Drug interactions with

- Some anti-cancer drugs
- Some antibiotics

Selenium

Selenium is an important trace element. It is found in vegetables, meat, fish, and Brazil nuts. Brazil nuts can vary in selenium content, but sometimes the concentration is so high that the U.S. National Institutes of Health advise that Brazil nuts should be only eaten occasionally. The Food Standards Agency recommends a safe upper level of 0.45 mg per day. Some formulations exceed this dose.

How does it work?

Selenium is an antioxidant and may prevent cell damage. It also helps produce thyroid hormone.

How good is it?

We don't know.

Side effects

- Can lead to nausea, vomiting, nail changes, irritability, weight loss, depression, confusion, liver and skin changes

Drug interactions with

- Drugs to lower cholesterol
- Vitamin preparations

Omega-3 Fatty Acids

Omega-3 acids are mainly derived from fish—they are used to prevent heart and joint disease. They are also used in depression. Omega-3 fatty acids have two main components: docosahexaenoic acid (DHA) and eicosapentaenoic acid (EPA). The pills are often large, and some people find them hard to swallow. Avoid preparations which have added vitamin A. This could cause vitamin A poisoning.

How does it work?

We don't know.

How good is it?

They may be worth taking with antidepressants. They may help prevent relapse in bipolar disorder. There is not enough evidence to recommend them as an alternative to antidepressants or mood stabilizers.

Side-effects

- Unknown

Drug interactions with

- Blood thinning drugs

Psychosis

Choices are limited. Rauwolfia, a plant originating from India, has been used, but is not as good as antipsychotic medicines. Reserpine, a drug developed from rauwolfia, can cause depression and is no longer used in the UK.

Omega-3s may be tried with antipsychotic treatment, but there is no good evidence that they help. Many antipsychotics can cause weight gain and lead to a higher risk of heart and blood pressure problems. Omega-3s may reduce these changes, but success is not guaranteed.

Movement Disorders

Many older antipsychotics could cause abnormal movements, known as tardive dyskinesia. If this occurs, the dose of the antipsychotic can be lowered, or an alternative antipsychotic given.

Complementary remedies may help—vitamin E, melatonin, and ginkgo biloba.

Vitamin E may prevent the movements getting worse. However, the potential benefits need to be offset against long-term use, particularly if high doses of vitamin E are considered.

Melatonin has also been tried, but the research is inconclusive.

A recent study found that *Gingko biloba* can reduce tardive dyskinesia and that the effect may last for some time, even after *Ginkgo biloba* has been stopped. As mentioned above, there may be health risks because of a potentially increased bleeding risk.

Addictions

The choice is limited. Valerian has been suggested to improve sleep in people withdrawing from drugs like valium. But no good research has been done. Passion flower was effective when combined with clonidine in one small study, and St John's wort may reduce alcohol craving.

Other remedies include:

- Kudzu
- Iboga

Kudzu

Kudzu, or Japanese arroweed flowers have a pleasant fragrance. They have been used for many medical purposes, including menopausal problems. It has also been used for alcohol problems.

How does it work?

It may reduce anxiety caused by alcohol withdrawal.

How good is it?

One study showed reduction in alcohol use in heavy drinkers. Another study failed to show any effect on craving.

Side-effects

- None reported

Drug interactions with

- Blood thinning drugs
- Oral contraceptives (the pill)
- Drugs for diabetes

Iboga

Iboga is a West African shrub producing ibogaine. This causes hallucinations and has been used widely for religious rites. It became famous as a treatment for opiate addiction in the 60s. However, it can have serious life-threatening side-effects. Until these safety concerns are clarified it cannot be recommended.

How does it work?

It probably affects several chemical transmitters in the brain.

How good is it?

It may help in withdrawal and in staying away from drugs.

Side-effects

Between 1990 and 2006, twelve deaths after ibogaine use have been reported. The risk of death may be as high as one in 300 treatments. It is not known how many deaths have occurred, and may have gone unreported because of the underground nature of ibogaine treatment.

Drug interactions with

- Drugs which affect the same neurotransmitters

Section 25.2

Physical Therapies for Mental Health

Physical Treatments

Which complementary and alternative medicines (CAMs) can be used for mental health problems?

Many treatments have been used, some more successfully than others. Your choice should be guided by their safety and effectiveness. If they are safe and do not interfere with other treatments, then anything that makes you feel good can be used.

How good are they?

Very little research has been done into these treatments. Research is expensive and many of the studies are too small to give a clear answer. Most research has been done on treatments for depression, anxiety, and insomnia.

Who can I speak to about CAMs?

Finding an expert can be difficult. Your doctor, nurse or pharmacist can give you some guidance, or may be able to suggest someone who knows more. It is best to choose a CAM therapist with a recognized qualification, who is member of a regulated society.

How to use CAMs safely?

- Keep an open mind about the different options available.

- If in doubt, seek advice from your doctor, nurse or pharmacist.

- Tell the therapist about any illness, seizures or allergies, or if you plan to become pregnant or breast-feed.

- Discuss your concerns about conventional treatments.
- Ask about your therapist's qualification and experience.
- Ask about the side-effects of treatment.
- Seek medical advice if you experience unusual symptoms.
- Make special time for your treatment sessions.

Acupuncture

Acupuncture involves piercing the skin with fine needles. There are two types:

- Traditional Chinese acupuncture involves placing the needles along assumed energy channels or meridians. This is done in order to restore a disturbed energy balance which is theoretically responsible for illness.

- The Western medical approach uses similar techniques without using the energy concept. In the West, acupuncture is mainly used as a treatment for pain. Its use for mental health problems is still in its infancy

How is the strength of acupuncture determined?

The dose of acupuncture can be varied by the needle sites, the depth and duration of insertion, the number of needles, and the number of sessions. The dose can also be increased by manual stimulation of the needles, or electrical stimulation. This is where the dose is increased by running a small electric current through the needles. Moxibustion is when the needles are heated by burning mugwort.

Which mental health problems can be treated with acupuncture?

Anxiety, depression, stress, and insomnia can all be treated. If you don't feel an improvement after several sessions, or your symptoms become severe, you should seek medical help.

How well does it work?

Anxiety: Acupuncture seems to reduce anxiety. Most research has studied its effect on conditions such as tooth extraction, withdrawal from alcohol addiction, and diseases such as cancer. It can help calm people down in these situations.

Depression: We don't really know whether it works, as only a few small studies have been done and the results are conflicting. Acupuncture could possibly be combined with antidepressants in some cases. Electro-acupuncture may be the most effective method. This seems to have a similar effect on muscles as exercise, and exercise has been shown to improve mood.

Stress: Anxiety, agitation, and low mood may be improved.

Insomnia: About one in ten people feel tired after acupuncture. It comes as no surprise that acupuncture has been used to treat insomnia, and some studies suggest that it may work. The main drawback is that the insomnia may come back once the treatment is stopped.

What about addiction and acupuncture?

Acupuncture is used to treat withdrawal symptoms, but on its own does not seem to help people overcome their addiction to smoking, drinking, or drugs. More research needs to be done to understand how acupuncture could help people with addiction problems.

Side-effects of acupuncture?

If you are sensitive to pain, or if you have fibromyalgia or chronic fatigue with muscle pain, it may not help you. This is because your pain sensitivity could make the treatment uncomfortable or painful. However, one recent trial has shown that it may reduce pain in fibromyalgia.

Most people get very few side-effects. Some needle points require more caution than others, for instance, those in the chest. Common side-effects include bruising, bleeding, and pain. Some people can faint which is why the first session should be conducted lying down. Some people can also become very tired. If this happens to you, then do not drive after the sessions. Similarly, you should not drive to the first session in case this happens to you.

Infection can occur, but since acupuncture needles are only used once, this is unlikely. Some people get anxious or have a strong emotional reaction to the treatment. If this happens during the session, it might be best to stop and discuss what happened. Sometimes it can help to simply lower the dose. Tell your acupuncturist if you may be pregnant.

Are there serious side-effects?

Acupuncture involves needles, so it is possible to pierce organs, nerves, and blood vessels. In the worst case, needling over the chest or back could pierce the heart or lungs. Skilled therapists would avoid such injuries. However, if you get breathing difficulties after needling of the chest and upper back, you should consult a doctor immediately and explain that you had acupuncture.

Ear Acupuncture

Ear acupuncture, or auriculotherapy, involves inserting very fine needles into the surface of the ears. The needles are never inserted into the openings of the ear. Since ears are prone to infections, the skin area should be cleaned and disinfected. Ear acupuncture has been used to treat addiction and pain. Some people use needles which stay in the ear, sometimes for up to two weeks. These needles are more prone to infection, and people who suffer from heart valve disease must never use them. People who are treated with steroids, or have diabetes, also have a higher risk of infection.

TENS

TENS is short for transcutaneous electrical nerve stimulation. Electrodes are placed on the skin, so no needles are used. TENS is mainly used as a treatment for pain.

Aromatherapy

This is based on the healing properties of plant oils. These oils are diluted in a carrier oil. The oils are commonly used in oil burners, in bath water, or massaged into the skin. The aroma of the essential oil evaporates and stimulates the sense of smell. An aromatherapy massage is based on techniques to relieve tension and improve circulation. Practitioners believe this allows oil molecules to be absorbed into the blood stream during massage, and then passed through the body to the nervous system. People use aromatherapy for relaxation, sleep improvement, pain relief, and to help depression.

Its effects are weak, so it is best to use it in conjunction with conventional treatments. Aromatherapy is safe, but some oils should not be used if you are pregnant or have epilepsy, or in babies and young children. Some oils can lead to allergies or increased sensitivity to light.

Homeopathy

Homeopathy uses the principle of "like to cure like." This involves using extremely diluted substances to avoid toxicity. The medicines may be so diluted that very few, or no, molecules of the original substance are present in the tablets or solutions taken. Homeopathic medicines are prepared from minerals, plants, and animal substances. The more diluted the solution, the stronger the claimed effect. This is one of the most controversial aspects of homeopathy.

There is a lot of scepticism about the effectiveness of homeopathy, and using it as a substitute for conventional treatments is unwise. However, some people find it helps to combine homeopathic and conventional medicines. Homeopathic remedies are very safe because they are highly diluted.

Yoga

Yoga is a technique which is more than 5000 years old. *Yoga* means *union* in Sanskrit. It uses spiritual and physical exercises to heal mind and body. The exercises need to be adapted to suit the person. Yoga can have a calming and relaxing effect, and reduce agitation. It may be useful for anxiety and stress. Yoga has also been tested as a treatment of depression and epilepsy, but the findings are inconclusive.

Biofeedback

Biofeedback is a technique where bodily functions which are usually ignored, or perceived as automatic, are monitored in order to control them. These functions include heart or breathing rate, blood pressure, sweating, and muscle tension. Monitors are attached to measure and provide feedback of the chosen function. It can be used for agitation, anxiety, and stress, but it is difficult to draw firm conclusions about its effectiveness. One of the main criticisms is that it is costly and similar effects can be achieved through meditation or relaxation.

Relaxation

Relaxation is usually used to reduce agitation and arousal. One technique is progressive muscle relaxation. This involves tensing and relaxing different muscle groups. It is useful for problems associated with muscle tension, and can help in anxiety and asthma. Sessions take about 20 minutes. The exercises need to be done every day to work. Autogenic training is another technique and involves autosuggestion to control breathing, heart rate and muscle tone.

Meditation

Spiritual techniques can help in a variety of mental and physical health problems. Religious activity can improve your health. However, meditation can affect your mental health, and even cause psychotic episodes in vulnerable people. People suffering from psychotic disorders should use these techniques with caution.

Hypnosis

Hypnosis involves the induction of a trance or sleep-like state. Suggestions, targeting the problems, can then be given to help with the healing. Hypnosis can be tried for many different problems. However, it is important to choose an experienced and well-trained hypnotherapist. Hypnosis can be used alongside conventional medicine to treat schizophrenia, but people suffering from psychosis should use these techniques with caution.

Reiki/Therapeutic Touch

Reiki relates to spiritual life force and energy. Reiki therapists claim to channel energy from their hands to the client which leads to healing. Advanced Reiki therapy involves healing from a distance. Reiki therapy is controversial. If Reiki is not successful, some therapists may claim that this is because the client was blocking the energy. This could result in people wrongly blaming themselves for the therapy not working. The evidence for Reiki being effective is poor. Therapeutic touch is a concept related to Reiki, but there is no distance healing.

Reflexology

This treatment works on the principle that specific points in the feet, hands, and ears represent certain body systems or organs. Illness is seen as a sign that the person is out of balance, and that energy flows are disturbed. By applying pressure point massage, the energy flows and balance is restored. Reflexology can give a sense of well-being and relaxation and it may be help in stress, anxiety and poor sleep. If symptoms are severe, reflexology may not work. In such cases, it still can be a useful additional treatment.

Section 25.3

Spirituality and Mental Health

Introduction

Spirituality and psychiatry—on the face of it, they do not seem to
have much in common. But we are becoming increasingly aware of
ways in which some aspects of spirituality can offer real benefits for
mental health.

This section is for:

- anyone who has an interest in spirituality and mental health;

- anyone with a mental health problem;

- carers and relatives;

- professionals who may not be sure about how to explore spiritual
  issues with their clients/patients.

It looks at:

- how spirituality, mental health, and mental healthcare can connect;

- how to make a place for spiritual needs within a mental health
  service;

- how spirituality can help mental health.

You don't need to hold a formal religious belief, to take part in religious practices, or belong to an established faith tradition, to read
this information—or to experience spirituality.

What Is Spirituality?

Spirituality involves experiences of:

- a deep-seated sense of meaning and purpose in life;
- a sense of belonging;
- a sense of connection of the deeply personal with the universal;
- acceptance, integration and a sense of wholeness.

These experiences are part of being human—they are as clearly present in people with a learning disability as they are in anybody else.

Spirituality often becomes more important in times of distress, emotional stress, physical and mental illness, loss, bereavement, and the approach of death.

All health care tries to relieve pain and to cure—but good health care tries to do more. Spirituality emphasizes the healing of the person, not just the disease. It views life as a journey, where good and bad experiences can help you to learn, develop and mature.

How Is Spirituality Different from Religion?

Religious traditions certainly include individual spirituality, which is universal. But each religion has its own distinct community-based worship, beliefs, sacred texts, and traditions.

Spirituality is not tied to any particular religious belief or tradition. Although culture and beliefs can play a part in spirituality, every person has their own unique experience of spirituality—it can be a personal experience for anyone, with or without a religious belief. It's there for anyone. Spirituality also highlights how connected we are to the world and other people.

What Is Spiritual Health Care?

People with mental health problems have said that they want:

- meaningful activity such as creative art, work, or enjoying nature;
- to feel safe and secure;
- to be treated with dignity and respect;
- to feel that they belong, are valued, and trusted;
- time to express feelings to members of staff;
- the chance to make sense of their life—including illness and loss;
- permission/support to develop their relationship with God or the Absolute.

Someone with a religious belief may need:

- a time, a place, and privacy in which to pray and worship;
- the chance to explore spiritual (and sometimes religious) matters;
- to be reassured that the psychiatrist will not try to undermine their faith;
- encouragement to deepen their faith;
- to feel universally connected;
- sometimes—the need for forgiveness.

What Difference Can Spirituality Make?

Service users tell us that they have gained:

- better self-control, self-esteem, and confidence;
- faster and easier recovery (often through healthy grieving of losses and through recognizing their strengths);
- better relationships—with self, others, and with God/creation/ nature;
- a new sense of meaning, hope, and peace of mind. This has allowed them to accept and live with their continuing problems.

A Religious/Spiritual Assessment

A helpful way to begin can be to ask "Would you say you are spiritual or religious in any way? Please tell me how." Another useful question is, "What sustains you?" or "What keeps you going in difficult times?" The answer to this will usually reveal a person's main spiritual concerns and practices.

Sometimes, a professional may want to use a questionnaire. They will want to find out:

- what helpful knowledge or strengths do you have that can be encouraged?
- what support can your faith community offer?

A gentle, unhurried approach works best—at its best, exploring spiritual issues can be therapeutic in itself.

- **Setting the scene:** What is your life all about? Is there anything that gives you a sense of meaning or purpose?

- **The past:** Emotional stress is often caused by a loss, or the threat of loss. Have you had any major losses or bereavements? How has this affected you and how have you coped?

- **The present:** Do you feel that you belong and that you are valued? Do you feel safe and respected? Are you and other people able to communicate clearly and freely? Do you feel that there is a spiritual aspect to your current problem? Would it help to involve a chaplain, or someone from your faith community? What do I need to understand about your religious background?

- **The future:** What do the next few weeks hold for you? What about the next few months or years? Are you worried about death and dying, or about the possibility of an afterlife? Would you want to discuss this more? What are your main fears about the future? Do you feel the need for forgiveness about anything? What, if anything, gives you hope?

- **Remedies:** What kind of support would help you? How could you get it? Have you thought about self-help?

A spiritual assessment should be part of every mental health assessment. Depression and substance misuse, for example, can sometimes reflect a spiritual void in a person's life. Mental health professionals also need to be able to distinguish between a spiritual crisis and a mental illness, particularly when these overlap.

Spiritual Practices

These span a wide range, from the religious to secular—which may not be obviously spiritual. You may:

- belong to a faith tradition and take part in services or other activities with other people;

- take part in rituals, symbolic practices, and other forms of worship;

- go on pilgrimage and retreats;

- spend time in meditation and prayer;

- read scripture;

- listen to singing and/or playing sacred music, including songs, hymns, psalms, and devotional chants;

- give of yourself in acts of compassion (including work, especially teamwork);

- engage in deep reflection (contemplation);
- follow traditions of yoga, Tai Chi, and similar disciplined practices;
- spend time enjoying nature;
- spend time in contemplative reading (of literature, poetry, philosophy, etc.);
- appreciate the arts;
- be creative—in painting, sculpture, cookery, gardening, etc.;
- make and keep good family relationships;
- make and keep friendships, especially those with trust and intimacy;
- join in team sports or other activities that involve cooperation and trust.

Spiritual Values and Skills

Spiritual practices can help us to develop the better parts of ourselves. They can help us to become more creative, patient, persistent, honest, kind, compassionate, wise, calm, hopeful, and joyful. These are all part of the best health care.

Spiritual skills include:

- being honest—and able to see yourself as others see you;
- being able to stay focused in the present, to be alert, unhurried, and attentive;
- being able to rest, relax, and create a still, peaceful state of mind;
- developing a deeper sense of empathy for others;
- being able to be with someone who is suffering, while still being hopeful;
- learning better judgment, for example about when to speak or act, and when to remain silent or do nothing;
- learning how to give without feeling drained;
- being able to grieve and let go.

Spirituality emphasizes our connections to other people and the world, which creates the idea of reciprocity. This means that the giver and receiver both get something from what happens, that if you help another person, you help yourself. Many carers naturally develop spiritual skills and values over time as a result of their commitment to those for whom they care. Those being cared for, in turn, can often give help to others in distress.

The Place of Chaplaincy/Pastoral Care

Times have changed. Hospital chaplaincy now involves clergy and others from many faiths, denominations, and humanist organizations. Chaplains (also called spiritual advisors) are increasingly part of the teams that provide care both in and outside hospital.

A modern mental health chaplaincy or pastoral care department should:

- have access to a sacred space;
- get on well with local clergy and faith communities;
- provide information about local religious groups, their traditions and practices;
- be aware that, sometimes, an individual's engagement with religious beliefs and activities can be unhelpful and even damaging;
- be able to give advice on difficult issues, such as paranormal influences, spirit possession, and the ministry of deliverance;
- work closely with the mental health team so that spiritual needs can be recognized and helped;
- make sure that service users and patients know about them.

Education and Research

There is some evidence that people who belong to a faith community, or who hold religious or spiritual beliefs, have better mental health. So, spirituality is now covered in courses for mental health care students and practitioners.

About the Spirituality and Psychiatry Special Interest Group (SIG)

The Spirituality and Psychiatry Special Interest Group (SPSIG) of the Royal College of Psychiatrists was founded in 1999 to:

- help psychiatrists to share experiences and to explore spirituality in mental healthcare;

- to increase knowledge of the research linking spirituality with better health;
- to raise the profile of spirituality in patient care.

The SPSIG has now over 2500 psychiatrist members. It runs an active program of one-day events for members and holds occasional conferences open to the general public. Information about these meetings (and the texts of all the talks) can be found in the *SPSIG Newsletter* at the SPSIG website (http://www.rcpsych.ac.uk/college/specialinterest groups/spirituality.aspx).

How to Start .....?

Spirituality is deeply personal. Try to discover what works best for you. A three-part daily routine can be helpful:

- a regular quiet time (for prayer, reflection or meditation);
- study of religious and/or spiritual material;
- making supportive friendships with others with similar spiritual and/or religious aims and aspirations.

You can find out about spiritual practices and traditions from a wide range of religious organizations. Secular spiritual activities are increasingly available and popular. For example, many complementary therapies have a spiritual or holistic element that is not part of any particular religion. The internet, especially internet bookshops, the local yellow pages, health food shops, and bookstores are all good places to look.

Part Four

Pediatric Mental Health Concerns

Chapter 26

Mental Health Care for Children and Teens

Chapter Contents

Section 26.1

Taking Your Child to a Therapist

Sometimes kids, like adults, can benefit from therapy. Therapy can help kids develop problem-solving skills and also teach them the value of seeking help. Therapists can help kids and families cope with stress and a variety of emotional and behavioral issues.

Many kids need help dealing with school stress, such as homework, test anxiety, bullying, or peer pressure. Others need help to discuss their feelings about family issues, particularly if there's a major transition, such as a divorce, move, or serious illness.

Should My Child See a Therapist?

Significant life events—such as the death of a family member, friend, or pet; divorce or a move; abuse; trauma; a parent leaving on military deployment; or a major illness in the family—can cause stress that might lead to problems with behavior, mood, sleep, appetite, and academic or social functioning.

In some cases, it's not as clear what's caused a child to suddenly seem withdrawn, worried, stressed, sulky, or tearful. But if you feel your child might have an emotional or behavioral problem or needs help coping with a difficult life event, trust your instincts.

Signs that a child may benefit from seeing a psychologist or licensed therapist include:

- developmental delay in speech, language, or toilet training

- learning or attention problems (such as ADHD)

- behavioral problems (such as excessive anger, acting out, bed-wetting or eating disorders)

- a significant drop in grades, particularly if your child normally maintains high grades

- episodes of sadness, tearfulness, or depression

- social withdrawal or isolation

- being the victim of bullying or bullying other children

- decreased interest in previously enjoyed activities

- overly aggressive behavior (such as biting, kicking, or hitting)

- sudden changes in appetite (particularly in adolescents)

- insomnia or increased sleepiness

- excessive school absenteeism or tardiness

- mood swings (e.g., happy one minute, upset the next)

- development of or an increase in physical complaints (such as headache, stomachache, or not feeling well) despite a normal physical exam by your doctor

- management of a serious, acute, or chronic illness

- signs of alcohol, drug, or other substance use (such as solvents or prescription drug abuse)

- problems in transitions (following separation, divorce, or relocation)

- bereavement issues

- custody evaluations

- therapy following sexual, physical, or emotional abuse or other traumatic events

Kids who aren't yet school-age could benefit from seeing a developmental or clinical psychologist if there's a significant delay in achieving developmental milestones such as walking, talking, and potty training, and if there are concerns regarding autism or other developmental disorders.

Talk to Caregivers, Teachers, and the Doctor

It's also helpful to speak to caregivers and teachers who interact regularly with your child. Is your child paying attention in class and turning in assignments on time? What's his or her behavior like at recess and with peers? Gather as much information as possible to determine the best course of action.

Discuss your concerns with your child's doctor, who can offer perspective and evaluate your child to rule out any medical conditions that could be having an effect. The doctor also may be able to refer you to a qualified therapist for the help your child needs.

Finding the Right Therapist

How do you find a qualified clinician who has experience working with kids and teens? While experience and education are important, it's also important to find a counselor your child feels comfortable talking to. Look for one who not only has the right experience, but also the best approach to help your child in the current circumstances.

Your doctor can be a good source of a referral. Most doctors have working relationships with mental health specialists such as child psychologists or clinical social workers. Friends, colleagues, or family members might also be able to recommend someone.

Consider a number of factors when searching for the right therapist for your child. A good first step is to ask if the therapist is willing to meet with you for a brief consultation or to talk with you during a phone interview before you commit to regular visits. Not all therapists are able to do this, given their busy schedules. Most therapists charge a fee for this type of service; others consider it a complimentary visit.

Factors to Consider

Consider the following factors when evaluating a potential therapist:

- Is the therapist licensed to practice in your state? (You can check with the state board for that profession or check to see if the license is displayed in the office.)

- Is the therapist covered by your health insurance plan's mental health benefits? If so, how many sessions are covered by your plan? What will your co-pay be?

- What are his or her credentials?

- What type of experience does the therapist have?

- How long has the therapist worked with children and adolescents?

- Would your child find the therapist friendly?

- What is the cancellation policy if you're unable to keep an appointment?

- Is the therapist available by phone during an emergency?

- Who will be available to your child during the therapist's vacation or illness or during off-hours?

- What types of therapy does the therapist specialize in?

- Is the therapist willing to meet with you in addition to working with your child?

The right therapist-client match is critical, so you might need to meet with a few before you find one who clicks with both you and your child.

As with other medical professionals, therapists may have a variety of credentials and specific degrees. As a general rule, your child's therapist should hold a professional degree in the field of mental health (psychology, social work, or psychiatry) and be licensed by your state. Psychologists, social workers, and psychiatrists all diagnose and treat mental health disorders.

It's also a good idea to know what those letters that follow a therapist's name mean:

Psychiatrists: Psychiatrists (MDs or DOs) are medical doctors who have advanced training and experience in psychotherapy and pharmacology. They can also prescribe medications.

Clinical psychologists: Clinical psychologists (PhDs, PsyDs, or EdDs) are therapists who have a doctorate degree that includes advanced training in the practice of psychology, and many specialize in treating children and teens and their families. Psychologists may help clients manage medications but do not prescribe medication.

Clinical social workers: A licensed clinical social worker (LCSW) has a master's degree, specializes in clinical social work, and is licensed in the state in which he or she practices. An LICSW is also a licensed clinical social worker. A CSW is a certified social worker. Many social workers are trained in psychotherapy, but the credentials vary from state to state. Likewise, the designations (i.e., LCSW, LICSW, CSW) can vary from state to state.

Different Types of Therapy

There are many types of therapy. Therapists choose the strategies that are most appropriate for a particular problem and for the individual child and family. Therapists will often spend a portion of each session with the parents alone, with the child alone, and with the family together.

Any one therapist may use a variety of strategies, including:

- Cognitive behavioral therapy (CBT). This type of therapy is often helpful with kids and teens who are depressed, anxious, or having problems coping with stress. Cognitive behavioral therapy restructures negative thoughts into more positive, effective ways of thinking. It can include work on stress management strategies, relaxation training, practicing coping skills, and other forms of treatment.

- Psychoanalytic therapy is less commonly used with children but can be used with older kids and teens who may benefit from more in-depth analysis of their problems. This is the quintessential talk therapy and does not focus on short-term problem-solving in the same way as CBT and behavioral therapies.

- In some cases, kids benefit from individual therapy, one-on-one work with the therapist on issues they need guidance on, such as depression, social difficulties, or worry. In other cases, the right option is group therapy, where kids meet in groups of 6 to 12 to solve problems and learn new skills (such as social skills or anger management).

- Family therapy can be helpful in many cases, such as when family members aren't getting along; disagree or argue often; or when a child or teen is having behavior problems. Family therapy involves counseling sessions with some, or all, family members, helping to improve communication skills among them. Treatment focuses on problem-solving techniques and can help parents re-establish their role as authority figures.

Preparing for the First Visit

You may be concerned that your child will become upset when told of an upcoming visit with a therapist. Although this is sometimes the case, it's essential to be honest about the session and why your child (or family) will be going. The issue will come up during the session, but it's important for you to prepare your child for it.

Explain to young kids that this type of visit to the doctor doesn't involve a physical exam or shots. You may also want to stress that this type of doctor talks and plays with kids and families to help them solve problems and feel better. Kids might feel reassured to learn that the therapist will be helping the parents and other family members too.

Older kids and teens may be reassured to hear that anything they say to the therapist is confidential and cannot be shared with anyone else, including parents or other doctors, without their permission—the exception is if they indicate that they're having thoughts of suicide or otherwise hurting themselves or others.

Giving kids this kind of information before the first appointment can help set the tone, prevent your child from feeling singled out or isolated, and provide reassurance that the family will be working together on the problem.

Providing Additional Support

While your child copes with emotional issues, be there to listen and care, and offer support without judgment. Patience is critical, too, as many young children are unable to verbalize their fears and emotions.

Try to set aside some time to discuss your child's worries or concerns. To minimize distractions, turn off the TV and let voice mail answer your phone calls. This will let your child know that he or she is your first priority.

Other ways to communicate openly and problem-solve include:

- Talk openly and as frequently with your child as you can.

- Show love and affection to your child, especially during troubled times.

- Set a good example by taking care of your own physical and emotional needs.

- Enlist the support of your partner, immediate family members, your child's doctor, and teachers.

- Improve communication at home by having family meetings that end with a fun activity (e.g., playing a game, making ice-cream sundaes).

- No matter how hard it is, set limits on inappropriate or problematic behaviors. Ask the therapist for some strategies to encourage your child's cooperation.

- Communicate frequently with the therapist.

- Be open to all types of feedback from your child and from the therapist.

- Respect the relationship between your child and the therapist. If you feel threatened by it, discuss this with the therapist (it's nothing to be embarrassed about).

- Enjoy favorite activities or hobbies with your child.

By recognizing problems and seeking help early on, you can help your child—and your entire family—move through the tough times toward happier, healthier times ahead.

Section 26.2

Treatment of Children with Mental Illness

Excerpted from "Treatment of Children with Mental Illnesses," National Institute of Mental Health (www.nimh.nih.gov), November 23, 2011.

What should I do if I am concerned about mental, behavioral, or emotional symptoms in my child?

Talk to your child's doctor or health care provider. Ask questions and learn everything you can about the behavior or symptoms that worry you. If your child is in school ask the teacher if your child has been showing worrisome changes in behavior. Share this with your child's doctor or health care provider. Keep in mind that every child is different. Even normal development, such as when children develop language, motor, and social skills, varies from child to child. Ask if your child needs further evaluation by a specialist with experience in child behavioral problems. Specialists may include psychiatrists, psychologists, social workers, psychiatric nurses, and behavioral therapists. Educators may also help evaluate your child.

If you take your child to a specialist, ask, "Do you have experience treating the problems I see in my child?" Don't be afraid to interview more than one specialist to find the right fit. Continue to learn everything you can about the problem or diagnosis. The more you learn, the better you can work with your child's doctor and make decisions that feel right for you, your child, and your family.

How do I know if my child's problems are serious?

Not every problem is serious. In fact, many everyday stresses can cause changes in your child's behavior. For example, the birth of a sibling may cause a child to temporarily act much younger than he or she is. It is important to be able to tell the difference between typical behavior changes and those associated with more serious problems. Pay special attention to behaviors that include:

- Problems across a variety of settings, such as at school, at home, or with peers
- Changes in appetite or sleep
- Social withdrawal, or fearful behavior toward things your child normally is not afraid of
- Returning to behaviors more common in younger children, such as bed-wetting, for a long time
- Signs of being upset, such as sadness or tearfulness
- Signs of self-destructive behavior, such as head-banging, or a tendency to get hurt often
- Repeated thoughts of death

Can symptoms be caused by a death in the family, illness in a parent, family financial problems, divorce, or other events?

Yes. Every member of a family is affected by tragedy or extreme stress, even the youngest child. It's normal for stress to cause a child to be upset. Remember this if you see mental, emotional, or behavioral symptoms in your child. If it takes more than one month for your child to get used to a situation, or if your child has severe reactions, talk to your child's doctor.

Check your child's response to stress. Take note if he or she gets better with time or if professional care is needed. Stressful events are challenging, but they give you a chance to teach your child important ways to cope.

Will my child get better with time?

Some children get better with time. But other children need ongoing professional help. Talk to your child's doctor or specialist about problems that are severe, continuous, and affect daily activities. Also, don't delay seeking help. Treatment may produce better results if started early.

Are there treatment options for children?

Yes. Once a diagnosis is made, your child's specialist will recommend a specific treatment. It is important to understand the various treatment choices, which often include psychotherapy or medication. Talk about the options with a health care professional who has experience treating the illness observed in your child. Some treatment choices have been studied experimentally, and other treatments are a part of health care practice. In addition, not every community has every type of service or program.

What are psychotropic medications?

Psychotropic medications are substances that affect brain chemicals related to mood and behavior. In recent years, research has been conducted to understand the benefits and risks of using psychotropics in children. Still, more needs to be learned about the effects of psychotropics, especially in children under six years of age. While researchers are trying to clarify how early treatment affects a growing body, families and doctors should weigh the benefits and risks of medication. Each child has individual needs, and each child needs to be monitored closely while taking medications.

Are there treatments other than medications?

Yes. Psychosocial therapies can be very effective alone and in combination with medications. Psychosocial therapies are also called talk therapies or behavioral therapy, and they help people with mental illness change behavior. Therapies that teach parents and children coping strategies can also be effective.

Cognitive behavioral therapy (CBT) is a type of psychotherapy that can be used with children. It has been widely studied and is an effective treatment for a number of conditions, such as depression, obsessive-compulsive disorder, and social anxiety. A person in CBT learns to change distorted thinking patterns and unhealthy behavior. Children can receive CBT with or without their parents, as well as in a group setting. CBT can be adapted to fit the needs of each child. It is especially useful when treating anxiety disorders.

Additionally, therapies for ADHD are numerous and include behavioral parent training and behavioral classroom management. Visit the NIMH website (www.nimh.nih.gov) for more information about therapies for ADHD.

Some children benefit from a combination of different psychosocial approaches. An example is behavioral parent management training in combination with CBT for the child. In other cases, a combination of medication and psychosocial therapies may be most effective. Psychosocial therapies often take time, effort, and patience. However, sometimes children learn new skills that may have positive long-term benefits.

More information about treatment choices can be found in the psychotherapies and medications sections of the NIMH website (www.nimh.nih.gov).

Does medication affect young children differently than older children or adults?

Yes. Young children handle medications differently than older children and adults. The brains of young children change and develop rapidly. Studies have found that developing brains can be very sensitive to medications. There are also developmental differences in how children metabolize—how their bodies process—medications. Therefore, doctors should carefully consider the dosage or how much medication to give each child. Much more research is needed to determine the effects and benefits of medications in children of all ages. But keep in mind that serious untreated mental disorders themselves can harm brain development.

Also, it is important to avoid drug interactions. If your child takes medicine for asthma or cold symptoms, talk to your doctor or pharmacist. Drug interactions could cause medications to not work as intended or lead to serious side effects.

What medications are used for which kinds of childhood mental disorders?

Psychotropic medications include stimulants, antidepressants, antianxiety medications, antipsychotics, and mood stabilizers. Dosages approved by the U.S. Food and Drug Administration (FDA) for use in children depend on body weight and age. NIMH's medications booklet describes the types of psychotropic medications and includes a chart that lists the ages for which each medication is FDA-approved. See the FDA website (www.fda.gov) for the latest information on medication approvals, warnings, and patient information guides.

When the FDA approves a medication, it means the drug manufacturer provided the agency with information showing the medication is safe and effective in a particular group of people. Based on this information, the drug's label lists proper dosage, potential side effects, and approved age. Medications approved for children follow these guidelines.

Many psychotropic medications have not been studied in children, which means they have not been approved by the FDA for use in children. But doctors may prescribe medications as they feel appropriate, even if those uses are not included on the label. This is called off-label use. Research shows that off-label use of some medications works well in some children. Other medications need more study in children. In particular, the use of most psychotropic medications has not been adequately studied in preschoolers.

More studies in children are needed before we can fully know the appropriate dosages, how a medication works in children, and what effects a medication might have on learning and development.

What else can I do to help my child?

Children with mental illness need guidance and understanding from their parents and teachers. This support can help your child achieve his or her full potential and succeed in school. Before a child is diagnosed, frustration, blame, and anger may have built up within a family. Parents and children may need special help to undo these unhealthy interaction patterns. Mental health professionals can counsel the child and family to help everyone develop new skills, attitudes, and ways of relating to each other.

Parents can also help by taking part in parenting skills training. This helps parents learn how to handle difficult situations and behaviors. Training encourages parents to share a pleasant or relaxing activity with their child, to notice and point out what their child does well, and to praise their child's strengths and abilities. Parents may also learn to arrange family situations in more positive ways. Also, parents may benefit from learning stress-management techniques to help them deal with frustration and respond calmly to their child's behavior.

Sometimes, the whole family may need counseling. Therapists can help family members find better ways to handle disruptive behaviors and encourage behavior changes. Finally, support groups help parents and families connect with others who have similar problems and concerns. Groups often meet regularly to share frustrations and successes, to exchange information about recommended specialists and strategies, and to talk with experts.

How can families of children with mental illness get support?

Like other serious illnesses, taking care of a child with mental illness is hard on the parents, family, and other caregivers. Caregivers often must tend to the medical needs of their loved ones, and also deal with how it affects their own health. The stress that caregivers are under may lead to missed work or lost free time. It can strain relationships with people who may not understand the situation and lead to physical and mental exhaustion.

Stress from caregiving can make it hard to cope with your child's symptoms. One study shows that if a caregiver is under enormous stress, his or her loved one has more difficulty sticking to the treatment plan. It is important to look after your own physical and mental health. You may also find it helpful to join a local support group.

Section 26.3

Helping Children and Adolescents Cope with Violence and Disasters

Excerpted from "Helping Children and Adolescents Cope with Violence and Disasters: What Parents Can Do," National Institute of Mental Health (www.nimh.nih.gov), May 3, 2011.

Coping with Trauma after Violence and Disasters

Disasters cause major damage. Hurricanes Katrina and Rita were examples. They occurred in 2005. Many homes were destroyed. Whole communities were damaged. Many survivors were displaced. There were also many deaths.

Trauma is also caused by major acts of violence. The September 11, 2001 terrorist attacks were examples. Another example was the 1999 shootings at Columbine High School in Colorado. The Oklahoma City bombing in 1995 was also an example. These acts claim lives. They also threaten our sense of security.

Beyond these events, children may face many other traumas. Each year, some are injured, some see others harmed by violence, and some suffer sexual abuse. Some may also lose loved ones or witness other tragic events.

Children are very sensitive. They struggle to make sense of trauma. They also respond differently to traumas. They may have emotional reactions. They may hurt deeply. They may find it hard to recover from frightening experiences. They need support. Adult helpers can provide this support. This may help children resolve emotional problems.

What Is Trauma?

There are two types of trauma—physical and mental. Physical trauma includes the body's response to serious injury and threat. Mental trauma includes frightening thoughts and painful feelings. They are the mind's response to serious injury. Mental trauma can produce strong feelings. It can also produce extreme behavior; such as intense fear or helplessness, withdrawal or detachment, lack of concentration, irritability, sleep disturbance, aggression, hyper vigilance (intensely watching for more distressing events), or flashbacks (sense that the event is reoccurring).

A response could be fear. It could be fear that a loved one will be hurt or killed. It is believed that more direct exposures to traumatic events causes greater harm. For instance, in a school shooting, an injured student will probably be more severely affected emotionally than a student who was in another part of the building. However, second-hand exposure to violence can also be traumatic. This includes witnessing violence such as seeing or hearing about death and destruction after a building is bombed or a plane crashes.

How Parents Can Help

After violence or a disaster parents and family should follow these guidelines:

- Identify and address their own feelings—this will allow them to help others.

- Explain to children what happened.

- Let children know you love them and the event was not their fault. Let them know you will take care of them, but only if you can; be honest. Also assure them that it's okay for them to feel upset.

- Do: Allow children to cry; Allow sadness; Let children talk about feelings; let them write about feelings; let them draw pictures

- Don't: Expect children to be brave or tough; Make children discuss the event before they are ready; Get angry if children show strong emotions; Get upset if they begin bed-wetting, acting out, or thumb-sucking

- If children have trouble sleeping: Give them extra attention; Let them sleep with a light on; Let them sleep in your room (for a short time)

- Try to keep normal routines (such routines may not be normal for some children): Bed-time stories; Eating dinner together; Watching TV together; Reading books, exercising, playing games

- If you can't keep normal routines, make new ones together

- Help children feel in control: Let them choose meals, if possible; Let them pick out clothes, if possible; Let them make some decisions for themselves, when possible

How Children React to Trauma

Children's reactions to trauma can be immediate. Reactions may also appear much later. Reactions differ in severity. They also cover a range of behaviors. People from different cultures may have their own ways of reacting. Other reactions vary according to age.

One common response is loss of trust. Another is fear of the event reoccurring. Some children are more vulnerable to trauma's effects. Children with existing mental health problems may be more affected. Children who have experienced other traumatic events may be more affected.

Children Age 5 and Under

Children under five can react in a number of ways:

- Facial expressions of fear

- Clinging to parent or caregiver

- Crying or screaming

- Whimpering or trembling

- Moving aimlessly

- Becoming immobile

- Returning to behaviors common to being younger: Thumb sucking; Bedwetting; Being afraid of the dark.

Young children's reactions are strongly influenced by parent reactions to the event.

Children Age 6 to 11

Children between six and 11 have a range of reactions. They may exhibit these behaviors:

- Isolate themselves
- Become quiet around friends, family, and teachers
- Have nightmares or other sleep problems
- Become irritable or disruptive
- Have outbursts of anger
- Start fights
- Be unable to concentrate
- Refuse to go to school
- Complain of unfounded physical problems
- Develop unfounded fears
- Become depressed
- Become filled with guilt
- Feel numb emotionally
- Do poorly with school and homework

Adolescents Age 12 to 17

Children between 12 and 17 have various reactions:

- Flashbacks to the traumatic event (flashbacks are the mind reliving the event)
- Avoiding reminders of the event
- Drug, alcohol, tobacco use and abuse
- Antisocial behavior (disruptive, disrespectful, or destructive behavior)
- Physical complaints
- Nightmares or other sleep problems
- Isolation or confusion
- Depression
- Suicidal thoughts.

Adolescents may feel guilty about the event. They may feel guilt for not preventing injury or deaths. They may also have thoughts of revenge.

More about Trauma and Stress

Some children will have prolonged problems after a traumatic event. These may include grief, depression, anxiety and post-traumatic stress disorder (PTSD). Children may show a range of symptoms:

- Re-experiencing the event through play, through trauma-specific nightmares/dreams, in flashbacks and unwanted memories, or by distress over events that remind them of the trauma
- Avoidance of reminders of the event
- Lack of responsiveness
- Lack of interest in things that used to interest them
- A sense of having no future
- Increased sleep disturbances
- Irritability
- Poor concentration
- Be easily startled
- Behavior from earlier life stages.

If, after a month in a safe environment children are not able to perform normal routines or new symptoms develop, contact a health professional.

Some people are more sensitive to trauma. Factors that may influence how someone may respond include the following:

- Being directly involved in the trauma, especially as a victim
- Severe and/or prolonged exposure to the event
- Personal history of prior trauma
- Family or personal history of mental illness and severe behavioral problems
- Lack of social support
- Lack of caring family and friends
- On-going life stressors such as moving to a new home, or new school, divorce, job change, financial troubles.

Some symptoms may require immediate attention. Contact a mental health professional if these symptoms occur:

- Flashbacks
- Racing heart and sweating
- Being easily startled
- Being emotionally numb
- Being very sad or depressed
- Thoughts or actions to end life

Chapter 27

Attention Deficit Hyperactivity Disorder (ADHD)

What is attention deficit hyperactivity disorder?

Attention deficit hyperactivity disorder (ADHD) is one of the most common childhood disorders and can continue through adolescence and adulthood. Symptoms include difficulty staying focused and paying attention, difficulty controlling behavior, and hyperactivity (over-activity). ADHD has three subtypes:

- Predominantly hyperactive-impulsive

  - Most symptoms (six or more) are in the hyperactivity-impulsivity categories.

  - Fewer than six symptoms of inattention are present, although inattention may still be present to some degree.

- Predominantly inattentive

  - The majority of symptoms (six or more) are in the inattention category and fewer than six symptoms of hyperactivity-impulsivity are present, although hyperactivity-impulsivity may still be present to some degree.

  - Children with this subtype are less likely to act out or have difficulties getting along with other children. They may sit quietly, but they are not paying attention to what they are

Excerpted from "Attention Deficit Hyperactivity Disorder (ADHD)," National Institute of Mental Health (www.nimh.nih.gov), September 22, 2011.

doing. Therefore, the child may be overlooked, and parents and teachers may not notice that he or she has ADHD.

- Combined hyperactive-impulsive and inattentive
  - Six or more symptoms of inattention and six or more symptoms of hyperactivity-impulsivity are present.
  - Most children have the combined type of ADHD.

Treatments can relieve many of the disorder's symptoms, but there is no cure. With treatment, most people with ADHD can be successful in school and lead productive lives. Researchers are developing more effective treatments and interventions, and using new tools such as brain imaging, to better understand ADHD and to find more effective ways to treat and prevent it.

What are the symptoms of ADHD in children?

Inattention, hyperactivity, and impulsivity are the key behaviors of ADHD. It is normal for all children to be inattentive, hyperactive, or impulsive sometimes, but for children with ADHD, these behaviors are more severe and occur more often. To be diagnosed with the disorder, a child must have symptoms for six or more months and to a degree that is greater than other children of the same age. Children who have symptoms of inattention may display these characteristics:

- Be easily distracted, miss details, forget things, and frequently switch from one activity to another

- Have difficulty focusing on one thing

- Become bored with a task after only a few minutes, unless they are doing something enjoyable

- Have difficulty focusing attention on organizing and completing a task or learning something new

- Have trouble completing or turning in homework assignments, often losing things (for example, pencils, toys, assignments) needed to complete tasks or activities

- Not seem to listen when spoken to

- Daydream, become easily confused, and move slowly

- Have difficulty processing information as quickly and accurately as others

- Struggle to follow instructions

Children who have symptoms of hyperactivity may display these characteristics:

- Fidget and squirm in their seats
- Talk nonstop
- Dash around, touching or playing with anything and everything in sight
- Have trouble sitting still during dinner, school, and story time
- Be constantly in motion
- Have difficulty doing quiet tasks or activities

Children who have symptoms of impulsivity may display these characteristics:

- Be very impatient
- Blurt out inappropriate comments, show their emotions without restraint, and act without regard for consequences
- Have difficulty waiting for things they want or waiting their turns in games
- Often interrupt conversations or others' activities

What causes ADHD?

Scientists are not sure what causes ADHD, although many studies suggest that genes play a large role. Like many other illnesses, ADHD probably results from a combination of factors. In addition to genetics, researchers are looking at possible environmental factors, and are studying how brain injuries, nutrition, and the social environment might contribute to ADHD.

Genes: Inherited from our parents, genes are the "blueprints" for who we are. Results from several international studies of twins show that ADHD often runs in families. Researchers are looking at several genes that may make people more likely to develop the disorder. Knowing the genes involved may one day help researchers prevent the disorder before symptoms develop. Learning about specific genes could also lead to better treatments.

Children with ADHD who carry a particular version of a certain gene have thinner brain tissue in the areas of the brain associated with attention. This National Institute of Mental Health (NIMH) research showed that the difference was not permanent, however, and as children with this gene grew up, the brain developed to a normal level of thickness. Their ADHD symptoms also improved.

Environmental factors: Studies suggest a potential link between cigarette smoking and alcohol use during pregnancy and ADHD in children. In addition, preschoolers who are exposed to high levels of lead, which can sometimes be found in plumbing fixtures or paint in old buildings, may have a higher risk of developing ADHD.

Brain injuries: Children who have suffered a brain injury may show some behaviors similar to those of ADHD. However, only a small percentage of children with ADHD have suffered a traumatic brain injury.

Sugar: The idea that refined sugar causes ADHD or makes symptoms worse is popular, but more research discounts this theory than supports it. In one study, researchers gave children foods containing either sugar or a sugar substitute every other day. The children who received sugar showed no different behavior or learning capabilities than those who received the sugar substitute. Another study in which children were given higher than average amounts of sugar or sugar substitutes showed similar results.

Food additives: Recent British research indicates a possible link between consumption of certain food additives like artificial colors or preservatives, and an increase in activity. Research is under way to confirm the findings and to learn more about how food additives may affect hyperactivity.

How is ADHD diagnosed?

No single test can diagnose a child as having ADHD. Instead, a licensed health professional needs to gather information about the child, and his or her behavior and environment. A family may want to first talk with the child's pediatrician. Some pediatricians can assess the child themselves, but many will refer the family to a mental health specialist with experience in childhood mental disorders such as ADHD. The pediatrician or mental health specialist will first try to rule out other possibilities for the symptoms. For example, certain situations, events, or health conditions may cause temporary behaviors in a child that seem like ADHD.

Between them, the referring pediatrician and specialist will determine if a child is impacted by these things:

- Undetected seizures that could be associated with other medical conditions

- Middle ear infection that is causing hearing problems

- Undetected hearing or vision problems

- Medical problems that affect thinking and behavior

- Learning disabilities

- Anxiety or depression, or other psychiatric problems that might cause ADHD-like symptoms

- A significant and sudden change, such as the death of a family member, a divorce, or parent's job loss

A specialist will also check school and medical records for clues, to see if the child's home or school settings appear unusually stressful or disrupted, and gather information from the child's parents and teachers. Coaches, babysitters, and other adults who know the child well also may be consulted.

The specialist also will ask these questions:

- Are the behaviors excessive and long-term, and do they affect all aspects of the child's life?

- Do they happen more often in this child compared with the child's peers?

- Are the behaviors a continuous problem or a response to a temporary situation?

- Do the behaviors occur in several settings or only in one place, such as the playground, classroom, or home?

The specialist pays close attention to the child's behavior during different situations. Some situations are highly structured, some have less structure. Others would require the child to keep paying attention. Most children with ADHD are better able to control their behaviors in situations where they are getting individual attention and when they are free to focus on enjoyable activities. These types of situations are less important in the assessment. A child also may be evaluated to see how he or she acts in social situations and may be given tests of intellectual ability and academic achievement to see if he or she has a learning disability.

Finally, if after gathering all this information the child meets the criteria for ADHD, he or she will be diagnosed with the disorder.

How is ADHD treated?

Currently available treatments focus on reducing the symptoms of ADHD and improving functioning. Treatments include medication, various types of psychotherapy, education or training, or a combination of treatments.

Medications: The most common type of medication used for treating ADHD is called a stimulant. Although it may seem unusual to treat ADHD with a medication considered a stimulant, it actually has a calming effect on children with ADHD. Many types of stimulant medications are available. A few other ADHD medications are non-stimulants and work differently than stimulants. For many children, ADHD medications reduce hyperactivity and impulsivity and improve their ability to focus, work, and learn. Medication also may improve physical coordination.

However, a one-size-fits-all approach does not apply for all children with ADHD. What works for one child might not work for another. One child might have side effects with a certain medication, while another child may not. Sometimes several different medications or dosages must be tried before finding one that works for a particular child. Any child taking medications must be monitored closely and carefully by caregivers and doctors.

Stimulant medications come in different forms, such as a pill, capsule, liquid, or skin patch. Some medications also come in short-acting, long-acting, or extended release varieties. In each of these varieties, the active ingredient is the same, but it is released differently in the body. Long-acting or extended release forms often allow a child to take the medication just once a day before school, so they don't have to make a daily trip to the school nurse for another dose. Parents and doctors should decide together which medication is best for the child and whether the child needs medication only for school hours or for evenings and weekends, too.

A list of medications and the approved age for use is given in Table 27.1. ADHD can be diagnosed and medications prescribed by M.D.s (usually a psychiatrist) and in some states also by clinical psychologists, psychiatric nurse practitioners, and advanced psychiatric nurse specialists. Check with your state's licensing agency for specifics.

Table 27.1. Medications and Approved Ages for Treating ADHD

Trade Name	Generic Name	Approved Age
Adderall	amphetamine	3 and older
Adderall XR	amphetamine (extended release)	6 and older
Concerta	methylphenidate (long acting)	6 and older
Daytrana	methylphenidate patch	6 and older
Desoxyn	methamphetamine hydrochloride	6 and older
Dexedrine	dextroamphetamine	3 and older
Dextrostat	dextroamphetamine	3 and older
Focalin	dexmethylphenidate	6 and older
Focalin XR	dexmethylphenidate (extended release)	6 and older
Metadate ER	methylphenidate (extended release)	6 and older
Metadate CD	methylphenidate (extended release)	6 and older
Methylin	methylphenidate (oral solution and chewable tablets)	6 and older
Ritalin	methylphenidate	6 and older
Ritalin SR	methylphenidate (extended release)	6 and older
Ritalin LA	methylphenidate (long acting)	6 and older
Strattera	atomoxetine	6 and older
Vyvanse	lisdexamfetamine dimesylate	6 and older

*Not all ADHD medications are approved for use in adults.

NOTE: "extended release" means the medication is released gradually so that a controlled amount enters the body over a period of time. "Long acting" means the medication stays in the body for a long time.

Over time, this list will grow, as researchers continue to develop new medications for ADHD. Medication guides for each of these medications are available from the U.S. Food and Drug Administration (FDA).

Side effects of stimulant medications: The most commonly reported side effects are decreased appetite, sleep problems, anxiety, and irritability. Some children also report mild stomachaches or headaches. Most side effects are minor and disappear over time or if the dosage level is lowered.

- **Decreased appetite:** Be sure your child eats healthy meals. If this side effect does not go away, talk to your child's doctor. Also talk to the doctor if you have concerns about your child's growth or weight gain while he or she is taking this medication.

- **Sleep problems:** If a child cannot fall asleep, the doctor may prescribe a lower dose of the medication or a shorter-acting form. The doctor might also suggest giving the medication earlier in the day, or stopping the afternoon or evening dose. Adding a prescription for a low dose of an antidepressant or a blood pressure medication called clonidine sometimes helps with sleep problems. A consistent sleep routine that includes relaxing elements like warm milk, soft music, or quiet activities in dim light, may also help.

- **Less common side effects:** A few children develop sudden, repetitive movements or sounds called tics. These tics may or may not be noticeable. Changing the medication dosage may make tics go away. Some children also may have a personality change, such as appearing "flat" or without emotion. Talk with your child's doctor if you see any of these side effects.

Under medical supervision, stimulant medications are considered safe. Stimulants do not make children with ADHD feel high, although some kids report feeling slightly different or "funny." Although some parents worry that stimulant medications may lead to substance abuse or dependence, there is little evidence of this.

In 2007, the FDA required that all makers of ADHD medications develop Patient Medication Guides that contain information about the risks associated with the medications. The guides must alert patients that the medications may lead to possible cardiovascular (heart and blood) or psychiatric problems. The agency undertook this precaution when a review of data found that ADHD patients with existing heart conditions had a slightly higher risk of strokes, heart attacks, and/or sudden death when taking the medications.

The review also found a slight increased risk, about one in 1,000, for medication-related psychiatric problems, such as hearing voices, having hallucinations, becoming suspicious for no reason, or becoming manic (an overly high mood), even in patients without a history of psychiatric problems. The FDA recommends that any treatment plan for ADHD include an initial health history, including family history, and examination for existing cardiovascular and psychiatric problems.

One ADHD medication, the non-stimulant atomoxetine (Strattera), carries another warning. Studies show that children and teenagers who take atomoxetine are more likely to have suicidal thoughts than children and teenagers with ADHD who do not take it. If your child is taking atomoxetine, watch his or her behavior carefully. A child may develop serious symptoms suddenly, so it is important to pay attention to your child's behavior every day. Ask other people who spend a lot of time with your child to tell you if they notice changes in your child's behavior. Call a doctor right away if your child shows any unusual behavior. While taking atomoxetine, your child should see a doctor often, especially at the beginning of treatment, and be sure that your child keeps all appointments with his or her doctor.

Psychotherapy: Different types of psychotherapy are used for ADHD. Behavioral therapy aims to help a child change his or her behavior. It might involve practical assistance, such as help organizing tasks or completing schoolwork, or working through emotionally difficult events. Behavioral therapy also teaches a child how to monitor his or her own behavior. Learning to give oneself praise or rewards for acting in a desired way, such as controlling anger or thinking before acting, is another goal of behavioral therapy. Parents and teachers also can give positive or negative feedback for certain behaviors. In addition, clear rules, chore lists, and other structured routines can help a child control his or her behavior.

Therapists may teach children social skills, such as how to wait their turn, share toys, ask for help, or respond to teasing. Learning to read facial expressions and the tone of voice in others, and how to respond appropriately can also be part of social skills training.

Do medications cure ADHD?

Current medications do not cure ADHD. Rather, they control the symptoms for as long as they are taken. Medications can help a child pay attention and complete schoolwork. It is not clear, however, whether medications can help children learn or improve their academic skills. Adding behavioral therapy, counseling, and practical support can help children with ADHD and their families to better cope with everyday problems. Research funded by the National Institute of Mental Health (NIMH) has shown that medication works best when treatment is regularly monitored by the prescribing doctor and the dose is adjusted based on the child's needs.

How can parents help?

Parenting skills training helps parents learn how to use a system of rewards and consequences to change a child's behavior. Parents are taught to give immediate and positive feedback for behaviors they want to encourage, and ignore or redirect behaviors they want to discourage. In some cases, the use of time-outs may be used when the child's behavior gets out of control. In a time-out, the child is removed from the upsetting situation and sits alone for a short time to calm down.

Parents are also encouraged to share a pleasant or relaxing activity with the child, to notice and point out what the child does well, and to praise the child's strengths and abilities. They may also learn to structure situations in more positive ways. For example, they may restrict the number of playmates to one or two, so that their child does not become overstimulated. Or, if the child has trouble completing tasks, parents can help their child divide large tasks into smaller, more manageable steps. Also, parents may benefit from learning stress-management techniques to increase their own ability to deal with frustration, so that they can respond calmly to their child's behavior.

Sometimes, the whole family may need therapy. Therapists can help family members find better ways to handle disruptive behaviors and to encourage behavior changes. Finally, support groups help parents and families connect with others who have similar problems and concerns. Groups often meet regularly to share frustrations and successes, to exchange information about recommended specialists and strategies, and to talk with experts.

How can parents help kids with ADHA stay organized and follow directions?

Schedule: Keep the same routine every day, from wake-up time to bedtime. Include time for homework, outdoor play, and indoor activities. Keep the schedule on the refrigerator or on a bulletin board in the kitchen. Write changes on the schedule as far in advance as possible.

Organize everyday items: Have a place for everything, and keep everything in its place. This includes clothing, backpacks, and toys.

Use homework and notebook organizers: Use organizers for school material and supplies. Stress to your child the importance of writing down assignments and bringing home the necessary books.

Be clear and consistent: Children with ADHD need consistent rules they can understand and follow.

Give praise or rewards when rules are followed: Children with ADHD often receive and expect criticism. Look for good behavior, and praise it.

Chapter 28

Autism Spectrum Disorder

What is autism spectrum disorder (ASD)?

Autism is a group of developmental brain disorders, collectively called autism spectrum disorder (ASD). The term spectrum refers to the wide range of symptoms, skills, and levels of impairment, or disability, that children with ASD can have. Some children are mildly impaired by their symptoms, but others are severely disabled.

Five disorders, sometimes called pervasive developmental disorders (PDDs), are classified as ASD according to the *Diagnostic and Statistical Manual of Mental Disorders, Fourth Edition - Text Revision* (*DSM-IV-TR*):

- Autistic disorder (classic autism)

- Asperger's disorder (Asperger syndrome)

- Pervasive developmental disorder not otherwise specified (PDD-NOS)

- Rett's disorder (Rett syndrome)

- Childhood disintegrative disorder (CDD)

What are the symptoms of ASD?

Symptoms of autism spectrum disorder (ASD) vary from one child to the next, but in general, they fall into three areas:

Excerpted from "A Parent's Guide to Autism Spectrum Disorder," National Institute of Mental Health (www.nimh.nih.gov), October 26, 2011.

- Social impairment

- Communication difficulties

- Repetitive and stereotyped behaviors

Children with ASD do not follow typical patterns when developing social and communication skills. Parents are usually the first to notice unusual behaviors in their child. Often, certain behaviors become more noticeable when comparing children of the same age.

In some cases, babies with ASD may seem different very early in their development. Even before their first birthday, some babies become overly focused on certain objects, rarely make eye contact, and fail to engage in typical back-and-forth play and babbling with their parents. Other children may develop normally until the second or even third year of life, but then start to lose interest in others and become silent, withdrawn, or indifferent to social signals. Loss or reversal of normal development is called regression and occurs in some children with ASD.

What is social impairment?

Some children with ASD may make little eye contact. They may tend to look and listen less to people in their environment or fail to respond to other people. They do not readily seek to share their enjoyment of toys or activities by pointing or showing things to others. They often respond unusually when others show anger, distress, or affection.

Recent research suggests that children with ASD do not respond to emotional cues in human social interactions because they may not pay attention to the social cues that others typically notice. For example, one study found that children with ASD focus on the mouth of the person speaking to them instead of on the eyes, which is where children with typical development tend to focus. A related study showed that children with ASD appear to be drawn to repetitive movements linked to a sound, such as hand-clapping during a game of pat-a-cake. More research is needed to confirm these findings, but such studies suggest that children with ASD may misread or not notice subtle social cues—a smile, a wink, or a grimace—that could help them understand social relationships and interactions. For these children, a question such as, "Can you wait a minute?" always means the same thing, whether the speaker is joking, asking a real question, or issuing a firm request. Without the ability to interpret another person's tone of voice as well as gestures, facial expressions, and other nonverbal communications, children with ASD may not properly respond.

Likewise, it can be hard for others to understand the body language of children with ASD. Their facial expressions, movements, and gestures are often vague or do not match what they are saying. Their tone of voice may not reflect their actual feelings either. Many older children with ASD speak with an unusual tone of voice and may sound sing-song or flat and robotlike.

Children with ASD also may have trouble understanding another person's point of view. For example, by school age, most children understand that other people have different information, feelings, and goals than they have. Children with ASD may lack this understanding, leaving them unable to predict or understand other people's actions.

What communication issues appear in ASD?

According to the American Academy of Pediatrics' developmental milestones, by the first birthday, typical toddlers can say one or two words, turn when they hear their name, and point when they want a toy. When offered something they do not want, toddlers make it clear with words, gestures, or facial expressions that the answer is "no."

For children with ASD, reaching such milestones may not be so straightforward. For example, some children with autism may display these characteristics:

- Fail or be slow to respond to their name or other verbal attempts to gain their attention

- Fail or be slow to develop gestures, such as pointing and showing things to others

- Coo and babble in the first year of life, but then stop doing so

- Develop language at a delayed pace

- Learn to communicate using pictures or their own sign language

- Speak only in single words or repeat certain phrases over and over, seeming unable to combine words into meaningful sentences

- Repeat words or phrases that they hear, a condition called echolalia

- Use words that seem odd, out of place, or have a special meaning known only to those familiar with the child's way of communicating

Even children with ASD who have relatively good language skills often have difficulties with the back and forth of conversations. For example, because they find it difficult to understand and react to social cues, children with Asperger syndrome often talk at length about a favorite subject, but they won't allow anyone else a chance to respond or notice when others react indifferently.

Children with ASD who have not yet developed meaningful gestures or language may simply scream or grab or otherwise act out until they are taught better ways to express their needs. As these children grow up, they can become aware of their difficulty in understanding others and in being understood. This awareness may cause them to become anxious or depressed.

What are repetitive and stereotyped behaviors?

Children with ASD often have repetitive motions or unusual behaviors. These behaviors may be extreme and very noticeable, or they can be mild and discreet. For example, some children may repeatedly flap their arms or walk in specific patterns, while others may subtly move their fingers by their eyes in what looks to be a gesture. These repetitive actions are sometimes called stereotypy or stereotyped behaviors.

Children with ASD also tend to have overly focused interests. Children with ASD may become fascinated with moving objects or parts of objects, like the wheels on a moving car. They might spend a long time lining up toys in a certain way, rather than playing with them. They may also become very upset if someone accidentally moves one of the toys. Repetitive behavior can also take the form of a persistent, intense preoccupation. For example, they might be obsessed with learning all about vacuum cleaners, train schedules, or lighthouses. Children with ASD often have great interest in numbers, symbols, or science topics.

How is ASD treated?

While there's no proven cure yet for autism spectrum disorder (ASD), treating ASD early, using school-based programs, and getting proper medical care can greatly reduce ASD symptoms and increase your child's ability to grow and learn new skills.

Research has shown that intensive behavioral therapy during the toddler or preschool years can significantly improve cognitive and language skills in young children with ASD. There is no single best treatment for all children with ASD, but the American Academy of Pediatrics recently noted common features of effective early intervention programs:

- Starting as soon as a child has been diagnosed with ASD

- Providing focused and challenging learning activities at the proper developmental level for the child for at least 25 hours per week and 12 months per year

- Having small classes to allow each child to have one-on-one time with the therapist or teacher and small group learning activities

- Having special training for parents and family

- Encouraging activities that include typically developing children, as long as such activities help meet a specific learning goal

- Measuring and recording each child's progress and adjusting the intervention program as needed

- Providing a high degree of structure, routine, and visual cues, such as posted activity schedules and clearly defined boundaries, to reduce distractions

- Guiding the child in adapting learned skills to new situations and settings and maintaining learned skills

- Using a curriculum that focuses on

  - Language and communication

  - Social skills, such as joint attention (looking at other people to draw attention to something interesting and share in experiencing it)

  - Self-help and daily living skills, such as dressing and grooming

  - Research-based methods to reduce challenging behaviors, such as aggression and tantrums

  - Cognitive skills, such as pretend play or seeing someone else's point of view

  - Typical school-readiness skills, such as letter recognition and counting.

One type of a widely accepted treatment is applied behavior analysis (ABA). The goals of ABA are to shape and reinforce new behaviors, such as learning to speak and play, and reduce undesirable ones. ABA, which can involve intensive, one-on-one child-teacher interaction for up to 40 hours a week, has inspired the development of other, similar interventions that aim to help those with ASD reach their full potential. ABA-based interventions include verbal behavior and pivotal response training:

- **Verbal behavior:** Focuses on teaching language using a sequenced curriculum that guides children from simple verbal behaviors (echoing) to more functional communication skills through techniques such as errorless teaching and prompting

- **Pivotal response training:** Aims at identifying pivotal skills, such as initiation and self-management, that affect a broad range of behavioral responses. This intervention incorporates parent and family education aimed at providing skills that enable the child to function in inclusive settings.

Other types of early interventions include these:

- **Developmental, Individual Difference, Relationship-based(DIR)/Floortime Model:** Aims to build healthy and meaningful relationships and abilities by following the natural emotions and interests of the child. One particular example is the Early Start Denver Model, which fosters improvements in communication, thinking, language, and other social skills and seeks to reduce atypical behaviors. Using developmental and relationship-based approaches, this therapy can be delivered in natural settings such as the home or pre-school.

- **TEACCH (Treatment and Education of Autistic and related Communication handicapped Children):** Emphasizes adapting the child's physical environment and using visual cues (for example, having classroom materials clearly marked and located so that students can access them independently). Using individualized plans for each student, TEACCH builds on the child's strengths and emerging skills.

- **Interpersonal synchrony:** Targets social development and imitation skills, and focuses on teaching children how to establish and maintain engagement with others.

For children younger than age three, these interventions usually take place at home or in a child care center. Because parents are a child's earliest teachers, more programs are beginning to train parents to continue the therapy at home.

Students with ASD may benefit from some type of social skills training program. While these programs need more research, they generally seek to increase and improve skills necessary for creating positive social interactions and avoiding negative responses. For example, Children's Friendship Training focuses on improving children's conversation and interaction skills and teaches them how to make friends, be a good sport, and respond appropriately to teasing.

Are children with ASD eligible for special education services?

Start by speaking with your child's teacher, school counselor, or the school's student support team to begin an evaluation. Each state has a Parent Training and Information Center and a Protection and Advocacy Agency that can help you get an evaluation. A team of professionals conducts the evaluation using a variety of tools and measures. The evaluation will look at all areas related to your child's abilities and needs.

Once your child has been evaluated, he or she has several options, depending on the specific needs. If your child needs special education services and is eligible under the Individuals with Disabilities Education Act (IDEA), the school district (or the government agency administering the program) must develop an individualized education plan, or IEP specifically for your child within 30 days.

IDEA provides free screenings and early intervention services to children from birth to age three. IDEA also provides special education and related services from ages three to 21. Information is available from the U.S. Department of Education (www.ed.gov).

If your child is not eligible for special education services—not all children with ASD are eligible—he or she can still get free public education suited to his or her needs, which is available to all public-school children with disabilities under Section 504 of the Rehabilitation Act of 1973, regardless of the type or severity of the disability.

The U.S. Department of Education's Office for Civil Rights enforces Section 504 in programs and activities that receive Federal education funds. More information on Section 504 is available on the Department of Education website.

More information about U.S. Department of Education programs for children with disabilities is available on their website.

During middle and high school years, your child's teachers will begin to discuss practical issues such as work, living away from a parent or caregiver's home, and hobbies. These lessons should include gaining work experience, using public transportation, and learning skills that will be important in community living.

Are medications used to treat ASD?

Some medications can help reduce symptoms that cause problems for your child in school or at home. Many other medications may be prescribed off-label, meaning they have not been approved by the U.S.

Food and Drug Administration (FDA) for a certain use or for certain people. Doctors may prescribe medications off-label if they have been approved to treat other disorders that have similar symptoms to ASD, or if they have been effective in treating adults or older children with ASD. Doctors prescribe medications off-label to try to help the youngest patients, but more research is needed to be sure that these medicines are safe and effective for children and teens with ASD.

At this time, the only medications approved by the FDA to treat aspects of ASD are the antipsychotics risperidone (Risperdal) and aripripazole (Abilify). These medications can help reduce irritability—meaning aggression, self-harming acts, or temper tantrums—in children ages five to 16 who have ASD.

Some medications that may be prescribed off-label for children with ASD include the following:

- Antipsychotic medications are more commonly used to treat serious mental illnesses such as schizophrenia. These medicines may help reduce aggression and other serious behavioral problems in children, including children with ASD. They may also help reduce repetitive behaviors, hyperactivity, and attention problems.

- Antidepressant medications, such as fluoxetine (Prozac) or sertraline (Zoloft), are usually prescribed to treat depression and anxiety but are sometimes prescribed to reduce repetitive behaviors. Some antidepressants may also help control aggression and anxiety in children with ASD. However, researchers still are not sure if these medications are useful; a recent study suggested that the antidepressant citalopram (Celexa) was no more effective than a placebo (sugar pill) at reducing repetitive behaviors in children with ASD.

- Stimulant medications, such as methylphenidate (Ritalin), are safe and effective in treating people with attention deficit hyperactivity disorder (ADHD). Methylphenidate has been shown to effectively treat hyperactivity in children with ASD as well. But not as many children with ASD respond to treatment, and those who do have shown more side effects than children with ADHD and not ASD.

All medications carry a risk of side effects. For details on the side effects of common psychiatric medications, visit the National Institute of Mental Health website at www.nimh.nih.gov.

Chapter 29

Bipolar Disorder in Children and Teens

What is bipolar disorder?

Bipolar disorder, also known as manic-depressive illness, is a brain disorder that causes unusual shifts in mood and energy. It can also make it hard for someone to carry out day-to-day tasks, such as going to school or hanging out with friends. Symptoms of bipolar disorder are severe. They are different from the normal ups and downs that everyone goes through from time to time. They can result in damaged relationships, poor school performance, and even suicide. But bipolar disorder can be treated, and people with this illness can lead full and productive lives.

Bipolar disorder often develops in a person's late teens or early adult years, but some people have their first symptoms during childhood. At least half of all cases start before age 25.

What are common symptoms of bipolar disorder in children and teens?

Youth with bipolar disorder experience unusually intense emotional states that occur in distinct periods called *mood episodes*. An overly joyful or overexcited state is called a manic episode, and an extremely sad or hopeless state is called a depressive episode. Sometimes, a mood

Excerpted from "Bipolar Disorder in Children and Teens: A Parent's Guide," National Institute of Mental Health (www.nimh.nih.gov), August 31, 2010.

episode includes symptoms of both mania and depression. This is called a mixed state. People with bipolar disorder also may be explosive and irritable during a mood episode. Extreme changes in energy, activity, sleep, and behavior go along with these changes in mood.

Symptoms of mania include mood changes such as being in an overly silly or joyful mood that's unusual for your child. It is different from times when he or she might usually get silly and have fun. Another symptom is having an extremely short temper. This is an irritable mood that is unusual. Behavioral changes associated with mania include sleeping little but not feeling tired; talking a lot and having racing thoughts; having trouble concentrating, attention jumping from one thing to the next in an unusual way; talking and thinking about sex more often; and behaving in risky ways more often, seeking pleasure a lot, and doing more activities than usual.

Symptoms of depression include mood changes such as being in a sad mood that lasts a long time, losing interest in activities they once enjoyed, and feeling worthless or guilty. Behavioral changes associated with depression include complaining about pain more often, such as headaches, stomach aches, and muscle pains; eating a lot more or less and gaining or losing a lot of weight; sleeping problems or oversleeping when these were not problems before; losing energy; and recurring thoughts of death or suicide.

It's normal for almost every child or teen to have some of these symptoms sometimes. These passing changes should not be confused with bipolar disorder. Symptoms of bipolar disorder are not like the normal changes in mood and energy that everyone has now and then. Bipolar symptoms are more extreme and tend to last for most of the day, nearly every day, for at least one week. Also, depressive or manic episodes include moods very different from a child's normal mood, and the behaviors described above may start at the same time. Sometimes the symptoms of bipolar disorder are so severe that the child needs to be treated in a hospital.

In addition to mania and depression, bipolar disorder can cause a range of moods. Depression range includes severe depression, moderate depression, and mild low mood. Moderate depression may cause less extreme symptoms, and mild low mood is called dysthymia when it is chronic or long-term. Sometimes, a child may have more energy and be more active than normal, but not show the severe signs of a full-blown manic episode. When this happens, it is called hypomania, and it generally lasts for at least four days in a row. Hypomania causes noticeable changes in behavior, but does not harm a child's ability to function in the way mania does.

What affects a child's risk of getting bipolar disorder?

Bipolar disorder tends to run in families. Children with a parent or sibling who has bipolar disorder are four to six times more likely to develop the illness, compared with children who do not have a family history of bipolar disorder. However, most children with a family history of bipolar disorder will not develop the illness. Compared with children whose parents do not have bipolar disorder, children whose parents have bipolar disorder may be more likely to have symptoms of anxiety disorders and attention deficit hyperactivity disorder (ADHD).

Several studies show that youth with anxiety disorders are more likely to develop bipolar disorder than youth without anxiety disorders. However, anxiety disorders are very common in young people. Most children and teens with anxiety disorders do not develop bipolar disorder.

At this time, there is no way to prevent bipolar disorder. The National Institute of Mental Health (NIMH) is currently studying how to limit or delay the first symptoms in children with a family history of the illness.

How does bipolar disorder affect children and teens differently than adults?

Bipolar disorder that starts during childhood or during the teen years is called early-onset bipolar disorder. Early-onset bipolar disorder seems to be more severe than the forms that first appear in older teens and adults. Youth with bipolar disorder are different from adults with bipolar disorder. Young people with the illness appear to have more frequent mood switches, are sick more often, and have more mixed episodes.

Watch out for any sign of suicidal thinking or behaviors. Take these signs seriously. On average, people with early-onset bipolar disorder have greater risk for attempting suicide than those whose symptoms start in adulthood. One large study on bipolar disorder in children and teens found that more than one-third of study participants made at least one serious suicide attempt. Some suicide attempts are carefully planned and others are not. Either way, it is important to understand that suicidal feelings and actions are symptoms of an illness that must be treated.

How is bipolar disorder detected in children and teens?

No blood tests or brain scans can diagnose bipolar disorder. However, a doctor may use tests like these to help rule out other possible causes for your child's symptoms. For example, the doctor may recommend testing for problems in learning, thinking, or speech and language. A careful medical exam may also detect problems that commonly co-occur with bipolar disorder and need to be treated, such as substance abuse.

Doctors who have experience with diagnosing early-onset bipolar disorder, such as psychiatrists, psychologists, or other mental health specialists, will ask questions about changes in your child's mood. They will also ask about sleep patterns, activity or energy levels, and if your child has had any other mood or behavioral disorders. The doctor may also ask whether there is a family history of bipolar disorder or other psychiatric illnesses, such as depression or alcoholism. Doctors usually diagnose mental disorders using guidelines from the *Diagnostic and Statistical Manual of Mental Disorders*, or *DSM*.

Researchers are also working on whether certain symptoms mean a child should be diagnosed with bipolar disorder. For example, scientists are studying children with very severe, chronic irritability and symptoms of ADHD, but no clear episodes of mania. Some experts think these children should be diagnosed with mania. At the same time, there is scientific evidence that suggests these irritable children are different from children with bipolar disorder in the following key areas: the outcome of their illness, family history, and brain function.

When you talk to your child's doctor or a mental health specialist, be sure to ask questions. Getting answers helps you understand the terms they use to describe your child's symptoms.

What illnesses often co-exist with bipolar disorder in children and teens?

Several illnesses may develop in people with bipolar disorder.

- **Alcoholism:** Adults with bipolar disorder are at very high risk of developing a substance abuse problem. Young people with bipolar disorder may have the same risk.

- **ADHD:** Many children with bipolar disorder have a history of ADHD. One study showed that ADHD is more common in people whose bipolar disorder started during childhood, compared with people whose bipolar disorder started later in life. Children who have co-occurring ADHD and bipolar disorder may have difficulty concentrating and controlling their activity. This may happen even when they are not manic or depressed.

- **Anxiety disorders:** Anxiety disorders, such as separation anxiety and generalized anxiety disorder, also commonly co-occur with bipolar disorder. This may happen in both children and adults. Children who have both types of disorders tend to develop bipolar disorder at a younger age and have more hospital stays related to mental illness.

- **Other mental disorders:** Some mental disorders cause symptoms similar to bipolar disorder. Two examples are major depression (sometimes called unipolar depression) and ADHD. If you look at symptoms only, there is no way to tell the difference between major depression and a depressive episode in bipolar disorder. For this reason, be sure to tell a diagnosing doctor of any past manic symptoms or episodes your child may have had. In contrast, ADHD does not have episodes. ADHD symptoms may resemble mania in some ways, but they tend to be more constant than in a manic episode of bipolar disorder.

What treatments are available for children and teens with bipolar disorder?

To date, there is no cure for bipolar disorder. However, treatment with medications, psychotherapy (talk therapy), or both may help people get better. It's important for you to know that children sometimes respond differently to psychiatric medications than adults do. To treat children and teens with bipolar disorder, doctors often rely on information about treating adults. This is because there haven't been many studies on treating young people with the illness, although several have been started recently.

One large study with adults funded by NIMH is the Systematic Treatment Enhancement Program for Bipolar Disorder (visit STEP-BD for more information). This study found that treating adults with medications and intensive psychotherapy for about nine months helped them get better. These adults got better faster and stayed well longer than adults treated with less intensive psychotherapy for six weeks. Combining medication treatment and psychotherapies may help young people with early-onset bipolar disorder as well. However, it's important for you to know that children sometimes respond differently to psychiatric medications than adults do.

Where can families of children with bipolar disorder get help?

As with other serious illnesses, taking care of a child with bipolar disorder is incredibly hard on the parents, family, and other caregivers. Caregivers often must tend to the medical needs of their child while dealing with how it affects their own health. The stress that caregivers are under may lead to missed work or lost free time. It can strain relationships with people who do not understand the situation and lead to physical and mental exhaustion.

Stress from caregiving can make it hard to cope with your child's bipolar symptoms. One study shows that if a caregiver is under a lot of stress, his or her loved one has more trouble sticking to the treatment plan, which increases the chance for a major bipolar episode. It is important to take care of your own physical and mental health. You may also find it helpful to join a local support group. If your child's illness prevents you from attending a local support group, try an online support group.

What if my child is in crisis?

If you think your child is in crisis:

- Call your doctor

- Call 911 or go to a hospital emergency room to get immediate help or ask a friend or family member to help you do these things

- Call the toll-free, 24-hour hotline of the National Suicide Prevention Lifeline at 800-273-TALK (800-273-8255); TTY: 800-799-4TTY (4889) to talk to a trained counselor

- Make sure your child is not left alone.

Chapter 30

Depression in Children and Teens

Depression Information for Students

Depression can occur during adolescence, a time of great personal change. You may be facing changes in where you go to school, your friends, your after-school activities, as well as in relationships with your family members. You may have different feelings about the type of person you want to be, your future plans, and may be making decisions for the first time in your life.

Many students don't know where to go for mental health treatment or believe that treatment won't help. Others don't get help because they think depression symptoms are just part of the typical stresses of school or being a teen. Some students worry what other people will think if they seek mental health care.

This information addresses common questions about depression and how it can affect high school students.

What is depression?

Depression is a common but serious mental illness typically marked by sad or anxious feelings. Most students occasionally feel sad or

---

This chapter begins with excerpts from "Depression and High School Students," 2011, and it continues with information for college students excerpted from "Depression and College Students," September 29, 2011. It concludes with facts about current research excerpted from "Depression in Children and Adolescents (Fact Sheet)," April 25, 2011. All three publications were produced by the National Institute of Mental Health (www.nimh.nih.gov).

anxious, but these emotions usually pass quickly—within a couple of days. Untreated depression lasts for a long time and interferes with your day-to-day activities.

What are the symptoms of depression?

Different people experience different symptoms of depression. If you are depressed, you may feel sad, anxious, empty, hopeless, guilty, worthless, helpless, irritable, or restless. You may also experience one or more of the following symptoms:

- Loss of interest in activities you used to enjoy
- Lack of energy
- Problems concentrating, remembering information, or making decisions
- Problems falling sleep, staying asleep, or sleeping too much
- Loss of appetite or eating too much
- Thoughts of suicide or suicide attempts
- Aches, pains, headaches, cramps, or digestive problems that do not go away.

Depression in adolescence frequently co-occurs with other disorders such as anxiety, disruptive behavior, eating disorders or substance abuse. It can also lead to increased risk for suicide.

Are there different types of depression?

Yes. The most common depressive disorders are called major depressive disorder and dysthymic disorder:

- Major depressive disorder is also called major depression. The symptoms of major depression are disabling and interfere with everyday activities such as studying, eating, and sleeping. People with this disorder may have only one episode of major depression in their lifetimes. But more often, depression comes back repeatedly.

- Dysthymic disorder is also called dysthymia. Dysthymia is mild, chronic depression. The symptoms of dysthymia last for a long time—two years or more. Dysthymia is less severe than major depression, but it can still interfere with everyday activities. People with dysthymia may also experience one or more episodes of major depression during their lifetimes.

Other types of depression include psychotic depression, which is severe depression accompanied by some form of psychosis, such as hallucinations and delusions, and seasonal affective disorder—depression that begins during the winter months and lifts during spring and summer.

What causes depression?

Depression does not have a single cause. Several factors can lead to depression. Some people carry genes that increase their risk of depression. But not all people with depression have these genes, and not all people with these genes have depression. Environment—your surroundings and life experiences—also affects your risk for depression. Any stressful situation may trigger depression. And high school students encounter a number of stressful situations!

How is depression treated?

A number of very effective treatments for depression are available. The most common treatments are antidepressants and psychotherapy. A National Institute of Mental Health (NIMH)–funded clinical trial of 439 teens with major depression found that a combination of medication and psychotherapy was the most effective treatment option. A doctor or mental health care provider can help you find the treatment that's right for you.

What are antidepressants?

Antidepressants work on brain chemicals called neurotransmitters, especially serotonin and norepinephrine. Other antidepressants work on the neurotransmitter dopamine. Scientists have found that these particular chemicals are involved in regulating mood, but they are unsure of the exact ways that they work.

What is psychotherapy?

Psychotherapy involves talking with a mental health care professional to treat a mental illness. Types of psychotherapy often used to treat depression include cognitive-behavioral therapy (CBT), which helps people change negative styles of thinking and behavior that may contribute to depression, and interpersonal therapy (IPT), which helps people understand and work through troubled personal relationships that may cause or worsen depression.

Depending on the type and severity of your depression, a mental health professional may recommend short-term therapy, lasting 10 to 20 weeks, or longer-term therapy.

How can I help myself if I am depressed?

If you have depression, you may feel exhausted, helpless, and hopeless. But it is important to realize that these feelings are part of the depression and do not reflect your real circumstances. Treatment can help you feel better. There are also things you can do to help yourself feel better:

- Engage in mild physical activity or exercise
- Participate in activities that you used to enjoy
- Break up large projects into smaller tasks and do what you can
- Spend time with or call your friends and family
- Expect your mood to improve gradually with treatment
- Remember that positive thinking will replace negative thoughts as your depression responds to treatment.

How can I help a friend who is depressed?

If you think a friend may have depression, you can help him or her get diagnosed and treated. Make sure he or she talks to an adult and gets evaluated by a doctor or mental health provider. If your friend seems unable or unwilling to seek help, offer to go with him or her and tell your friend that his or her health and safety is important to you.

Encourage your friend to stay in treatment or seek a different treatment if he or she does not begin to feel better after six to eight weeks. Other things you can do include the following:

- Offer emotional support, understanding, patience, and encouragement
- Talk to your friend, not necessarily about depression, and listen carefully
- Never discount the feelings your friend expresses, but point out realities and offer hope
- Never ignore comments about suicide
- Report comments about suicide to your friend's parents, therapist, or doctor
- Invite your friend out for walks, outings, and other activities—keep trying if your friend declines, but don't push him or her to take on too much too soon

- Remind your friend that with time and treatment, the depression will lift.

What if I or someone I know is in crisis?

If you are thinking about harming yourself or having thoughts of suicide, or if you

- Call your doctor or mental health care provider.

- Call 911 or go to a hospital emergency room to get immediate help, or ask a friend or family member to help you do these things.

- Call your campus suicide or crisis hotline.

- Call the National Suicide Prevention Lifeline's toll-free, 24-hour hotline at 800-273-TALK (800-273-8255) or TTY: 800-799-4TTY (800-799-4889) to talk to a trained counselor.

- If you are in crisis, make sure you are not left alone.

- If someone else is in crisis, make sure he or she is not left alone.

Additional Depression Information for College Students

Many people experience the first symptoms of depression during their college years. Unfortunately, many college students who have depression aren't getting the help they need. They may not know where to go for help, or they may believe that treatment won't help. Others don't get help because they think their symptoms are just part of the typical stress of college, or they worry about being judged if they seek mental health care.

In reality most colleges offer free or low-cost mental health services to students. Depression is a medical illness and treatments can be very effective. Early diagnosis and treatment of depression can relieve depression symptoms, prevent depression from returning, and help students succeed in college and after graduation.

How does depression affect college students?

In 2009, the American College Health Association-National College Health Assessment (ACHA-NCHA)—a nationwide survey of college students at 2- and 4-year institutions—found that nearly 30 percent of college students reported feeling "so depressed that it was difficult to function" at some time in the past year.

Depression can affect your academic performance in college. Studies suggest that college students who have depression are more likely to smoke. Research suggests that students with depression do not necessarily drink alcohol more heavily than other college students. But students with depression, especially women, are more likely to drink to get drunk and experience problems related to alcohol abuse, such as engaging in unsafe sex. It is not uncommon for students who have depression to self-medicate with street drugs.

Depression is also a major risk factor for suicide. Better diagnosis and treatment of depression can help reduce suicide rates among college students. In the Fall 2009 ACHA–NCHA survey, about six percent of college students reported seriously considering suicide, and about one percent reported attempting suicide in the previous year. Suicide is the third leading cause of death for teens and young adults ages 15 to 24. Students should also be aware that the warning signs can be different in men versus women.

What causes of depression are of special concern to college students?

Depression does not have a single cause. Several factors can lead to depression. Some people carry genes that increase their risk of depression. Environment—your surroundings and life experiences, such as stress, also affects your risk for depression.

Common stresses of college include living away from family for the first time, missing family or friends, feeling alone or isolated, experiencing conflict in relationships, facing new and sometimes difficult school work, and worrying about finances.

If I think I may have depression, where can I get help?

Most colleges provide mental health services through counseling centers, student health centers, or both. Check out your college website for information.

- Counseling centers offer students free or very low-cost mental health services. Some counseling centers provide short-term or long-term counseling or psychotherapy, also called talk therapy. These centers may also refer you to mental health care providers in the community for additional services.

- Student health centers provide basic health care services to students at little or no cost. A doctor or health care provider may be able to diagnose and treat depression or refer you to other mental health services.

If your college does not provide all of the mental health care you need, your insurance may cover additional mental health services. Many college students have insurance through their colleges, parents, or employers. If you are insured, contact your insurance company to find out about your mental health care coverage.

Researching Depression in Children and Adolescents

About 11 percent of adolescents have a depressive disorder by age 18 according to the National Comorbidity Survey-Adolescent Supplement (NCS-A). Girls are more likely than boys to experience depression. The risk for depression increases as a child gets older. According to the World Health Organization, major depressive disorder is the leading cause of disability among Americans age 15 to 44.

Because normal behaviors vary from one childhood stage to another, it can be difficult to tell whether a child who shows changes in behavior is just going through a temporary "phase" or is suffering from depression.

What We Now Know

- Youth who have depression may show signs that are slightly different from the typical adult symptoms of depression. Children who are depressed may complain of feeling sick, refuse to go to school, cling to a parent or caregiver, or worry excessively that a parent may die. Older children and teens may sulk, get into trouble at school, be negative or grouchy, or feel misunderstood.

- Findings from large-scale effectiveness trials funded by the National Institute of Mental Health (NIMH) are helping doctors and their patients make better individual treatment decisions. For example, the Treatment for Adolescents with Depression Study (TADS) found that combination treatment of medication and psychotherapy works best for most teens with depression.

- The Treatment of SSRI [selective serotonin re-uptake inhibitor]-Resistant Depression in Adolescents (TORDIA) study found that teens who did not respond to a first antidepressant medication are more likely to get better if they switch to a treatment that includes both medication and psychotherapy.

- The Treatment of Adolescent Suicide Attempters (TASA) study found that a new treatment approach that includes medication plus a specialized psychotherapy designed specifically to reduce suicidal thinking and behavior may reduce suicide attempts in severely depressed teens.

- Depressed teens with coexisting disorders such as substance abuse problems are less likely to respond to treatment for depression. Studies focusing on conditions that frequently co-occur and how they affect one another may lead to more targeted screening tools and interventions.

- With medication, psychotherapy, or combined treatment, most youth with depression can be effectively treated. Youth are more likely to respond to treatment if they receive it early in the course of their illness.

- Although antidepressants are generally safe, the U.S. Food and Drug Administration has placed a "black box" warning label—the most serious type of warning—on all antidepressant medications. The warning says there is an increased risk of suicidal thinking or attempts in youth taking antidepressants. Youth and young adults should be closely monitored especially during initial weeks of treatment.

- Studies focusing on depression in teens and children are pinpointing factors that appear to influence risk, treatment response, and recovery. Given the chronic nature of depression, effective intervention early in life may help reduce future burden and disability.

- Multi-generational studies have revealed a link between depression that runs in families and changes in brain structure and function, some of which may precede the onset of depression. This research is helping to identify biomarkers and other early indicators that may lead to better treatment or prevention.

- Advanced brain imaging techniques are helping scientists identify specific brain circuits that are involved in depression and yielding new ways to study the effectiveness of treatments.

Chapter 31

Learning Disabilities

What are learning disabilities?

Learning disabilities are caused by a difference in brain structure that is present at birth and is often hereditary. They affect the way the brain processes information. This processing is the main function involved in learning.

Learning disabilities can impact how someone learns to read, write, hear, speak, and calculate. There are many kinds of learning disabilities and they can affect people differently.

Learning disabilities do not reflect IQ (intelligence quotient) or how smart a person is. Instead, a person with a learning disability has trouble performing specific types of skills or completing a task.

Learning disabilities are not the same as mental or physical disabilities, such as intellectual and developmental disabilities, deafness, or blindness. But, learning disabilities may occur together with mental or physical disabilities.

Children with learning disabilities cannot be identified on the basis of acuity (such as vision or hearing) or other physical signs, nor can they be diagnosed solely based on neurological findings. Learning disabilities are widely regarded as variations on normal development and are only considered disabilities when they interfere significantly with school performance and adaptive functions.

"Learning Disabilities," National Institute of Child Health and Human Development (www.nichd.nih.gov), March 24, 2010.

What are the signs and symptoms of learning disabilities?

A delay in achieving certain developmental milestones, when most other aspects of development are normal, could be a sign of a learning disability. Such delays may include problems with language, motor delays, or problems with socialization.

If you think your child may have a learning disability, talk to your child's health care provider or educator to discuss options for evaluation and treatment. These professionals can screen for potential difficulties, but it is essential that someone specializing in the diagnosis of learning disabilities do a full evaluation to confirm the presence of a learning disability.

What are some types of learning disabilities?

Learning disabilities include a variety of disorders that affect the ability to learn. Some examples include (but are not limited to):

- Reading disability is a reading and language-based learning disability, also commonly called dyslexia. For most children with learning disabilities receiving special education services, the primary area of difficulty is reading. People with reading disabilities often have problems recognizing words that they already know. They may also be poor spellers and may have problems with decoding skills. Other symptoms may include trouble with handwriting and problems understanding what they read. About 15 percent to 20 percent of people in the United States have a language-based disability, and of those, most have dyslexia.

- Dyscalculia is a learning disability related to math. Those with dyscalculia may have difficulty understanding math concepts and solving even simple math problems.

- Dysgraphia is a learning disability related to handwriting. People with this condition may have problems forming letters as they write or may have trouble writing within a defined space.

- Information-processing disorders are learning disorders related to a person's ability to use the information that they take in through their senses—seeing, hearing, tasting, smelling, and touching. These problems are not related to an inability to see or hear. Instead, the conditions affect the way the brain recognizes, responds to, retrieves, and stores sensory information.

- Language-related learning disabilities are problems that interfere with age-appropriate communication, including speaking, listening, reading, spelling, and writing.

What is the treatment for learning disabilities?

While there is no direct cure for a learning disability, early screening and intervention from specialists can often provide great benefits. Early intervention can prevent learning difficulties, thus reducing the number of children requiring special education services.

Under the 2004 reauthorization of the Individuals with Disabilities Education Improvement Act, legislators made significant changes in how people with learning disabilities could be identified as eligible for special education services. This reauthorization allows for the optional use of the Response to Intervention (RTI) approach to determine whether a child has a specific learning disability and may receive special education services. There is evidence that the IQ-discrepancy model normally used is ineffective in identifying all students with learning disabilities; therefore many schools are implementing an RTI approach.

RTI is a tiered approach to educational intervention; the most common is a three-tier model. The first tier provides high quality reading instruction to all students, with careful progress monitoring by teachers in the classrooms. Tier 2 is the same high quality instruction but with increased intensity for those not progressing well enough. If students do not progress with this more intensive instruction, they are identified for Tier 3, which is targeted special education intervention. Tier 3 students would have full evaluations and the establishment of an Individualized Education Program (IEP).

Most children with learning disabilities are eligible for special assistance at school. An IEP should be developed for students who need special education and related services. An IEP includes specific academic, communication, motor, learning, functional, and socialization goals for a child based on his or her educational needs.

A number of parents' organizations, both national and local, provide information on therapeutic and educational services and how to get these services for a child. Visit http://www.nlm.nih.gov/medlineplus/learningdisorders.html for a listing of these organizations.

Chapter 32

Pediatric Autoimmune Neuropsychiatric Disorders Associated with Strepto-coccal Infections (PANDAS)

Overview

PANDAS, is an abbreviation for pediatric autoimmune neuropsychiatric disorders associated with streptococcal infections. The term is used to describe a subset of children who have obsessive compulsive disorder (OCD) and/or tic disorders such as Tourette syndrome, and in whom symptoms worsen following streptococcal infections such as strep throat and scarlet fever.

The children usually have dramatic, "overnight" onset of symptoms, including motor or vocal tics, obsessions, and/or compulsions. In addition to these symptoms, children may also become moody, irritable, or show concerns about separating from parents or loved ones. This abrupt onset is generally preceded by a strep throat infection.

What is the mechanism behind this phenomenon? At present, it is unknown but researchers at the National Institute of Mental Health (NIMH) are pursuing a theory that the mechanism is similar to that of rheumatic fever, an autoimmune disorder triggered by strep throat infections. In every bacterial infection, the body produces antibodies against the invading bacteria, and the antibodies help eliminate the bacteria from the body. However in rheumatic fever, the antibodies mistakenly recognize and attack the heart valves, joints, and/or certain

"PANDAS: Frequently Asked Questions about Pediatric Autoimmune Neuro-psychiatric Disorders Associated with Streptococcal Infections," National Institute of Mental Health (www.nimh.nih.gov), September 23, 2009.

parts of the brain. This phenomenon is called molecular mimicry, which means that proteins on the cell wall of the strep bacteria are similar in some way to the proteins of the heart valve, joints, or brain. Because the antibodies set off an immune reaction which damages those tissues, the child with rheumatic fever can get heart disease (especially mitral valve regurgitation), arthritis, and/or abnormal movements known as Sydenham chorea or St. Vitus dance.

In PANDAS, it is believed that something very similar to Sydenham chorea occurs. One part of the brain that is affected in PANDAS is the basal ganglia, which is believed to be responsible for movement and behavior. Thus, the antibodies interact with the brain to cause tics and/or OCD, instead of Sydenham chorea.

Frequently Asked Questions

Is there a test for PANDAS?

No. The diagnosis of PANDAS is a clinical diagnosis, which means that there are no lab tests that can diagnose PANDAS. Instead clinicians use five diagnostic criteria for the diagnosis of PANDAS (see below). At the present time the clinical features of the illness are the only means of determining whether or not a child might have PANDAS.

What are the diagnostic criteria for PANDAS?

- Presence of obsessive-compulsive disorder and/or a tic disorder
- Pediatric onset of symptoms (age three years to puberty)
- Episodic course of symptom severity
- Association with group A beta-hemolytic streptococcal infection (a positive throat culture for strep or history of scarlet fever)
- Association with neurological abnormalities (motoric hyperactivity, or adventitious movements, such as choreiform movements).

What is an episodic course of symptoms?

Children with PANDAS seem to have dramatic ups and downs in their OCD and/or tic severity. Tics or OCD which are almost always present at a relatively consistent level do not represent an episodic course. Many kids with OCD or tics have good days and bad days, or even good weeks and bad weeks. However, patients with PANDAS have a very sudden onset or worsening of their symptoms, followed by a slow, gradual improvement. If they get another strep infection, their symptoms suddenly worsen again. The increased symptom severity usually persists for at least several weeks, but may last for several months or longer. The tics or OCD then seem to gradually fade away, and the children often enjoy a few weeks or several months without problems. When they have another strep throat infection the tics or OCD return just as suddenly and dramatically as they did previously.

Are there any other symptoms associated with PANDAS episodes?

Yes. Children with PANDAS often experience one or more of the following symptoms in conjunction with their OCD and/or tics:

- Attention deficit hyperactivity disorder (ADHD) symptoms (hyperactivity, inattention, fidgety)

- Separation anxiety (child is clingy and has difficulty separating from his/her caregivers; for example, the child may not want to be in a different room in the house from his/her parents)

- Mood changes (irritability, sadness, emotional lability)

- Sleep disturbance

- Night- time bed wetting and/or day- time urinary frequency

- Fine/gross motor changes (for example, changes in handwriting)

- Joint pains

My child has had strep throat before, and he has tics and/ or OCD. Does that mean he has PANDAS?

No. Many children have OCD and/or tics, and almost all school aged children get strep throat at some point in their lives. In fact, the average grade-school student will have two to three strep throat infections each year. PANDAS is considered when there is a very close relationship between the abrupt onset or worsening or OCD and/or tics, and a preceding strep infection. If strep is found in conjunction with two or three episodes of OCD/tics, then it may be that the child has PANDAS.

Could an adult have PANDAS?

No. By definition, PANDAS is a pediatric disorder. It is possible that adolescents and adults may have immune mediated OCD, but this is not known.

My child has PANDAS. Should he have his tonsils removed?

The National Institutes of Health (NIH) does not recommend tonsillectomies for children with PANDAS, as there is no evidence that they are helpful. If a tonsillectomy is recommended because of frequent episodes of tonsillitis, it would be useful to discuss the pros and cons of the procedure with your child's doctor, because of the role that the tonsils play in fighting strep infections.

What exactly is an anti-streptococcal antibody titer?

The anti-streptococcal antibody titer determines whether there is immunologic evidence of a previous strep infection. Two different strep tests are commercially available: the antistrepolysin O (ASO) titer, which rises three to six weeks after a strep infection, and the antistreptococcal DNAase B (antiDNAse-B) titer, which rises six to eight weeks after a strep infection.

What does an elevated anti-streptococcal antibody titer mean? Is this bad for my child?

An elevated anti-strep titer (such as ASO or antiDNAse-B) means the child has had a strep infection sometime within the past few months, and his body created antibodies to fight the strep bacteria. Some children create lots of antibodies and have very high titers (up to 2,000), while others have more modest elevations. The height of the titer elevation doesn't matter. Further, elevated titers are not a bad thing. They are measuring a normal, healthy response—the production of antibodies to fight off an infection. The antibodies stay in the body for some time after the infection is gone, but the amount of time that the antibodies persist varies greatly between different individuals. Some children have positive antibody titers for many months after a single infection.

When is a strep titer considered to be abnormal or elevated?

The lab at NIH considers strep titers between 0–400 to be normal. Other labs set the upper limit at 150 or 200. Since each lab measures titers in different ways, it is important to know the range used by the laboratory where the test was done—just ask where they draw the line between negative or positive titers.

It is important to note that some grade-school aged children have chronically elevated titers. These may actually be in the normal range for that child, as there is a lot of individual variability in titer values. Because of this variability, doctors will often draw a titer when the child is sick, or shortly thereafter, and then draw another titer several weeks later to see if the titer is rising—if so, this is strong evidence that the illness was due to strep. (Of course, a less expensive way to make this determination is to take a throat culture at the time that the child is ill.)

Should an elevated strep titer be treated with antibiotics?

No. Elevated titers indicate that a patient has had a past strep exposure but the titers cannot tell you precisely when the strep infection occurred. Children may have positive titers for many months after one infection. Since these elevated titers are merely a marker of a prior infection and not proof of an ongoing infection it is not appropriate to give antibiotics for elevated titers. Antibiotics are recommended only when a child has a positive rapid strep test or positive strep throat culture.

What are the treatment options for children with PANDAS?

The treatments for children with PANDAS are the same as if they had other types of OCD or tic disorders. Children with OCD, regardless of whether or not their illness is strep triggered, benefit from cognitive behavioral therapy and/or anti-obsessional medications. A recent study showed that the combination of an SSRI medication (such as fluoxetine) and cognitive behavioral therapy was the best treatment for OCD, and that medication alone or cognitive behavioral therapy alone were better than no treatment, or use of a placebo (sugar pill). It often takes time for these treatments to work, so the sooner therapy is started, the better it is for the child.

Children with strep triggered tics should be helped by the same tic medications that doctors use to treat other tic disorders. Your child's primary physician can help you decide which type of specialist your child may need to see to receive these treatments.

Can penicillin be used to treat PANDAS or prevent future PANDAS symptom exacerbations?

Penicillin and other antibiotics kill streptococcus and other types of bacteria. The antibiotics treat the sore throat or pharyngitis caused by the strep by getting rid of the bacteria. However, in PANDAS, it appears that antibodies produced by the body in response to the strep infection are the cause of the problem, not the bacteria themselves. Therefore one could not expect antibiotics such as penicillin to treat the symptoms of PANDAS. Researchers at the NIMH have been investigating the use of antibiotics as a form of prophylaxis or prevention of future problems. At this time, however, there isn't enough evidence to recommend the long-term use of antibiotics.

What about treating PANDAS with plasma exchange or immunoglobulin (IVIG)?

The results of a controlled trial of plasma exchange (also known as plasmapheresis) and immunoglobulin (IVIG) for the treatment of children in the PANDAS subgroup was published in *The Lancet*, Vol. 354, October 2, 1999. All of the children participating in the study had clear evidence of a strep infection as the trigger of their OCD and tics, and all were severely ill at the time of treatment. The study showed that plasma exchange and IVIG were both effective for the treatment of severe, strep triggered OCD and tics, and that there were persistent benefits of the interventions. However, there were a number of side-effects associated with the treatments, including nausea, vomiting, headaches, and dizziness. In addition, there is a risk of infection with any invasive procedure, such as these. Thus, the treatments should be reserved for severely ill patients, and administered by a qualified team of health care professionals. The NIH is not currently conducting any trials with immunomodulatory therapies, and so is not able to offer either or the treatments.

Of note, a separate study was conducted to evaluate the effectiveness of plasma exchange in the treatment of chronic OCD (Nicolson et al.: An Open Trial of Plasma Exchange in Childhood Onset Obsessive-compulsive Disorder Without Poststreptococcal Exacerbations. *J Am Acad Child Adolesc Psychiatry* 2000, 39[10]: 1313–1315. None of those children benefited, suggesting that plasma exchange or IVIG is not helpful for children who do not have strep triggered OCD or tics.

Part Five

Other Populations with Distinctive Mental Health Concerns

Chapter 33

Mental Health Issues among Men

Chapter Contents

Section 33.1

Mental Health for Men

"Men's Health: Mental Health for Men," Office on Women's Health
(www.womehshealth.gov), January 10, 2011.

Men's Mental Health

Mental health helps us face the challenges in our life, makes us feel comfortable, supports our physical health, and more. But day-to-day stress and difficult times can wear down our mental health. Major changes like losing a job, the death of a loved one, going off to combat, or coming out as gay can be especially hard. And even happy times—like becoming a father—can take a toll on your emotions.

Today, we know a lot more about ways to promote mental health. Try some simple steps, like making sure to get enough sleep, getting social support, exercising, and finding healthy ways to cope when you feel stressed.

If you are struggling with your mental health, you are not alone. In fact, about one out of four American adults suffers from a mental health condition each year. Experts don't know exactly what causes mental illnesses, but a combination of genes and life events often is involved. It's important to remember that mental health disorders are real medical illnesses that can't be willed or wished away.

This section describes some common mental health conditions experienced by men. These include alcohol and drug abuse, anxiety disorders, post-traumatic stress disorder (PTSD), and body image and eating disorders.

Alcohol and Drug Abuse

Alcohol and drug use in men often begin early in their lives, during the teen or young adult years. The reasons men begin drinking too much or using drugs vary, and the path from casual, social use to abuse and addiction is complex. What we do know is that abusing alcohol and drugs is very harmful—not only to you, but to the people in your life.

Anything more than moderate drinking can be risky. For a man, moderate drinking is considered two drinks a day. Years of heavy drinking can lead to heart disease, cancer, and other health problems. Binge drinking, which is drinking five or more drinks at one time, can be especially dangerous.

Consider these risks of drinking too much or using drugs:

- Depression, anxiety, suicide

- Accidents

- Violence, often against loved ones

- Risky sexual behavior, such as unprotected sex or sex with multiple partners

- Employment problems

- Health problems, including cancer and HIV

- Addiction, which is a disease described by uncontrollable cravings and physical dependence

In the moment, it may seem like a good idea to use drugs or alcohol to get high, relax, or escape. But alcohol and drug abuse can soon cause serious problems. Fortunately, substance abuse disorders are also treatable. If you have a problem with drugs or alcohol, seek help from your doctor or a treatment facility. With treatment, it's possible to not only regain your health, but also restore the relationships that matter to you.

Anxiety Disorders and PTSD

It's natural to feel worried or nervous at times, like before a work presentation or having an operation. But for people with anxiety disorders, everyday situations cause much more worry than most people feel. Often, people with these disorders know their anxiety is extreme, but they can't make the anxious feelings go away. Common types of anxiety disorders include generalized anxiety disorder, obsessive-compulsive disorder (OCD), panic disorder, and phobias.

Post-traumatic stress disorder (PTSD) is one of the more common anxiety disorders. Its symptoms include feeling like you are reliving a dangerous experience. Men who serve in combat may develop PTSD. But it also can come from living through any dangerous experience, like an accident or hurricane. Men who have PTSD may experience it differently from women. For example, women with PTSD may feel very jumpy, but men are more likely to feel angry or have problems with alcohol or drugs.

Social phobia, which makes a person feel very strong fear in social situations, also often affects men. It can come up when you need to speak in a large group, for example, and can cause both emotional and physical symptoms, like feeling sick to your stomach.

Body Image and Eating Disorders

Did you know that men, like women, can struggle with body image issues or an eating disorder? Men may feel a lot of pressure to have a "perfect," muscular body and may focus too much on exercise and dieting. This focus can wind up hurting a man's body, job, and relationships. But medicines and counseling can help men with eating and body image disorders lead healthy lives.

Eating Disorders

Eating disorders involve extreme emotions, attitudes, and behaviors around weight and food. The most common eating disorder for men is binge eating disorder. With binge eating disorder, people eat a lot of food even if they feel full. They sometimes may try to make up for their overeating episodes by dieting. Other eating disorders that affect men include anorexia and bulimia.

Body Image Issues

People with body image issues may feel unhappy with how they look and feel self-conscious about their bodies. If these feelings are extreme, the person may have body dysmorphic disorder (BDD). People with BDD have extreme concern over what they see as flaws. Men and women are affected equally, but may focus on different parts of the body. Men tend to worry more about their skin, hair, nose, muscles, and genitals.

Obsession with food or how you look can be very painful. If you have eating or body image issues, don't let shame or embarrassment keep you from seeking help.

Muscle Mistakes

Some men try to pump up their muscles by taking anabolic steroids. But using steroids in this way can harm your physical and mental health—and it's illegal. Also, injecting steroids raises your risk of getting HIV and hepatitis.

Sometimes, men try natural supplements like creatine to build muscle. Keep in mind that "natural" doesn't necessarily mean safe. Make sure to discuss any supplements with your doctor before taking them.

Section 33.2

Men and Depression

"Men and Depression," National Institute of Mental Health
(www.nimh.nih.gov), October 4, 2011.

Are you tired and irritable all the time? Have you lost interest in your work, family, or hobbies? Are you having trouble sleeping and feeling angry or aggressive, sad, or worthless? Have you been feeling like this for weeks or months? If so, you may have depression.

What is depression?

Everyone feels sad or irritable sometimes, or has trouble sleeping occasionally. But these feelings and troubles usually pass after a couple of days. When a man has depression, he has trouble with daily life and loses interest in anything for weeks at a time.

Men and women both get depression. But men can experience it differently than women. Men may be more likely to feel very tired and irritable and lose interest in their work, family, or hobbies. They may be more likely to have difficulty sleeping than women who have depression. And although women with depression are more likely to attempt suicide, men are more likely to die by suicide.

Many men do not recognize, acknowledge, or seek help for their depression. They may be reluctant to talk about how they are feeling. But depression is a real and treatable illness. It can affect any man at any age. With the right treatment, most men with depression can get better and gain back their interest in work, family, and hobbies.

What are the different forms of depression?

Major depression: Severe symptoms that interfere with a man's ability to work, sleep, study, eat, and enjoy most aspects of life. An episode of major depression may occur only once in a person's lifetime. But more often, a person can have several episodes.

Dysthymic disorder (dysthymia): Depressive symptoms that last a long time (two years or longer) but are less severe than those of major depression.

Minor depression: Similar to major depression and dysthymia, but symptoms are less severe and may not last as long.

What are the signs and symptoms of depression in men?

Different people have different symptoms. Some symptoms of depression include the following:

- Feeling sad or "empty"
- Feeling hopeless, irritable, anxious, or angry
- Loss of interest in work, family, or once-pleasurable activities, including sex
- Feeling very tired
- Not being able to concentrate or remember details
- Not being able to sleep, or sleeping too much
- Overeating, or not wanting to eat at all
- Thoughts of suicide, suicide attempts
- Aches or pains, headaches, cramps, or digestive problems
- Inability to meet the responsibilities of work, caring for family, or other important activities.

What causes depression in men?

Several factors may contribute to depression in men:

- **Genes:** Men with a family history of depression may be more likely to develop it than those whose family members do not have the illness.
- **Brain chemistry and hormones:** The brains of people with depression look different on scans than those of people without the illness. Also, the hormones that control emotions and mood can affect brain chemistry.
- **Stress:** Loss of a loved one, a difficult relationship or any stressful situation may trigger depression in some men.

Most of the time, it is likely a combination of these factors.

How is depression treated?

The first step to getting the right treatment is to visit a doctor or mental health professional. He or she can do an exam or lab tests to rule out other conditions that may have the same symptoms as depression. He or she can also tell if certain medications you are taking may be affecting your mood.

The doctor needs to get a complete history of symptoms. Tell the doctor when the symptoms started, how long they have lasted, how bad they are, whether they have occurred before, and if so, how they were treated. Tell the doctor if there is a history of depression in your family.

Medication: Medications called antidepressants can work well to treat depression. But they can take several weeks to work. Antidepressants can have side effects such as headache; nausea, feeling sick to your stomach; difficulty sleeping and nervousness; agitation or restlessness; and sexual problems.

Most side effects lessen over time. Talk to your doctor about any side effects you may have.

It's important to know that although antidepressants can be safe and effective for many people, they may present serious risks to some, especially children, teens, and young adults. A black box—the most serious type of warning that a prescription drug can have—has been added to the labels of antidepressant medications. These labels warn people that antidepressants may cause some people to have suicidal thoughts or make suicide attempts, especially those who become agitated when they first start taking the medication and before it begins to work. Anyone taking antidepressants should be monitored closely, especially when they first start taking them.

For most people, though, the risks of untreated depression far outweigh those of antidepressant medications when they are used under a doctor's supervision. Careful monitoring by a professional will also minimize any potential risks.

Therapy: Several types of therapy can help treat depression. Some therapies are just as effective as medications for certain types of depression. Therapy helps by teaching new ways of thinking and behaving, and changing habits that may be contributing to the depression. Therapy can also help men understand and work through difficult situations or relationships that may be causing their depression or making it worse.

How can I help a loved one who is depressed?

If you know someone who has depression, first help him find a doctor or mental health professional and make an appointment. Offer him support, understanding, patience, and encouragement. Talk to him, and listen carefully. Never ignore comments about suicide, and report them to his therapist or doctor. Invite him out for walks, outings, and other activities. If he says no, keep trying, but don't push him to take on too much too soon. Encourage him to report any concerns about medications to his health care provider. Ensure that he gets to his doctor's appointments. Remind him that with time and treatment, the depression will lift.

How can I help myself if I am depressed?

As you continue treatment, gradually you will start to feel better. Remember that if you are taking an antidepressant, it may take several weeks for it to start working. Try to do things that you used to enjoy before you had depression. Go easy on yourself. Here are some other things that may help:

- See a professional as soon as possible. Research shows that getting treatment sooner rather than later can relieve symptoms quicker and reduce the length of time treatment is needed.

- Break up large tasks into small ones, and do what you can as you can. Don't try to do too many things at once.

- Spend time with other people and talk to a friend or relative about your feelings.

- Do not make important decisions until you feel better. Discuss decisions with others who know you well.

Where can I go for help?

If you are unsure where to go for help, ask your family doctor. You can also check the phone book for mental health professionals or check with your insurance carrier to find someone who participates in your plan. Hospital doctors can help in an emergency.

What if I or someone I know is in crisis?

Men with depression are at risk for suicide. If you or someone you know is in crisis, get help quickly.

- Call your doctor.

- Call 911 for emergency services or go to the nearest hospital emergency room.

- Call the toll-free, 24-hour hotline of the National Suicide Prevention Lifeline at 800-273-TALK (800-273-8255); TTY: 800-799-4TTY (800-799-4889).

Chapter 34

Mental Health Issues among Women

Chapter Contents

Section 34.1

Premenstrual Syndrome and Premenstrual Dysphoric Disorder

From "Premenstrual Syndrome (PMS) Fact Sheet," Office on Women's
Health (www.womenshealth.gov), May 18, 2010.

What is premenstrual syndrome (PMS)?

Premenstrual syndrome (PMS) is a group of symptoms linked to the
menstrual cycle. PMS symptoms occur one to two weeks before your period (menstruation or monthly bleeding) starts. The symptoms usually
go away after you start bleeding. PMS can affect menstruating women of
any age and the effect is different for each woman. For some people, PMS
is just a monthly bother. For others, it may be so severe that it makes it
hard to even get through the day. PMS goes away when your monthly
periods stop, such as when you get pregnant or go through menopause.

What causes PMS?

The causes of PMS are not clear, but several factors may be involved. Changes in hormones during the menstrual cycle seem to be
an important cause. These changing hormone levels may affect some
women more than others. Chemical changes in the brain may also be
involved. Stress and emotional problems, such as depression, do not
seem to cause PMS, but they may make it worse. Some other possible
causes include low levels of vitamins and minerals, eating a lot of salty
foods, which may cause you to retain (keep) fluid, and drinking alcohol
and caffeine, which may alter your mood and energy level.

What are the symptoms of PMS?

Symptoms vary from woman to woman. PMS often includes both
physical and emotional symptoms, including acne; swollen or tender
breasts; feeling tired; trouble sleeping; upset stomach, bloating, constipation, or diarrhea; headache or backache; appetite changes or food cravings; joint or muscle pain; trouble with concentration or memory; tension,
irritability, mood swings, or crying spells; and anxiety or depression.

452

How do I know if I have PMS?

Your doctor may diagnose PMS based on which symptoms you have, when they occur, and how much they affect your life. If you think you have PMS, keep track of which symptoms you have and how severe they are for a few months. Record your symptoms each day on a calendar. Take this with you when you see your doctor about your PMS.

Your doctor will also want to make sure you don't have one of the following conditions that shares symptoms with PMS:

- Depression
- Anxiety
- Menopause
- Chronic fatigue syndrome (CFS)
- Irritable bowel syndrome (IBS)
- Problems with the endocrine system, which makes hormones

What is the treatment for PMS?

Many things have been tried to ease the symptoms of PMS. No treatment works for every woman. You may need to try different ones to see what works for you. Some treatment options include lifestyle changes, medications, and alternative therapies.

Lifestyle changes: If your PMS isn't so bad that you need to see a doctor, some lifestyle changes may help you feel better. Below are some steps you can take that may help ease your symptoms.

- Exercise regularly. Each week, you should get two hours and 30 minutes of moderate-intensity physical activity; one hour and 15 minutes of vigorous-intensity aerobic physical activity; or a combination of moderate and vigorous-intensity activity; and muscle-strengthening activities on two or more days.
- Eat healthy foods, such as fruits, vegetables, and whole grains.
- Avoid salt, sugary foods, caffeine, and alcohol, especially when you're having PMS symptoms.
- Get enough sleep. Try to get about eight hours of sleep each night.
- Find healthy ways to cope with stress. Talk to your friends, exercise, or write in a journal. Some women also find yoga, massage, or relaxation therapy helpful.
- Don't smoke.

Medications: Over-the-counter pain relievers may help ease physical symptoms, such as cramps, headaches, backaches, and breast tenderness. Here are some examples:

- Ibuprofen (for instance, Advil, Motrin, Midol Cramp)
- Ketoprofen (for instance, Orudis KT)
- Naproxen (for instance, Aleve)
- Aspirin

In more severe cases of PMS, prescription medicines may be used to ease symptoms. One approach has been to use drugs that stop ovulation, such as birth control pills. Women on the pill report fewer PMS symptoms, such as cramps and headaches, as well as lighter periods.

Alternative therapies: Certain vitamins and minerals have been found to help relieve some PMS symptoms. These include the following:

- Folic acid (400 micrograms)
- Calcium with vitamin D (see Table 34.1 for amounts)
- Magnesium (400 milligrams)
- Vitamin B6 (50 to 100 mg)
- Vitamin E (400 international units)

Table 34.1. Amounts of calcium you need each day

Ages	Milligrams per day
9–18	1300
19–50	1000
51 and older	1200

Pregnant or nursing women need the same amount of calcium as other women of the same age.

Some women find their PMS symptoms relieved by taking supplements such as black cohosh, chasteberry, or evening primrose oil.

Talk with your doctor before taking any of these products. Many have not been proven to work and they may interact with other medicines you are taking.

What is premenstrual dysphoric disorder (PMDD)?

A brain chemical called serotonin may play a role in premenstrual dysphoric disorder (PMDD), a severe form of PMS. The main symptoms, which can be disabling, include the following:

- Feelings of sadness or despair, or even thoughts of suicide
- Feelings of tension or anxiety
- Panic attacks
- Mood swings or frequent crying
- Lasting irritability or anger that affects other people
- Lack of interest in daily activities and relationships
- Trouble thinking or focusing
- Tiredness or low energy
- Food cravings or binge eating
- Trouble sleeping
- Feeling out of control
- Physical symptoms, such as bloating, breast tenderness, headaches, and joint or muscle pain

You must have five or more of these symptoms to be diagnosed with PMDD. Symptoms occur during the week before your period and go away after bleeding starts.

Making some lifestyle changes may help ease PMDD symptoms. See "What is the treatment for PMS?" above to learn more.

Antidepressants called selective serotonin reuptake inhibitors (SSRIs) have also been shown to help some women with PMDD. These drugs change serotonin levels in the brain. The Food and Drug Administration (FDA) has approved three SSRIs for the treatment of PMDD:

- Sertraline (Zoloft)
- Fluoxetine (Sarafem)
- Paroxetine HCl (Paxil CR)

Yaz (drospirenone and ethinyl estradiol) is the only birth control pill approved by the FDA to treat PMDD. Individual counseling, group counseling, and stress management may also help relieve symptoms.

Section 34.2

Women and Depression

Excerpted from "Women and Depression: Discovering Hope," National Institute of Mental Health (NIMH), October 4, 2011. The complete text of this document, including references, is available online at http://www.nimh.nih.gov/health/publications/women-and-depression-discovering-hope/complete-index.shtml

What is depression?

Everyone occasionally feels blue or sad, but these feelings are usually fleeting and pass within a couple of days. When a woman has a depressive disorder, it interferes with daily life and normal functioning, and causes pain for both the woman with the disorder and those who care about her. Depression is a common but serious illness and most who have it need treatment to get better.

Depression affects both men and women, but more women than men are likely to be diagnosed with depression in any given year. Efforts to explain this difference are ongoing, as researchers explore certain factors (biological, social, etc.) that are unique to women.

Many women with a depressive illness never seek treatment. But the vast majority, even those with the most severe depression, can get better with treatment.

What causes depression in women?

Scientists are examining many potential causes for and contributing factors to women's increased risk for depression. It is likely that genetic, biological, chemical, hormonal, environmental, psychological, and social factors all intersect to contribute to depression.

Genetics: If a woman has a family history of depression, she may be more at risk of developing the illness. However, this is not a hard and fast rule. Depression can occur in women without family histories of depression, and women from families with a history of depression may not develop depression themselves. Genetics research indicates that the risk for developing depression likely involves the combination of multiple genes with environmental or other factors.

Chemicals and hormones: Brain chemistry appears to be a signifi-cant factor in depressive disorders. Modern brain-imaging technologies, such as magnetic resonance imaging (MRI), have shown that the brains of people suffering from depression look different than those of people without depression. The parts of the brain responsible for regulating mood, thinking, sleep, appetite and behavior don't appear to be function-ing normally. In addition, important neurotransmitters—chemicals that brain cells use to communicate—appear to be out of balance. But these images do not reveal why the depression has occurred.

Scientists are also studying the influence of female hormones, which change throughout life. Researchers have shown that hormones di-rectly affect the brain chemistry that controls emotions and mood. Specific times during a woman's life are of particular interest, including puberty; the times before menstrual periods; before, during, and just after pregnancy (postpartum); and just prior to and during menopause (perimenopause).

Premenstrual dysphoric disorder: Some women may be suscep-tible to a severe form of premenstrual syndrome called premenstrual dysphoric disorder (PMDD). Women affected by PMDD typically ex-perience depression, anxiety, irritability, and mood swings the week before menstruation, in such a way that interferes with their normal functioning. Women with debilitating PMDD do not necessarily have unusual hormone changes, but they do have different responses to these changes. They may also have a history of other mood disorders and differences in brain chemistry that cause them to be more sensi-tive to menstruation-related hormone changes. Scientists are explor-ing how the cyclical rise and fall of estrogen and other hormones may affect the brain chemistry that is associated with depressive illness.

Postpartum depression: Women are particularly vulnerable to depression after giving birth, when hormonal and physical changes and the new responsibility of caring for a newborn can be overwhelming. Many new mothers experience a brief episode of mild mood changes known as the "baby blues," but some will suffer from postpartum de-pression, a much more serious condition that requires active treatment and emotional support for the new mother. One study found that post-partum women are at an increased risk for several mental disorders, including depression, for several months after childbirth.

Some studies suggest that women who experience postpartum de-pression often have had prior depressive episodes. Some experience it during their pregnancies, but it often goes undetected. Research suggests that visits to the doctor may be good opportunities for screening for depression both during pregnancy and in the postpartum period.

Menopause: Hormonal changes increase during the transition between premenopause to menopause. While some women may transition into menopause without any problems with mood, others experience an increased risk for depression. This seems to occur even among women without a history of depression. However, depression becomes less common for women during the post-menopause period.

Stress: Stressful life events such as trauma, loss of a loved one, a difficult relationship, or any stressful situation—whether welcome or unwelcome—often occur before a depressive episode. Additional work and home responsibilities, caring for children and aging parents, abuse, and poverty also may trigger a depressive episode. Evidence suggests that women respond differently than men to these events, making them more prone to depression. In fact, research indicates that women respond in such a way that prolongs their feelings of stress more so than men, increasing the risk for depression. However, it is unclear why some women faced with enormous challenges develop depression, and some with similar challenges do not.

How does depression affect adolescent girls?

Before adolescence, girls and boys experience depression at about the same frequency. By adolescence, however, girls become more likely to experience depression than boys.

Research points to several possible reasons for this imbalance. The biological and hormonal changes that occur during puberty likely contribute to the sharp increase in rates of depression among adolescent girls. In addition, research has suggested that girls are more likely than boys to continue feeling bad after experiencing difficult situations or events, suggesting they are more prone to depression. Another study found that girls tended to doubt themselves, doubt their problem-solving abilities, and view their problems as unsolvable more so than boys. The girls with these views were more likely to have depressive symptoms as well. Girls also tended to need a higher degree of approval and success to feel secure than boys.

Finally, girls may undergo more hardships, such as poverty, poor education, childhood sexual abuse, and other traumas than boys. One study found that more than 70 percent of depressed girls experienced a difficult or stressful life event prior to a depressive episode, as compared with only 14 percent of boys.

How does depression affect older women?

As with other age groups, more older women than older men experience depression, but rates decrease among women after menopause. Evidence suggests that depression in post-menopausal women generally occurs in women with prior histories of depression. In any case, depression is not a normal part of aging.

The death of a spouse or loved one, moving from work into retirement, or dealing with a chronic illness can leave women and men alike feeling sad or distressed. After a period of adjustment, many older women can regain their emotional balance, but others do not and may develop depression. When older women do suffer from depression, it may be overlooked because older adults may be less willing to discuss feelings of sadness or grief, or they may have less obvious symptoms of depression. As a result, their doctors may be less likely to suspect or spot it.

For older adults who experience depression for the first time later in life, other factors, such as changes in the brain or body, may be at play. For example, older adults may suffer from restricted blood flow, a condition called ischemia. Over time, blood vessels become less flexible. They may harden and prevent blood from flowing normally to the body's organs, including the brain. If this occurs, an older adult with no family or personal history of depression may develop what some doctors call "vascular depression." Those with vascular depression also may be at risk for a coexisting cardiovascular illness, such as heart disease or a stroke.

Is it safe to take antidepressant medication during pregnancy?

At one time, doctors assumed that pregnancy was accompanied by a natural feeling of well being, and that depression during pregnancy was rare, or never occurred at all. However, recent studies have shown that women can have depression while pregnant, especially if they have a prior history of the illness. In fact, a majority of women with a history of depression will likely relapse during pregnancy if they stop taking their antidepressant medication either prior to conception or early in the pregnancy, putting both mother and baby at risk.

However, antidepressant medications do pass across the placental barrier, potentially exposing the developing fetus to the medication. Some research suggests the use of selective serotonin reuptake inhibitors (SSRIs) during pregnancy is associated with miscarriage and/or birth defects, but other studies do not support this. Some studies have indicated that fetuses exposed to SSRIs during the third trimester may be born with withdrawal symptoms such as breathing problems, jitteriness, irritability, difficulty feeding, or hypoglycemia. In 2004, the U.S. Food and Drug Administration (FDA) issued a warning against the use of SSRIs in the late third trimester, suggesting that clinicians gradually taper expectant mothers off SSRIs in the third trimester to avoid any ill effects on the baby.

Although some studies suggest that exposure to SSRIs in pregnancy may have adverse effects on the infant, generally they are mild and short-lived, and no deaths have been reported. On the flip side, women who stop taking their antidepressant medication during pregnancy increase their risk for developing depression again and may put both themselves and their infant at risk.

In light of these mixed results, women and their doctors need to consider the potential risks and benefits to both mother and fetus of taking an antidepressant during pregnancy, and make decisions based on individual needs and circumstances. In some cases, a woman and her doctor may decide to taper her antidepressant dose during the last month of pregnancy to minimize the newborn's withdrawal symptoms, and after delivery, return to a full dose during the vulnerable postpartum period.

[For more information on antidepressants, see Chapter 22—Mental Health Medications; for more information on depression during pregnancy, see the next section of this chapter, Section 34.3—Pregnancy and Depression.]

Is it safe to take antidepressant medication while breast-feeding?

Antidepressants are excreted in breast milk, usually in very small amounts. The amount an infant receives is usually so small that it does not register in blood tests. Few problems are seen among infants nursing from mothers who are taking antidepressants. However, as with antidepressant use during pregnancy, both the risks and benefits to the mother and infant should be taken into account when deciding whether to take an antidepressant while breastfeeding.

What if I or someone I know is in crisis?

Women are more likely than men to attempt suicide. If you are thinking about harming yourself or attempting suicide, tell someone who can help immediately.

- Call your doctor.
- Call 911 for emergency services.

- Go to the nearest hospital emergency room.

- Call the toll-free, 24-hour hotline of the National Suicide Prevention Lifeline at 800-273-TALK (800-273-8255); TTY: 800-799-4TTY (4889) to be connected to a trained counselor at a suicide crisis center nearest you.

Section 34.3

Pregnancy and Depression

As many as one out of five women have symptoms of depression during pregnancy. For some women, those symptoms are severe. In pregnancy, women who have been depressed before are at higher risk of depression than other women.

Depression is a serious medical condition. It poses risks for the woman and her baby. But a range of treatments are available. These include therapy, support groups and medications.

It is usually best for a team of health care professionals to work with a pregnant woman who is depressed or who has a history of depression. Team members include:

- The provider who is caring for her during her pregnancy

- A mental health professional

- The provider who will take care of the baby after birth

Together, the team and the woman decide what is best for her and her baby.

Often a pregnant woman wonders whether antidepressant drugs, such as Zoloft and Prozac, will harm her baby or herself. There are no simple answers. Each woman and her health care providers must work together to make the best decision for her and her baby. The drugs used to treat depression have both risks and benefits.

Important: If you are taking an antidepressant and find that you are pregnant, do not stop taking your medication without first talking to your health provider. Call him or her as soon as you discover that you are expecting. It may be unhealthy to stop taking an antidepressant suddenly.

What Is Depression?

Depression is an illness that involves the body, mood, and thought. It affects the way a woman feels about herself and the way she thinks about things. This information addresses two types of depression:

Major depression is a serious illness that interferes with a person's ability to work, study, sleep, eat, and enjoy oneself. It may appear once in a person's life, but more often occurs several times.

Milder forms of depression are less severe. Persons may still have long-term symptoms. They are able to conduct day-to-day activities, but they don't always function well or feel good. They may also have episodes of major depression.

The Risks of Untreated Depression during Pregnancy

Depression, especially if it isn't treated, carries serious risks for the pregnant woman and her baby. These risks include:

- Poor prenatal care
- Preeclampsia, a type of high blood pressure that occurs during pregnancy
- Poor weight gain
- Unhealthy eating habits
- Use of drugs or alcohol to self-medicate
- Suicide

Depressed mothers are often less able to care for themselves or their children, or to bond with their children.

Babies born to women with depression may be more irritable, less active, and less attentive than other babies. They may also be born prematurely or have low birthweight.

What Are the Symptoms of Depression?

A woman who is depressed feels sad or "blue" and has other symptoms that last for two weeks or longer. The other symptoms include the following:

- Trouble sleeping
- Sleeping too much
- Lack of interest
- Feelings of guilt
- Loss of energy
- Difficulty concentrating
- Changes in appetite
- Restlessness, agitation or slowed movement
- Thoughts or ideas about suicide

It may be hard to diagnose depression during pregnancy. Some of its symptoms are similar to those normally found in pregnancy. For instance, changes in appetite and trouble sleeping are common when a woman is pregnant. Other medical conditions have symptoms similar to those for depression. For instance, a woman who has anemia or a thyroid problem may lack energy but not be depressed. If you have any of the symptoms listed, talk to your health care provider. He or she will check to see what might be causing your symptoms.

Treatment without Medication

Depression can be treated in several ways. Support groups may help. Some women go to therapy or counseling with a mental health professional (such as a social worker, psychotherapist, or psychiatrist). For women with mild forms of depression, individual or group therapy may be all the treatment they need.

Some people suffer from a type of depression that comes on during the fall or winter, when there is less sunlight. This is called seasonal affective disorder (SAD). This condition is treated with light therapy. In her home, the patient looks into a box with special light bulbs. The health provider recommends how many times a day and for how long the patient needs to use the light box.

Another form of treatment is electroconvulsive therapy (ECT). During this treatment, electric current is passed through the brain. ECT may be recommended in cases of severe depression.

Medication: Antidepressants

Most antidepressants can be categorized into one of two groups. (Use of trade names is for identification only and does not imply endorsement.)

- **Group 1:** Selective Serotonin Uptake Inhibitors (SSRIs). This group of drugs includes: Prozac (fluoxetine); Lexapro (escitalopram); Zoloft (sertraline); Celexa (citalopram); Effexor (venlafaxine); Paxil (paroxetine); Cymbalta (duloxetine)

- **Group 2:** Tricyclic antidepressants (TCAs). This group of drugs includes: Elavil (amitriptyline); Tofranil (imipramine); Pamelor (Aventyl, nortriptyline)

If a woman is taking an antidepressant and wants to get pregnant, she should talk to her health care provider beforehand. Together, they will decide whether she should keep taking the medication, change the medication, gradually reduce the dose or stop taking it.

What Research Tells Us about Antidepressants

It's challenging to study and understand the risks of any drug given to pregnant women. During pregnancy, two patients—the mother and the fetus—are exposed to the drug. Medications that are safe for a woman are sometimes risky for a fetus. Because of this, researchers have not studied many drugs during pregnancy. Here is what we know from research.

Several drugs have been used for many years without any obvious signs of serious risk to the baby. For instance, TCAs have been around for many years, so we have more information about them than about SSRIs. SSRIs are a newer group of drugs than TCAs. Researchers are continuing to study them.

Some antidepressants, but not all, have been linked to problems for the baby. Examples include heart problems, low birthweight, and high blood pressure in the arteries that supply blood to the lungs (pulmonary hypertension).

Women who are depressed are very likely to become ill again if they stop taking their medications.

Some women benefit from a combination of therapy and antidepressants.

Choosing an Antidepressant

This decision is difficult because we don't know all the answers. No drug is entirely safe. A woman and her health care team must look at her case and carefully weigh:

- The risks and benefits of various drugs
- The risks and benefits of other types of treatment

- The risk of untreated depression for the woman and her baby

St. John's Wort and Other Herbal Remedies

St. John's wort is an herb that some people use to treat depression. According to the National Center for Complementary and Alternative Medicine, some research has shown that St. John's wort may be useful for treating mild to moderate depression. Other studies have shown that it is does not help one type of major depression.

Herbal products, such as St. John's wort, vary in strength and quality from product to product. We need more research to help us know whether St. John's wort is useful and safe for treating depression in pregnant women.

Important: We know very little about the effect of St. John's wort on the fetus. Do no take this herb or other herbal remedies without first speaking to your health provider.

Resources

The Organization of Teratology Information Services (OTIS, http://www.otispregnancy.org), (866) 626-6847. Provides fact sheets on pregnancy and specific antidepressants, including Prozac and Zoloft.

Depression During and After Pregnancy (http://www.mchb.hrsa.gov/pregnancyandbeyond/depression), a resource for women, their families and friends, provided by the U.S. Department of Health and Human Services.

Depression During and After Pregnancy (http://mchlibrary.info/KnowledgePaths/kp_postpartum.html), provided by the Maternal and Child Health Library.

Section 34.4

Postpartum Depression and Postpartum Psychosis

Whether you're becoming a mom for the first time or the fourth, the days and weeks immediately following your baby's birth can be as overwhelming as they are joyful and exciting.

Many women experience major mood shifts after childbirth, ranging from brief, mild baby blues to the longer-lasting, deeper clinical depression known as postpartum depression.

Feelings of sadness and depression are more common after childbirth than many people may realize. It's important for new mothers—and those who love them—to understand the symptoms of postpartum depression and to reach out to family, friends, and medical professionals for help.

With the proper support and treatment, mothers who are experiencing any degree of postpartum depression can go on to be healthy, happy parents.

Baby Blues

Up to 80% of women experience something called the baby blues, feelings of sadness and emotional surges that begin in the first days after childbirth. With the baby blues, a woman might feel happy one minute and tearful or overwhelmed the next. She might feel sad, blue, irritable, discouraged, unhappy, tired, or moody. Baby blues usually last only a few days—but can linger as long as a week or two.

Why It Happens

These emotional surges are believed to be a natural effect of the hormone shifts that occur with pregnancy and childbirth. Levels of estrogen and progesterone that increased during pregnancy drop suddenly after delivery, and this can affect mood. These female hormones return to their pre-pregnancy levels within a week or so. As hormone levels normalize, baby blues usually resolve on their own without medical treatment.

What to Do

Getting proper rest, nutrition, and support are quite important—since being exhausted or sleep deprived or feeling stressed can reinforce and fuel feelings of sadness and depression.

To cope with baby blues, new moms should try to accept help in the first days and weeks after labor and delivery. Let family and friends help with errands, food shopping, household chores, or child care. Let someone prepare a meal or watch the baby while you relax with a shower, bath, or a nap.

Get plenty of rest and eat nutritious foods. Talking to people close to you, or to other new mothers, can help you feel supported and remind you that you're not alone. You don't have to stifle the tears if you feel the need to cry a bit—but try not to dwell on sad thoughts. Let the baby blues run their course and pass.

When to Call the Doctor

If baby blues linger longer than a week or two, talk to your doctor to discuss whether postpartum depression may be the cause of your emotional lows.

Postpartum Depression

For some women, the feelings of sadness or exhaustion run deeper and last longer than baby blues. About 10% of new mothers experience postpartum depression, which is a true clinical depression triggered by childbirth.

Postpartum depression usually begins two to three weeks after giving birth, but can start any time during the first few days, weeks, or months post-delivery.

A woman with postpartum depression may feel sad, tearful, despairing, discouraged, hopeless, worthless, or alone. She also may:

- have trouble concentrating or completing routine tasks;
- lose her appetite or not feel interested in food;
- feel indifferent to her baby or not feel attached or bonded;

- feel overwhelmed by her situation and feel that there is no hope of things getting better;

- feel like she is just going through the motions of her day without being able to feel happy, interested, pleased, or joyful about anything.

Feelings and thoughts like these are painful for a woman to experience—especially during a time that is idealized as being full of happiness. Many women are reluctant to tell someone when they feel this way. But postpartum depression is a medical condition that requires attention and treatment.

Sometimes new mothers are reluctant to tell others about their depression. It's common for them to have thoughts like, "I'm not supposed to feel this way. I have this wonderful new baby. I should feel grateful and happy—what's wrong with me?" These thoughts make women think that depression is a personal failing. But it's not—postpartum depression is a medical condition, and it responds to treatment.

Why It Happens

Postpartum depression can affect any woman—but some may be more at risk for developing it. Women who have battled depression at another time in their lives or have one or more relatives who have had depression might have a genetic tendency to develop postpartum depression.

Most postpartum depression is thought to be related to fluctuating hormone levels that affect mood and energy. Levels of estrogen and progesterone that increased during pregnancy drop suddenly after delivery. In some cases a woman's thyroid hormone may decrease, too.

These rapid hormone shifts affect the brain's mood chemistry in a way that can lead to sadness, low mood, and depression that lingers. Stress hormones may have an added effect on mood. Some women might experience this more than others.

When to Call the Doctor

If feelings of sadness or depression are strong, if they linger throughout most of the day for days in a row, or if they last longer that a week or two, talk to your doctor. A new mother who feels like giving up, who feels that life is not worth living, or who has suicidal thoughts or feelings needs to tell her doctor right away.

Postpartum depression can last for several months or even longer if it goes untreated. With proper treatment, a woman can feel like herself again. Treatment may include talk therapy, medication, or both. In addition, proper diet, exercise, rest, and social support can be very helpful. Some women find yoga to be beneficial. Some research suggests that expressing thoughts and emotions through certain writing techniques can help relieve symptoms of depression.

It may take several weeks for a woman to begin to feel better once she is being treated for depression, though some begin to feel better sooner. Ask your doctor about how soon to expect improvements and ways to take care of yourself in the meantime.

Postpartum Psychosis

A more serious and rare condition is postpartum psychosis. It affects about 1 in 1,000 women who give birth and occurs within the first month after labor and delivery. It may include hallucinations, such as hearing voices or seeing things, or feelings of paranoia.

With postpartum psychosis, a woman can have irrational ideas about her baby—such as that the baby is possessed or that she has to hurt herself or her child. This condition can be extremely serious and disabling, and new mothers who are experiencing these symptoms need medical attention right away.

Why It Happens

Women who have other psychiatric illnesses, such as bipolar disorder or schizoaffective disorder, may be at greater risk of developing postpartum psychosis.

When to Call the Doctor

Postpartum psychosis requires immediate medical attention and, often, a brief hospitalization. If you or someone you know is experiencing symptoms, don't delay getting medical attention.

Understanding the Changes after Childbirth

New mothers experience many layers of change in the days and weeks immediately following labor and delivery. In addition to the sudden drop in estrogen and progesterone—which can affect mood—other huge physical, emotional, and domestic changes can affect how a new mom feels.

Physical Changes

Pregnancy brings many physical changes, and labor and delivery are physically intense and challenging. It takes time for the body to recover, and a new mother might feel exhausted, emotionally drained, or uncomfortable after delivery.

Personal and Emotional Changes

A woman's role and responsibilities may change quite a bit when she becomes a new mother. It can take time to adjust—even if she felt prepared for the change. Some women may feel isolated, worried, or scared.

Some new mothers face added stresses related to difficult circumstances or lack of support. Enduring a tough relationship, a precarious financial situation, or some other major life event at the same time—like a move or a job loss—can add stress.

Pregnancy-related stress—such as difficulty conceiving or complications during pregnancy or labor—can add to a new mom's feeling of being depleted. Sometimes (but not always) these stresses can pave the way for depression.

Changes in Routines and Responsibilities

A newborn brings special demands on a mother's time, attention, and energy. For first-time mothers, there can be lots to learn about meeting the baby's most basic needs, like sleeping, feeding, bathing, and soothing. There are lots of new routines to establish.

The baby's sleeping, waking, and feeding schedules can make it hard for a new mom to get the sleep and rest required to help handle all these new stresses and responsibilities. And without a good night's sleep, even small things can seem overwhelming.

Getting Help and Helping Yourself

Tell your doctor if you're having trouble with postpartum moods, thoughts, or feelings. Let someone else you trust know, too. This might be your partner, a friend, or a family member. This is a time to reach out and accept help and support from people close to you.

In addition to getting treatment for postpartum depression, small things you do can make it easier to get through a difficult time. You might find it helpful to:

- Take time for yourself. Schedule a babysitter for a regular time. This way you'll be sure to get time for yourself and know that it's coming.

- Focus on little things to look forward to during the day. This might be a hot shower, relaxing bath, walk around the block, or visit with a friend.

- Read something uplifting. Since depression may make it difficult to concentrate, choose something light and positive that can be read a bit at a time.

- Indulge in other simple pleasures. Page through a magazine, listen to music you enjoy, sip a cup of tea.

- Be with others. Create opportunities to spend time with other adults, like family and friends, who can provide some comfort and good company.

- Ask for help. Don't shy away from asking for emotional support or help with caring for the baby or tackling household chores.

- Accept help. Accepting help doesn't make you helpless—by reaching out you help yourself and your baby.

- Rest. Give your child a quiet place to sleep, and try to rest when the baby does.

- Get moving. A daily walk can help lift mood. (Check with your doctor before starting any new exercise program.)

- Be patient. Know that it may take time to feel better and take one day at a time.

- Be optimistic. Try to think of small things you're grateful for.

- Join a support group. Ask your doctor or women's center about resources in your community.

Helping Someone with Postpartum Depression

If you're concerned that your partner or someone else you know is experiencing postpartum depression, it's important to encourage her to talk to her doctor and to a mental health professional. Sometimes a woman is reluctant to seek help or may not recognize her own symptoms right away.

Consider giving the new mom some information on postpartum depression, and offer to read through it together. You might offer to make an appointment for her and go with her if she wants.

Once she's receiving the care she needs, support, love, and friendship are good medicine, too. Here are a few things that you can continue do for her:

- Check in with her regularly to see how she's doing.

- Listen when she wants to talk.

- Go for a walk with her (every day if possible!).

- Make her a nutritious meal (regularly!).

- Give her some breaks from housework and childcare responsibilities.

- Let her take a nap or a relaxing bath while you care for her baby.

- Be patient, be kind.

- Believe in her—and remind her of her true qualities and strengths.

Brighter Days Ahead

Like all forms of depression, postpartum depression creates a cloud of negative feelings and thoughts over a woman's view of herself, those around her, her situation, and the future. Under the cloud of depression, a woman might see herself as helpless or worthless. She might view her situation as overwhelming or hopeless. Things might seem disappointing, uninteresting, or without meaning. Keep in mind that the bleak negative perspective is part of depression.

With the right treatment and support, the cloud can be lifted. This can free a woman to feel like herself again, to regain her perspective and sense of her own strength, her energy, her joy, and her hope. With those things in place, it's easier to work with changes, to see solutions to life's challenges, and to enjoy life's pleasures again.

Section 34.5

Menopause and Mental Health

"Menopause and Mental Health," Office on Women's Health
(www.womenshealth.gov), September 29, 2010.

Problems and Causes

Midlife is often considered a period of increased risk for depression in women. Some women report mood swings, irritability, tearfulness, anxiety, and feelings of despair in the years leading up to menopause. But the reason for these emotional problems isn't always clear. Research shows that menopausal symptoms such as sleep problems, hot flashes, night sweats, and fatigue can affect mood and well-being. The drop in estrogen levels during perimenopause and menopause might also affect mood. Or it could be a combination of hormone changes and menopausal symptoms.

But changes in mood also can have causes that are unrelated to menopause. If you are having emotional problems that are interfering with your quality of life, it is important to discuss them with your doctor. Talk openly with your doctor about the other things going on in your life that might be adding to your feelings. Other things that could cause feelings of depression and/or anxiety during menopause include:

- Having depression before menopause
- Feeling negative about menopause and getting older
- Increased stress
- Having severe menopausal symptoms
- Smoking
- Not being physically active
- Not being happy in your relationship or not being in a relationship
- Not having a job
- Not having enough money

473

- Having low self-esteem (how you feel about yourself)

- Not having the social support you need

- Feeling disappointed that you can't have children anymore

Ways to Feel Better

If you need treatment for your symptoms, you and your doctor can work together to find a treatment that is best for you. Depression during the menopausal transition is treated in much the same way as depression that strikes at any other time life. If your mood is affecting your quality of life, here are a few things you can do:

- Try to get enough sleep. Go to bed and wake up at the same times every day. Keep your room cool and dark. Use your bed only for sleeping and sex. Avoid alcohol, caffeine, large meals, or physical activity before bed.

- Engage in physical activity for at least 30 minutes on most days of the week.

- Set limits for yourself, and look for positive ways to unwind and ease daily stress. Try relaxation techniques, reading a book, or spending some quiet time outdoors.

- Talk to your friends or go to a support group for women who are going through the same thing as you. You also can get counseling to talk through your problems and fears.

- Ask your doctor about therapy or medicines. Menopausal hormone therapy (MHT) can reduce symptoms that might be causing your moodiness. Antidepressants might also help. Note: MHT is not an antidepressant. If you are having signs of depression, ask your doctor about other treatments that can help.

Chapter 35

Mental Health Issues among Older Adults

Chapter Contents

Section 35.1

Depression in Late Life

Everyone Feels Sad or Blue Sometimes

It is a natural part of life. But when the sadness persists and interferes with everyday life, it may be depression. Depression is not a normal part of growing older. It is a treatable medical illness, much like heart disease or diabetes.

Depression is a serious illness affecting approximately 15 out of every 100 adults over age 65 in the United States. The disorder affects a much higher percentage of people in hospitals and nursing homes. When depression occurs in late life, it sometimes can be a relapse of an earlier depression. But when it occurs for the first time in older adults, it usually is brought on by another medical illness. When someone is already ill, depression can be both more difficult to recognize and more difficult to endure.

Depression Is Not a Passing Mood

Sadness associated with normal grief or everyday "blues" is different from depression. A sad or grieving person can continue to carry on with regular activities. The depressed person suffers from symptoms that interfere with his or her ability to function normally for a prolonged period of time.

Recognizing depression in the elderly is not always easy. It often is difficult for the depressed elder to describe how he or she is feeling. In addition, the current population of older Americans came of age at a time when depression was not understood to be a biological disorder and medical illness. Therefore, some elderly fear being labeled "crazy," or worry that their illness will be seen as a character weakness.

The depressed person or their family members may think that a change in mood or behavior is simply "a passing mood," and the person should just "snap out of it." But someone suffering from depression can not just "get over it." Depression is a medical illness that must be diagnosed and treated by trained professionals. Untreated, depression may last months or even years.

Untreated Depression Can

- Lead to disability
- Worsen symptoms of other illnesses
- Lead to premature death
- Result in suicide

When it is properly diagnosed and treated, more than 80 percent of those suffering from depression recover and return to their normal lives.

The most common symptoms of late-life depression include:

- Persistent sadness (lasting two weeks or more)
- Feeling slowed down
- Excessive worries about finances and health problems
- Frequent tearfulness
- Feeling worthless or helpless
- Weight changes
- Pacing and fidgeting
- Difficulty sleeping
- Difficulty concentrating
- Physical symptoms such as pain or gastrointestinal problems.

One important sign of depression is when people withdraw from their regular social activities. Rather than explaining their symptoms as a medical illness, often depressed persons will give different explanations such as:

- " It's too much trouble,"
- " I don't feel well enough," or
- " I don't have the energy."

For the same reasons, they often neglect their personal appearance, or may begin cooking and eating less. Like many illnesses, there are varying levels and types of depression. A person may not feel "sad" about anything, but may exhibit symptoms such as difficulty sleeping, weight loss, or physical pain with no apparent explanation. This person still may be clinically depressed. Those same symptoms also may be a sign of another problem—only a doctor can make the correct diagnosis.

It Can Happen to Anyone

Sometimes depression will occur for no apparent reason. In other words, nothing necessarily needs to "happen" in one's life for depression to occur. This can be because the disease often is caused by biological changes in the brain. However, in older adults, there usually are understandable reasons for the depression. As the brain and body age, a number of natural bio-chemical changes begin to take place. Changes as the result of aging, medical illnesses or genetics may put the older adult at a greater risk for developing depression.

Life Changes

Chronic or serious illness is the most common cause of depression in the elderly. But even when someone is struggling with a chronic illness such as arthritis, it is not natural to be depressed. Depression is defined as an illness if it lasts two weeks or more and if it affects one's ability to lead a normal life.

Many factors can contribute to the development of depression. Often people describe one specific event that triggered their depression, such as the death of a partner or loved one, or the loss of a job through layoff or retirement. What seems like a normal period of sadness or grief may lead to a prolonged, intense grief that requires medical attention.

The loss of a life-long partner or a friend is a frequent occurrence in later life. It is normal to grieve after such a loss. But it may be depression rather than bereavement if the grief persists, or is accompanied by any of the following symptoms:

- Guilt unconnected with the loved one's death

- Thoughts of one's own death

- Persistent feelings of worthlessness

- Inability to function at one's usual level

- Difficulty sleeping

- Weight loss

If any of these symptoms are triggered by a loss, a physician should be consulted.

Changes in the older adult's sensory abilities or environment may contribute to the development of depression. Examples of such changes include:

- Changes in vision and hearing
- Changes in mobility
- Retirement
- Moving from the family home
- Neighborhood changes

Other Illnesses

In the older population, medical illnesses are a common trigger for depression, and often depression will worsen the symptoms of other illnesses. The following illnesses are common causes of late-life depression:

- Cancer
- Parkinson's disease
- Heart disease
- Stroke
- Alzheimer's disease

In addition, certain medical illnesses may hide the symptoms of depression. When a depressed person is preoccupied with physical symptoms resulting from a stroke, gastrointestinal problems, heart disease or arthritis, he or she may attribute the depressive symptoms to an existing physical illness, or may ignore the symptoms entirely. For this reason, he or she may not report the depressive symptoms to his or her doctor, creating a barrier to becoming well.

Depression Is Treatable

Most depressed elderly people can improve dramatically from treatment. In fact, there are highly effective treatments for depression in late life. Common treatments prescribed by physicians include:

- Psychotherapy

- Antidepressant medications

- Electroconvulsive therapy (ECT).

Psychotherapy can play an important role in the treatment of depression with, or without, medication. This type of treatment is most often used alone in mild to moderate depression. There are many forms of short-term therapy (10–20 weeks) that have proven to be effective. It is important that the depressed person find a therapist with whom he or she feels comfortable and who has experience with older patients.

Antidepressants work by increasing the level of neurotransmitters in the brain. Neurotransmitters are the brain's "messengers." Many feelings, including pain and pleasure, are a result of the neurotransmitters' function. When the supply of neurotransmitters is imbalanced, depression may result.

A frequent reason some people do not respond to antidepressant treatment is because they do not take the medication properly. Missing doses or taking more than the prescribed amount of the medication compromises the effect of the antidepressant. Similarly, stopping the medication too soon often results in a relapse of depression. In fact, most patients who stop taking their medication before four to six months after recovery will experience a relapse of depression.

Usually, antidepressant medication is taken for at least six months to a year. Typically, it takes four to 12 weeks to begin seeing results from antidepressant medication. If after this period of time the depression does not subside, the patient should consult his or her physician. Antidepressant drugs are not habit-forming or addictive. And because depression is often a recurrent illness, it usually is necessary to stay on the medication for six months after recovery to prevent new episodes of depression.

Electroconvulsive therapy (ECT) is a treatment that unnecessarily evokes fear in many people. In reality, ECT is one of the most safe, fast-acting and effective treatments for severe depression. It can be life saving. ECT often is the best choice for the person who has a life-threatening depression that is not responding to antidepressant medication or for the person who cannot tolerate the medication.

After a thorough evaluation, a physician will determine the treatment best suited for a person's depression. The treatment of depression demands patience and perseverance for the patient and the physician. Sometimes several different treatments must be tried before full recovery. Each person has individual biological and psychological characteristics that require individualized care.

Suicide

Suicide is more common in older people than in any other age group. The population over age 65 accounts for more than 25 percent of the nation's suicides. In fact, white men over age 80 are six times more likely to commit suicide than the general population, constituting the largest risk group. Suicide attempts or severe thoughts or wishes by older adults must always be taken seriously.

It is appropriate and important to ask a depressed person:

- Do they feel as though life is no longer an option for them?
- Have they had thoughts about harming themselves?
- Are they planning to do it?
- Is there a collection of pills or guns in the house?
- Are they often alone?

Most depressed people welcome care, concern and support, but they are frightened and may resist help. In the case of a potentially suicidal elder, caring friends or family members must be more than understanding. They must actively intervene by removing pills and weapons from the home and calling the family physician, mental health professional or, if necessary, the police.

Caring for a Depressed Person

The first step in helping an elderly person who may be depressed is to make sure he or she gets a complete physical checkup. Depression may be a side effect of a pre-existing medical condition or of a medication. If the depressed older adult is confused or withdrawn, it is helpful for a caring family member or friend to accompany the person to the doctor and provide important information.

The physician may refer the older adult to a psychiatrist with geriatric training or experience. If a person is reluctant to see a psychiatrist, he or she may need assurance that an evaluation is necessary to determine if treatment is needed to reduce symptoms, improve functioning and enhance well-being.

It is important to remember that depression is a highly treatable medical condition and is not a normal part of growing older. Therefore, it is crucial to understand and recognize the symptoms of the illness. As with any medical condition, the primary care physician should be consulted if someone has symptoms that interfere with everyday life.

An older person who is diagnosed with depression also should know that there are trained professionals who specialize in treating the elderly (called "geriatric psychiatrists") who may be able to help.

Section 35.2

Anxiety and Older Adults

Overcoming Worry and Fear

Feeling anxious or nervous is a common emotion for people of all ages and a normal reaction to stress. Feeling anxious can help us handle problems and strange situations, and even avoid danger. It is normal to feel anxious about illnesses, new social interactions, and frightening events. But when one feels anxious often and the anxiety is overwhelming and affects daily tasks, social life, and relationships, it may be an illness.

Anxiety is a common illness among older adults, affecting as many as 10–20 percent of the older population, though it is often undiagnosed. Phobia—when an individual is fearful of certain things, places or events—is the most typical type of anxiety. Among adults, anxiety is the most common mental health problem for women, and the second most common for men, after substance abuse.

Older adults with anxiety disorders often go untreated for a number of reasons. Older adults often do not recognize or acknowledge their symptoms. When they do, they may be reluctant to discuss their feelings with their physicians. Some older adults may not seek treatment because they have suffered symptoms of anxiety for most of their lives and believe the feelings are normal. Both patients and physicians may miss a diagnosis of anxiety because of other medical conditions and prescription drug use, or particular situations that the patient is coping with. For example, the anxiety suffered by a recently widowed patient may be more than normal grieving. Complicated or chronic grief is often accompanied by persistent anxiety and grieving spouses may avoid reminders of the deceased.

Untreated anxiety can lead to cognitive impairment, disability, poor physical health, and a poor quality of life. Fortunately, anxiety is treatable with prescription drugs and therapy.

What Is Anxiety?

An anxiety disorder causes feelings of fear, worry, apprehension, or dread that are excessive or disproportional to the problems or situations that are feared. There are several types of anxiety disorders.

Specific phobias: A specific phobia is an intense, irrational fear of a place, thing or event that actually poses little or no threat. Some common specific phobias are heights, escalators, tunnels, highway driving, closed-in spaces, flying, and spiders. Agoraphobia is a fear of public places, leaving one's home, or being alone. Phobias more common to older adults include fear of death, disaster to family, and dental procedures. Facing, or thinking about, these situations or things can bring on severe anxiety or a panic attack (chest pain, heart palpitations, shortness of breath, dizziness, or nausea).

Social phobia (also called social anxiety disorder): Social phobia is when an individual feels overwhelmingly anxious and self-conscious in everyday social situations. An older adult might feel intense, persistent, and chronic fear of being judged by others and of doing things that will cause embarrassment. Some older persons suffer a social phobia because they are embarrassed about being unable to remember names or are ashamed of their appearance due to illness. A social anxiety disorder makes it hard to make and keep friends. Some with social phobia can be around others, but are anxious beforehand, very uncomfortable throughout the encounter, and, afterwards, worry how they were judged. Physical symptoms can include blushing, heavy sweating, trembling, nausea, and difficulty talking.

Generalized anxiety disorder (GAD): Those with GAD suffer constant worries, and there may be nothing or little to cause these worries. Those with GAD are overly concerned about health issues, money, family problems, or possible disaster. Those with GAD usually understand that they worry more than necessary. Older adults with GAD have difficulty relaxing, sleeping and concentrating, and startle easily. Symptoms include fatigue, chest pains, headaches, muscle tension, muscle aches, difficulty swallowing, trembling, twitching, irritability, sweating, nausea, lightheadedness, having to go to the bathroom frequently, feeling out of breath, and hot flashes.

Post-traumatic stress disorder (PTSD): PTSD develops after a traumatic event that involved physical harm or the threat of physical harm to the individual, a loved one, or even strangers. PTSD can result from traumatic incidents, such as a mugging, rape, abuse, car accidents, or natural disasters such as floods or earthquakes, in addition to resulting from experiences of war. Symptoms may emerge months or years after the event. Some older adults may relive a trauma 30 years or more after an event due to feeling helpless because of a new disability (for example, being confined to a wheel chair) or specific triggers that revive old memories (for example, news coverage of current wars).

A person with PTSD may startle easily, be emotionally numb with people with whom they were once close, have difficulty feeling affection, and lose interest in things they once enjoyed. Those suffering PTSD may be irritable, aggressive or violent. A person with PTSD can experience flashbacks, in which vivid thoughts of the trauma occur during the day or in nightmares during sleep. During a flashback, a person may believe the traumatic event is happening again.

Obsessive-compulsive disorder (OCD): While OCD is not common among older adults, some older people do suffer from persistent, upsetting thoughts that they control by performing certain rituals, such as repeatedly checking things, touching things in a particular order, or counting things. Some common fears include possible violence and harm to loved ones. Some with OCD are preoccupied with order and symmetry; others accumulate or hoard unneeded items.

Panic disorder: Those with panic disorder have sudden attacks of terror, and usually a pounding heart, chest pain, sweatiness, weakness, faintness, dizziness, or nausea. Panic attacks can occur at any time, even during sleep. An attack usually peaks within 10 minutes, but some symptoms may last much longer. Panic disorder is not common among older adults, however, an older adult with the disorder may refuse to be left alone. An older person experiencing a panic attack may think he or she is having a heart attack or stroke.

Why Should an Older Adult Be Concerned about Anxiety?

For older adults, depression often goes along with anxiety, and both can be debilitating, reducing overall health and quality of life. It is important to know the signs of both anxiety and depression and to talk with a physician about any concerns. Anxiety is also strongly linked to memory. Anxiety can interfere with memory, and significant anxiety can contribute to amnesia or flashbacks of a traumatic event.

What Leads to Anxiety Disorder?

A number of things can contribute to an anxiety disorder:

- Extreme stress or trauma
- Bereavement and complicated or chronic grief
- Alcohol, caffeine, drugs (prescription, over-the-counter, and illegal)
- A family history of anxiety disorders
- Other medical or mental illnesses or
- Neurodegenerative disorders (like Alzheimer's or other dementias)

The stresses and changes that sometimes go along with aging—poor health, memory problems, and losses—can cause an anxiety disorder. Common fears about aging can lead to anxiety. Many older adults are afraid of falling, being unable to afford living expenses and medication, being victimized, being dependent on others, being left alone, and death.

Older adults and their families should be aware that health changes can also bring on anxiety. Anxiety disorders commonly occur along with other physical or mental illnesses, including alcohol or substance abuse, which may hide the symptoms or make them worse.

It's also important to note that many older adults living with anxiety suffered an anxiety disorder (possibly undiagnosed and untreated) when they were younger.

A stressful event, such as the death of a loved one, can cause a mild, brief anxiety, but anxiety that lasts at least six months can get worse if not treated.

Signs of Anxiety Disorder

- Excessive worry or fear
- Refusing to do routine activities or being overly preoccupied with routine
- Avoiding social situations
- Overly concerned about safety
- Racing heart, shallow breathing, trembling, nausea, sweating
- Poor sleep
- Muscle tension, feeling weak and shaky

- Hoarding/collecting
- Depression
- Self-medication with alcohol or other central nervous system depressants

Depression and Anxiety

In older adults, anxiety and depression often occur together. It is important for older adults to tell their physicians if they are experiencing symptoms of either.

Symptoms of depression usually last more than two weeks:

- Disturbed sleep (sleeping too much or too little)
- Changes in appetite (weight loss or gain)
- Physical aches and pains
- Lack of energy or motivation
- Irritability and intolerance
- Loss of interest or pleasure
- Feelings of worthlessness or guilt
- Difficulties with concentration or decision-making
- Noticeable restlessness or slow movement
- Recurring thoughts of death or suicide
- Changed sex drive

Who Can Help?

Older adults who think they may be suffering from anxiety should share their concerns with their primary care physicians. A physician can help determine if the symptoms are due to an anxiety disorder, a medical condition, or both. If the physician diagnoses an anxiety disorder, the next step is to see a mental health care professional. Both patient and provider should work as a team to make a plan to treat the anxiety disorder.

What Are the Treatment Options?

Treatment can involve medication, therapy, stress reduction, coping skills, and family or other social support.

A mental health care provider can determine what type of disorder or combination of disorders the patient has, and if any other conditions, such as grief, depression, substance abuse, or dementia, are present.

Those who have been treated before for an anxiety disorder should tell their provider about previous treatment. If they received medication, they should indicate what was used, dosage, side effects, and whether the treatment was helpful. If the patient attended therapy sessions, he or she should describe the type, how many sessions, and whether it was helpful. Sometimes individuals must try several different treatments or combinations of treatments before they find the one that works best for them.

Medication

Medication will not cure anxiety disorders but will keep them under control while the person receives therapy. Medication must be prescribed by physicians, often psychiatrists or geriatric psychiatrists, who can also offer therapy or work as a team with psychologists, social workers, or counselors who provide therapy.

The main medications used for anxiety disorders are antidepressants, anti-anxiety drugs, and beta-blockers, which control some of the physical symptoms.

Antidepressants: Antidepressants are typically prescribed for most anxiety disorders. They work by altering the brain chemistry. Because symptoms usually start to fade after 4–6 weeks of antidepressants, it is important to take them long enough for them to work. Antidepressants include selective serotonin reuptake inhibitors (SSRIs), serotonin and norepinephrine reuptake inhibitors (SNRIs), tricyclics, and monoamine oxidase inhibitors (MAOIs).

Anti-anxiety drugs: Anti-anxiety drugs, also called anxiolytics, are sometimes prescribed when a quick-acting and/or short-term medication is needed. Buspirone is an anti-anxiety drug that has been shown to be effective for older adults. Benzodiazepines, another anti-anxiety drug, are effective but should be prescribed carefully to older adults because of risk of memory impairment, unsteadiness, and falls. When they are used, benzodiazepines are usually prescribed for short periods of time. Some people experience withdrawal symptoms if they stop taking them abruptly instead of tapering off. When taken regularly for a long time, benzodiazepines can be addictive but typically are not.

Beta-blockers: Beta-blockers can help relieve anxiety by preventing the physical symptoms that go along with certain anxiety disorders.

Taking Medication

- Learn about the effects (for example, when it should begin to help and in what way) and side effects.

- Tell your doctor about any other drugs (both prescription and over-the-counter), herbal supplements, or alternative therapies you are taking.

- Find out when and how the medication should be stopped. Some cannot be stopped abruptly and must be tapered down under a doctor's supervision.

- Some medications are only effective if taken regularly.

Therapy

Therapy or psychotherapy involves talking with a trained mental health professional, such as a psychiatrist, psychologist, social worker, or counselor, to discover what caused the anxiety disorder and how to deal with its symptoms.

In cognitive-behavioral therapy, therapists help people change the thinking patterns that contribute to their fears and the ways they react to anxiety-provoking situations. A therapist can teach new coping and relaxation skills and help resolve problems that cause anxiety. When a patient is ready to face his or her fears, a therapist can teach exposure techniques to desensitize the patient to the situations that trigger anxious feelings. Therapists also teach deep breathing and other relaxation techniques to relieve anxiety. Behavioral therapy is short-term therapy of 12 or fewer sessions.

What Else Can a Person Do to Relieve Anxiety?

- Acknowledge worries and address any fears that can be handled (for example, if an individual is worried about finances, a visit to a financial planner may be helpful)

- Talk with family, a friend or spiritual leader

- Adopt stress management techniques, meditation, prayer, and deep breathing from the lower abdomen

- Exercise

- Avoid things that can aggravate the symptoms of anxiety disorders:
  - Caffeine (coffee, tea, soda, chocolate)
  - Nicotine (smoking)
  - Over-eating
  - Over-the-counter cold medications
  - Certain illegal drugs
  - Certain herbal supplements
  - Alcohol (While alcohol might initially help a person relax, it eventually interferes with sleep and overall wellness, and can even contribute to anxiety, depression, and dementia.)
- Limit news of current events. It is important to stay current, but too much negative news can contribute to anxiety.
- Allow time for treatment to work

Concerned about an Older Family Member or Friend?

If you suspect an older adult you know might have a problem with anxiety, notice and ask about any changes in:

- Daily routines and activities. Is the person avoiding situations and activities he or she once enjoyed?
- Worries. Does he or she seem to worry excessively?
- Medication. Is he or she taking a new medication, either prescription or over-the-counter? Or has the dosage changed for one of the medications?
- Is he or she drinking more alcoholic drinks than previously?
- Mood. Is the older adult tearful, lacking emotion, or "just doesn't feel right."

When talking with an older adult who has an anxiety problem:
- Be calm and reassuring
- Acknowledge their fears but do not play along with them
- Be supportive without supporting their anxiety
- Encourage them to engage in social activities
- Offer assistance in getting them help from a physician or mental health professional

Section 35.3

Understanding Memory Loss

Excerpted from "Understanding Memory Loss,"
National Institute on Aging (www.nia.nih.gov), September 2010.

Introduction

We've all forgotten a name, where we put our keys, or if we locked the front door. It's normal to forget things once in a while. However, forgetting how to make change, use the telephone, or find your way home may be signs of a more serious memory problem.

Mary's Story

Mary couldn't find her car keys. She looked on the hook just inside the front door. They weren't there. She searched in her purse. No luck. Finally, she found them on her desk. Yesterday, she forgot her neighbor's name. Her memory was playing tricks on her. She was starting to worry about it. She decided to see her doctor. After a complete check-up, her doctor said that Mary was fine. Her forgetfulness was just a normal part of getting older. The doctor suggested that Mary take a class, play cards with friends, or help out at the local school to sharpen her memory.

Mild Forgetfulness vs. More Serious Memory Problems
Mild Forgetfulness

It is true that some of us get more forgetful as we age. It may take longer to learn new things, remember certain words, or find our glasses. These changes are often signs of mild forgetfulness, not serious memory problems.

See your doctor if you're worried about your forgetfulness. Tell him or her about your concerns. Be sure to make a follow-up appointment to check your memory in the next six months to a year. If you think you might forget, ask a family member, friend, or the doctor's office to remind you.

What can I do about mild forgetfulness?

You can do many things to help keep your memory sharp and stay alert. You can learn a new skill, volunteer in your community, at a school, or at your place of worship, or spend time with friends and family. You can use memory tools such as big calendars, to-do lists, and notes to yourself or put your wallet or purse, keys, and glasses in the same place each day. Other things that can help are getting lots of rest, exercising and eating well, avoiding drinking a lot of alcohol, and getting help if you feel depressed for weeks at a time.

Serious Memory Problems

Serious memory problems make it hard to do everyday things. For example, you may find it hard to drive, shop, or even talk with a friend. These are some signs of serious memory problems:

- Asking the same questions over and over again

- Getting lost in places you know well

- Not being able to follow directions

- Becoming more confused about time, people, and places

- Not taking care of yourself—eating poorly, not bathing, or being unsafe

What can I do about serious memory problems?

See your doctor if you are having any of the problems listed above. It's important to find out what might be causing a serious memory problem. Once you know the cause, you can get the right treatment.

Serious Memory Problems—Causes and Treatments

Many things can cause serious memory problems, such as blood clots, depression, and Alzheimer disease.

Medical Conditions

Certain medical conditions can cause serious memory problems. These problems should go away once you get treatment. Medical conditions that may cause memory problems include bad reactions to certain medicines; depression; not eating enough healthy foods, or too few vitamins and minerals in your body; drinking too much alcohol; blood clots or tumors in the brain; head injury, such as a concussion

491

from a fall or accident; and thyroid, kidney, or liver problems. These medical conditions are serious. See your doctor for treatment.

Emotional Problems

Some emotional problems in older people can cause serious memory problems. Feeling sad, lonely, worried, or bored can cause you to be confused and forgetful. Treatment for emotional problems may involve the following steps:

- You may need to see a doctor or counselor for treatment. Once you get help, your memory problems should get better.

- Being active, spending more time with family and friends, and learning new skills also can help you feel better and improve your memory.

Mild Cognitive Impairment

As some people grow older, they have more memory problems than other people their age. This condition is called mild cognitive impairment, or MCI. People with MCI can take care of themselves and do their normal activities. MCI memory problems may include losing things often, forgetting to go to events and appointments, and having more trouble coming up with words than other people of the same age.

Your doctor can do thinking, memory, and language tests to see if you have MCI. He or she also may suggest that you see a specialist for more tests. Because MCI may be an early sign of Alzheimer disease, it's really important to see your doctor or specialist every 6 to 12 months.

At this time, there is no proven treatment for MCI. Your doctor can check to see if you have any changes in your memory or thinking skills over time. You may want to try to keep your memory sharp. See the list under "What Can I Do about Mild Forgetfulness?" above for some ways to help your memory.

Alzheimer Disease

Alzheimer disease causes serious memory problems. The signs of Alzheimer disease begin slowly and get worse over time. This is because changes in the brain cause large numbers of brain cells to die.

It may look like simple forgetfulness at first, but over time, people with Alzheimer disease have trouble thinking clearly. They find it hard to do everyday things like shopping, driving, and cooking. As the illness gets worse, people with Alzheimer disease may need someone to take care of all their needs at home or in a nursing home. These needs may include feeding, bathing, and dressing.

Taking certain medicines can help a person in the early or middle stages of Alzheimer disease. These medicines can keep symptoms, such as memory loss, from getting worse for a time. The medicines can have side effects and may not work for everyone. Talk with your doctor about side effects or other concerns you may have.

Other medicines can help if you are worried, depressed, or having problems sleeping.

Vascular Dementia

Many people have never heard of vascular dementia. Like Alzheimer disease, it is a medical condition that causes serious memory problems. Unlike Alzheimer disease, signs of vascular dementia may appear suddenly. This is because the memory loss and confusion are caused by small strokes or changes in the blood supply to the brain. If the strokes stop, you may get better or stay the same for a long time. If you have more strokes, you may get worse.

To lower your chances of having more strokes you can take steps such as controling your high blood pressure, treating your high cholesterol, taking care of your diabetes, and stopping smoking.

Help for Serious Memory Problems

What can I do if I'm worried about my memory?

See your doctor. If your doctor thinks your memory problems are serious, you may need to have a complete health check-up. The doctor will review your medicines and may test your blood and urine. You also may need to take tests that check your memory, problem solving, counting, and language skills.

In addition, the doctor may suggest a brain scan. Pictures from the scan can show normal and problem areas in the brain. Once the doctor finds out what is causing your memory problems, ask about the best treatment for you.

What can family members do to help?

If your family member or friend has a serious memory problem, you can help the person live as normal a life as possible. You can help the person stay active, go places, and keep up everyday routines. You can remind the person of the time of day, where he or she lives, and what is happening at home and in the world. You also can help the person remember to take medicine or visit the doctor.

Some families use the following things to help with memory problems:

- Big calendars to highlight important dates and events

- Lists of the plans for each day

- Notes about safety in the home

- Written directions for using common household items (most people with Alzheimer disease can still read)

Section 35.4

Alzheimer Disease

Excerpted from "Alzheimer's Disease Fact Sheet,"
National institute on Aging (www.nia.nih.gov), September 20, 2011.

Alzheimer disease is an irreversible, progressive brain disease that slowly destroys memory and thinking skills, and eventually even the ability to carry out the simplest tasks. In most people with Alzheimer disease, symptoms first appear after age 60. Estimates vary, but experts suggest that as many as 5.1 million Americans may have Alzheimer disease.

Alzheimer disease is the most common cause of dementia among older people. Dementia is the loss of cognitive functioning—thinking, remembering, and reasoning—and behavioral abilities, to such an extent that it interferes with a person's daily life and activities. Dementia ranges in severity from the mildest stage, when it is just beginning to affect a person's functioning, to the most severe stage, when the person must depend completely on others for basic activities of daily living.

Alzheimer disease is named after Dr. Alois Alzheimer. In 1906, Dr. Alzheimer noticed changes in the brain tissue of a woman who had died of an unusual mental illness. Her symptoms included memory loss, language problems, and unpredictable behavior. After she died, he examined her brain and found many abnormal clumps (now called amyloid plaques) and tangled bundles of fibers (now called neurofibrillary tangles). Plaques and tangles in the brain are two of the main features of Alzheimer disease. The third is the loss of connections between nerve cells (neurons) in the brain.

Changes in the Brain in Alzheimer Disease

Although we still don't know how the Alzheimer disease process begins, it seems likely that damage to the brain starts a decade or more before problems become evident. During the preclinical stage of Alzheimer disease, people are free of symptoms but toxic changes are taking place in the brain. Abnormal deposits of proteins form amyloid plaques and tau tangles throughout the brain, and once-healthy neurons begin to work less efficiently. Over time, neurons lose their ability to function and communicate with each other, and eventually they die.

Before long, the damage spreads to a nearby structure in the brain called the hippocampus, which is essential in forming memories. As more neurons die, affected brain regions begin to shrink. By the final stage of Alzheimer disease, damage is widespread, and brain tissue has shrunk significantly.

Very Early Signs and Symptoms

Memory problems are typically one of the first warning signs of cognitive loss, possibly due to the development of Alzheimer disease. Some people with memory problems have a condition called amnestic mild cognitive impairment (MCI). People with this condition have more memory problems than normal for people their age, but their symptoms are not as severe as those seen in people with Alzheimer disease. Other recent studies have found links between some movement difficulties and MCI. Researchers also have seen links between MCI and some problems with the sense of smell. The ability of people with MCI to perform normal daily activities is not significantly impaired. However, more older people with MCI, compared with those without MCI, go on to develop Alzheimer disease.

A decline in other aspects of cognition, such as word-finding, vision/spatial issues, and impaired reasoning or judgment, may also signal the very early stages of Alzheimer disease. Scientists are looking to see whether brain imaging and biomarker studies, for example, of people with MCI and those with a family history of Alzheimer disease, can detect early changes in the brain like those seen in Alzheimer disease. Initial studies indicate that early detection using biomarkers and imaging may be possible, but findings will need to be confirmed by other

495

studies before these techniques can be used to help with diagnosis in everyday medical practice.

These and other studies offer hope that someday we may have tools that could help detect Alzheimer early, track the course of the disease, and monitor response to treatments.

Mild Alzheimer Disease

As Alzheimer disease progresses, memory loss worsens, and changes in other cognitive abilities are evident. Problems can include, for example, getting lost, trouble handling money and paying bills, repeating questions, taking longer to complete normal daily tasks, using poor judgment, and having some mood and personality changes. People often are diagnosed in this stage.

Moderate Alzheimer Disease

In this stage, damage occurs in areas of the brain that control language, reasoning, sensory processing, and conscious thought. Memory loss and confusion grow worse, and people begin to have problems recognizing family and friends. They may be unable to learn new things, carry out tasks that involve multiple steps (such as getting dressed), or cope with new situations. They may have hallucinations, delusions, and paranoia, and may behave impulsively.

Severe Alzheimer Disease

By the final stage, plaques and tangles have spread throughout the brain, and brain tissue has shrunk significantly. People with severe Alzheimer cannot communicate and are completely dependent on others for their care. Near the end, the person may be in bed most or all of the time as the body shuts down.

Causes of Alzheimer Disease

Scientists don't yet fully understand what causes Alzheimer disease, but it has become increasingly clear that it develops because of a complex series of events that take place in the brain over a long period of time. It is likely that the causes include some mix of genetic, environmental, and lifestyle factors. Because people differ in their genetic make-up and lifestyle, the importance of any one of these factors in increasing or decreasing the risk of developing Alzheimer disease may differ from person to person.

The Basics of Alzheimer Disease

Scientists are conducting studies to learn more about plaques, tangles, and other features of Alzheimer disease. They can now visualize beta-amyloid associated with plaques by imaging the brains of living individuals. Scientists are also exploring the very earliest steps in the disease process. Findings from these studies will help them understand the causes of Alzheimer disease.

One of the great mysteries of Alzheimer disease is why it largely strikes older adults. Research on how the brain changes normally with age is shedding light on this question. For example, scientists are learning how age-related changes in the brain may harm neurons and contribute to Alzheimer disease damage. These age-related changes include atrophy (shrinking) of certain parts of the brain, inflammation, the production of unstable molecules called free radicals, and mitochondrial dysfunction (a breakdown of energy production within a cell).

Genetics

Early-onset Alzheimer disease is a rare form of the disease. It occurs in people aged 30 to 60 and represents less than five percent of all people who have Alzheimer disease. Most cases of early-onset Alzheimer disease are familial Alzheimer disease, caused by changes in one of three known genes inherited from a parent.

Most people with Alzheimer disease have late-onset Alzheimer disease, which usually develops after age 60. Many studies have linked the apolipoprotein E (APOE) gene to late-onset Alzheimer disease. This gene has several forms. One of them, APOE ε4, seems to increase a person's risk of getting the disease. However, carrying the APOE ε4 form of the gene does not necessarily mean that a person will develop Alzheimer disease, and people carrying no APOE ε4 can also develop the disease.

Most experts believe that additional genes may influence the development of late-onset Alzheimer disease. Scientists around the world are searching for these genes, and have identified a number of common genes in addition to APOE ε4 that may increase a person's risk for late-onset Alzheimer disease.

For more about this area of research, see the "Alzheimer's Disease Genetics Fact Sheet," available at www.nia.nih.gov/alzheimers.

Environmental/Lifestyle Factors

Research also suggests that a host of factors beyond basic genetics may play a role in the development and course of Alzheimer disease.

There is a great deal of interest, for example, in associations between cognitive decline and vascular and metabolic conditions such as heart disease, stroke, high blood pressure, diabetes, and obesity. Understanding these relationships and testing them in clinical trials will help us understand whether reducing risk factors for these conditions may help with Alzheimer disease as well.

Further, a nutritious diet, physical activity, social engagement, and mentally stimulating pursuits can all help people stay healthy as they age. New research suggests the possibility that these and other factors also might help to reduce the risk of cognitive decline and Alzheimer disease. Clinical trials of specific interventions are underway to test some of these possibilities.

Diagnosing Alzheimer Disease

Alzheimer disease can be definitively diagnosed only after death, by linking clinical measures with an examination of brain tissue and pathology in an autopsy. But doctors now have several methods and tools to help them determine fairly accurately whether a person who is having memory problems Alzheimer disease. Doctors may take these steps:

- Ask questions about overall health, past medical problems, ability to carry out daily activities, and changes in behavior and personality

- Conduct tests of memory, problem solving, attention, counting, and language

- Carry out standard medical tests, such as blood and urine tests, to identify other possible causes of the problem

- Perform brain scans, such as computed tomography (CT) or magnetic resonance imaging (MRI), to distinguish Alzheimer disease from other possible causes for symptoms, like stroke or tumor

These tests may be repeated to give doctors information about how the person's memory is changing over time.

Early, accurate diagnosis is beneficial for several reasons. It can tell people whether their symptoms are from Alzheimer disease or another cause, such as stroke, tumor, Parkinson disease, sleep disturbances, side effects of medications, or other conditions that may be treatable and possibly reversible.

Beginning treatment early on in the disease process can help preserve function for some time, even though the underlying disease process cannot be changed. Having an early diagnosis also helps families plan for the future, make living arrangements, take care of financial and legal matters, and develop support networks.

In addition, an early diagnosis can provide greater opportunities for people to get involved in clinical trials. In a typical clinical trial, scientists test a drug or treatment to see if that intervention is effective and for whom it would work best.

Treating Alzheimer Disease

Alzheimer disease is complex, and it is unlikely that any one intervention will be found to delay, prevent, or cure it. That's why current approaches in treatment and research focus on several different aspects, including helping people maintain mental function, managing behavioral symptoms, and slowing or delaying the symptoms of disease.

Maintaining Mental Function

Four medications are approved by the U.S. Food and Drug Administration to treat Alzheimer disease. Donepezil (Aricept), rivastigmine (Exelon), and galantamine (Razadyne) are used to treat mild to moderate Alzheimer disease (donepezil can be used for severe Alzheimer disease as well). Memantine (Namenda) is used to treat moderate to severe Alzheimer disease. These drugs work by regulating neurotransmitters (the chemicals that transmit messages between neurons). They may help maintain thinking, memory, and speaking skills, and help with certain behavioral problems. However, these drugs don't change the underlying disease process, are effective for some but not all people, and may help only for a limited time.

Managing Behavioral Symptoms

Common behavioral symptoms of Alzheimer disease include sleeplessness, agitation, wandering, anxiety, anger, and depression. Scientists are learning why these symptoms occur and are studying new treatments—drug and non-drug—to manage them. Treating behavioral symptoms often makes people with Alzheimer disease more comfortable and makes their care easier for caregivers.

Slowing, Delaying, or Preventing Alzheimer Disease

Alzheimer disease research has developed to a point where scientists can look beyond treating symptoms to think about addressing underlying disease processes. In ongoing clinical trials, scientists are looking at many possible interventions, such as immunization therapy, cognitive training, physical activity, antioxidants, and the effects of cardiovascular and diabetes treatments.

Supporting Families and Caregivers

Caring for a person with Alzheimer disease can have high physical, emotional, and financial costs. The demands of day-to-day care, changing family roles, and difficult decisions about placement in a care facility can be hard to handle. Researchers have learned much about Alzheimer disease caregiving, and studies are helping to develop new ways to support caregivers.

Becoming well-informed about the disease is one important long-term strategy. Programs that teach families about the various stages of Alzheimer disease and about flexible and practical strategies for dealing with difficult caregiving situations provide vital help to those who care for people with Alzheimer disease.

Developing good coping skills and a strong support network of family and friends also are important ways that caregivers can help themselves handle the stresses of caring for a loved one with Alzheimer disease. For example, staying physically active provides physical and emotional benefits.

Some Alzheimer disease caregivers have found that participating in a support group is a critical lifeline. These support groups allow caregivers to find respite, express concerns, share experiences, get tips, and receive emotional comfort.

Chapter 36

Lesbian, Gay, Bisexual, and Transsexual (LGBT) Mental Health Issues

Chapter Contents

Section 36.1

Sexual Orientation and the Psychological Impact of Prejudice and Discrimination

Since 1975, the American Psychological Association has called on psychologists to take the lead in removing the stigma of mental illness that has long been associated with lesbian, gay, and bisexual orientations. The discipline of psychology is concerned with the well-being of people and groups and therefore with threats to that well-being. The prejudice and discrimination that people who identify as lesbian, gay, or bisexual regularly experience have been shown to have negative psychological effects. This text is designed to provide accurate information for those who want to better understand sexual orientation and the impact of prejudice and discrimination on those who identify as lesbian, gay, or bisexual.

What is sexual orientation?

Sexual orientation refers to an enduring pattern of emotional, romantic, and/or sexual attractions to men, women, or both sexes. Sexual orientation also refers to a person's sense of identity based on those attractions, related behaviors, and membership in a community of others who share those attractions. Research over several decades has demonstrated that sexual orientation ranges along a continuum, from exclusive attraction to the other sex to exclusive attraction to the same sex. However, sexual orientation is usually discussed in terms of three categories: heterosexual (having emotional, romantic, or sexual attractions to members of the other sex), gay/lesbian (having emotional, romantic, or sexual attractions to members of one's own sex), and bisexual (having emotional, romantic, or sexual attractions to both men and women). This range of behaviors and attractions has been described in various cultures and nations throughout the world.

Many cultures use identity labels to describe people who express these attractions. In the United States the most frequent labels are lesbians (women attracted to women), gay men (men attracted to men), and bisexual people (men or women attracted to both sexes). However, some people may use different labels or none at all.

Sexual orientation is distinct from other components of sex and gender, including biological sex (the anatomical, physiological, and genetic characteristics associated with being male or female), gender identity (the psychological sense of being male or female), and social gender role (the cultural norms that define feminine and masculine behavior). [Note: This text focuses on sexual orientation. Another American Psychological Association publication, "Answers to Your Questions about Transgender Individuals and Gender Identity" addresses gender identity. Visit www.apa.org for more information.]

Sexual orientation is commonly discussed as if it were solely a characteristic of an individual, like biological sex, gender identity, or age. This perspective is incomplete because sexual orientation is defined in terms of relationships with others. People express their sexual orientation through behaviors with others, including such simple actions as holding hands or kissing. Thus, sexual orientation is closely tied to the intimate personal relationships that meet deeply felt needs for love, attachment, and intimacy. In addition to sexual behaviors, these bonds include nonsexual physical affection between partners, shared goals and values, mutual support, and ongoing commitment. Therefore, sexual orientation is not merely a personal characteristic within an individual. Rather, one's sexual orientation defines the group of people in which one is likely to find the satisfying and fulfilling romantic relationships that are an essential component of personal identity for many people.

How do people know if they are lesbian, gay, or bisexual?

According to current scientific and professional understanding, the core attractions that form the basis for adult sexual orientation typically emerge between middle childhood and early adolescence. These patterns of emotional, romantic, and sexual attraction may arise without any prior sexual experience. People can be celibate and still know their sexual orientation—be it lesbian, gay, bisexual, or heterosexual.

Different lesbian, gay, and bisexual people have very different experiences regarding their sexual orientation. Some people know that they are lesbian, gay, or bisexual for a long time before they actually pursue relationships with other people. Some people engage in sexual activity (with same-sex and/or other-sex partners) before assigning a clear label to their sexual orientation. Prejudice and discrimination make it difficult for many people to come to terms with their sexual orientation identities, so claiming a lesbian, gay, or bisexual identity may be a slow process.

What causes a person to have a particular sexual orientation?

There is no consensus among scientists about the exact reasons that an individual develops a heterosexual, bisexual, gay, or lesbian orientation. Although much research has examined the possible genetic, hormonal, developmental, social, and cultural influences on sexual orientation, no findings have emerged that permit scientists to conclude that sexual orientation is determined by any particular factor or factors. Many think that nature and nurture both play complex roles; most people experience little or no sense of choice about their sexual orientation.

What role do prejudice and discrimination play in the lives of lesbian, gay, and bisexual people?

Lesbian, gay, and bisexual people in the United States encounter extensive prejudice, discrimination, and violence because of their sexual orientation. Intense prejudice against lesbians, gay men, and bisexual people was widespread throughout much of the 20th century. Public opinion studies over the 1970s, 1980s, and 1990s routinely showed that, among large segments of the public, lesbian, gay, and bisexual people were the target of strongly held negative attitudes. More recently, public opinion has increasingly opposed sexual orientation discrimination, but expressions of hostility toward lesbians and gay men remain common in contemporary American society. Prejudice against bisexuals appears to exist at comparable levels. In fact, bisexual individuals may face discrimination from some lesbian and gay people as well as from heterosexual people.

Sexual orientation discrimination takes many forms. Severe anti-gay prejudice is reflected in the high rate of harassment and violence directed toward lesbian, gay, and bisexual individuals in American society. Numerous surveys indicate that verbal harassment and abuse are nearly universal experiences among lesbian, gay, and bisexual people. Also, discrimination against lesbian, gay, and bisexual people in employment and housing appears to remain widespread. The HIV/AIDS pandemic is another area in which prejudice and discrimination against lesbian, gay, and bisexual people have had negative effects.

Early in the pandemic, the assumption that HIV/AIDS was a "gay disease" contributed to the delay in addressing the massive social upheaval that AIDS would generate. Gay and bisexual men have been disproportionately affected by this disease. The association of HIV/AIDS with gay and bisexual men and the inaccurate belief that some people held that all gay and bisexual men were infected served to further stigmatize lesbian, gay, and bisexual people.

What is the psychological impact of prejudice and discrimination?

Prejudice and discrimination have social and personal impact. On the social level, prejudice and discrimination against lesbian, gay, and bisexual people are reflected in the everyday stereotypes of members of these groups. These stereotypes persist even though they are not supported by evidence, and they are often used to excuse unequal treatment of lesbian, gay, and bisexual people. For example, limitations on job opportunities, parenting, and relationship recognition are often justified by stereotypic assumptions about lesbian, gay, and bisexual people.

On an individual level, such prejudice and discrimination may also have negative consequences, especially if lesbian, gay, and bisexual people attempt to conceal or deny their sexual orientation. Although many lesbians and gay men learn to cope with the social stigma against homosexuality, this pattern of prejudice can have serious negative effects on health and well-being. Individuals and groups may have the impact of stigma reduced or worsened by other characteristics, such as race, ethnicity, religion, or disability. Some lesbian, gay, and bisexual people may face less of a stigma. For others, race, sex, religion, disability, or other characteristics may exacerbate the negative impact of prejudice and discrimination.

The widespread prejudice, discrimination, and violence to which lesbians and gay men are often subjected are significant mental health concerns. Sexual prejudice, sexual orientation discrimination, and antigay violence are major sources of stress for lesbian, gay, and bisexual people. Although social support is crucial in coping with stress, antigay attitudes and discrimination may make it difficult for lesbian, gay, and bisexual people to find such support.

Is homosexuality a mental disorder?

No, lesbian, gay, and bisexual orientations are not disorders. Research has found no inherent association between any of these sexual orientations and psychopathology. Both heterosexual behavior and homosexual behavior are normal aspects of human sexuality. Both have been documented in many different cultures and historical eras. Despite the persistence of stereotypes that portray lesbian, gay, and bisexual people as disturbed, several decades of research and clinical experience have led all mainstream medical and mental health organizations in this country to conclude that these orientations represent normal forms of human experience. Lesbian, gay, and bisexual relationships are normal forms of human bonding. Therefore, these mainstream organizations long ago abandoned classifications of homosexuality as a mental disorder.

What about therapy intended to change sexual orientation from gay to straight?

All major national mental health organizations have officially expressed concerns about therapies promoted to modify sexual orientation. To date, there has been no scientifically adequate research to show that therapy aimed at changing sexual orientation (sometimes called reparative or conversion therapy) is safe or effective. Furthermore, it seems likely that the promotion of change therapies reinforces stereotypes and contributes to a negative climate for lesbian, gay, and bisexual persons. This appears to be especially likely for lesbian, gay, and bisexual individuals who grow up in more conservative religious settings.

Helpful responses of a therapist treating an individual who is troubled about her or his same-sex attractions include helping that person actively cope with social prejudices against homosexuality, successfully resolve issues associated with and resulting from internal conflicts, and actively lead a happy and satisfying life. Mental health professional organizations call on their members to respect a person's (client's) right to self-determination; be sensitive to the client's race, culture, ethnicity, age, gender, gender identity, sexual orientation, religion, socioeconomic status, language, and disability status when working with that client; and eliminate biases based on these factors.

What is "coming out" and why is it important?

The phrase "coming out" is used to refer to several aspects of lesbian, gay, and bisexual persons' experiences: self-awareness of same-sex attractions; the telling of one or a few people about these attractions; widespread disclosure of same-sex attractions; and identification with the lesbian, gay, and bisexual community. Many people hesitate to come out because of the risks of meeting prejudice and discrimination. Some choose to keep their identity a secret; some choose to come out in limited circumstances; some decide to come out in very public ways.

Coming out is often an important psychological step for lesbian, gay, and bisexual people. Research has shown that feeling positively about one's sexual orientation and integrating it into one's life fosters greater well-being and mental health. This integration often involves disclosing one's identity to others; it may also entail participating in the gay community. Being able to discuss one's sexual orientation with others also increases the availability of social support, which is crucial to mental health and psychological well-being. Like heterosexuals, lesbians, gay men, and bisexual people benefit from being able to share their lives with and receive support from family, friends, and acquaintances. Thus, it is not surprising that lesbians and gay men who feel they must conceal their sexual orientation report more frequent mental health concerns than do lesbians and gay men who are more open; they may even have more physical health problems.

What about sexual orientation and coming out during adolescence?

Adolescence is a period when people separate from their parents and families and begin to develop autonomy. Adolescence can be a period of experimentation, and many youths may question their sexual feelings. Becoming aware of sexual feelings is a normal developmental task of adolescence. Sometimes adolescents have same-sex feelings or experiences that cause confusion about their sexual orientation. This confusion appears to decline over time, with different outcomes for different individuals.

Some adolescents desire and engage in same-sex behavior but do not identify as lesbian, gay, or bisexual, sometimes because of the stigma associated with a nonheterosexual orientation. Some adolescents experience continuing feelings of same-sex attraction but do not engage in any sexual activity or may engage in heterosexual behavior for varying lengths of time. Because of the stigma associated with same-sex attractions, many youths experience same-sex attraction for many years before becoming sexually active with partners of the same sex or disclosing their attractions to others.

For some young people, this process of exploring same-sex attractions leads to a lesbian, gay, or bisexual identity. For some, acknowledging this identity can bring an end to confusion. When these young people receive the support of parents and others, they are often able to live satisfying

507

and healthy lives and move through the usual process of adolescent development. The younger a person is when she or he acknowledges a nonheterosexual identity, the fewer internal and external resources she or he is likely to have. Therefore, youths who come out early are particularly in need of support from parents and others.

Young people who identify as lesbian, gay, or bisexual may be more likely to face certain problems, including being bullied and having negative experiences in school. These experiences are associated with negative outcomes, such as suicidal thoughts, and high-risk activities, such as unprotected sex and alcohol and drug use. On the other hand, many lesbian, gay, and bisexual youths appear to experience no greater level of health or mental health risks. Where problems occur, they are closely associated with experiences of bias and discrimination in their environments. Support from important people in the teen's life can provide a very helpful counterpart to bias and discrimination.

Support in the family, at school, and in the broader society helps to reduce risk and encourage healthy development. Youth need caring and support, appropriately high expectations, and the encouragement to participate actively with peers. Lesbian, gay, and bisexual youth who do well despite stress—like all adolescents who do well despite stress—tend to be those who are socially competent, who have good problem-solving skills, who have a sense of autonomy and purpose, and who look forward to the future.

In a related vein, some young people are presumed to be lesbian, gay, or bisexual because they don't abide by traditional gender roles (i.e., the cultural beliefs about what is appropriate "masculine" and "feminine" appearance and behavior). Whether these youths identify as heterosexual or as lesbian, gay, or bisexual, they encounter prejudice and discrimination based on the presumption that they are lesbian, gay, or bisexual. The best support for these young people is school and social climates that do not tolerate discriminatory language and behavior.

At what age should lesbian, gay, or bisexual youths come out?

There is no simple or absolute answer to this question. The risks and benefits of coming out are different for youths in different circumstances. Some young people live in families where support for their sexual orientation is clear and stable; these youths may encounter less risk in coming out, even at a young age. Young people who live in less supportive families may face more risks in coming out. All young people who come out may experience bias, discrimination, or even violence in their schools, social groups, work places, and faith communities. Supportive families, friends, and schools are important buffers against the negative impacts of these experiences.

What is the nature of same-sex relationships?

Research indicates that many lesbians and gay men want and have committed relationships. For example, survey data indicate that between 40% and 60% of gay men and between 45% and 80% of lesbians are currently involved in a romantic relationship. Further, data from the 2000 U.S. Census indicate that of the 5.5 million couples who were living together but not married, about one in nine (594,391) had partners of the same sex. Although the census data are almost certainly an underestimate of the actual number of cohabiting same-sex couples, they indicate that there are 301,026 male same-sex households and 293,365 female same-sex households in the United States.

Stereotypes about lesbian, gay, and bisexual people have persisted, even though studies have found them to be misleading. For instance, one stereotype is that the relationships of lesbians and gay men are dysfunctional and unhappy. However, studies have found same-sex and heterosexual couples to be equivalent to each other on measures of relationship satisfaction and commitment.

A second stereotype is that the relationships of lesbians, gay men, and bisexual people are unstable. However, despite social hostility toward same-sex relationships, research shows that many lesbians and gay men form durable relationships. For example, survey data indicate that between 18% and 28% of gay couples and between 8% and 21% of lesbian couples have lived together 10 or more years. It is also reasonable to suggest that the stability of same-sex couples might be enhanced if partners from same-sex couples enjoyed the same levels of support and recognition for their relationships as heterosexual couples do, i.e., legal rights and responsibilities associated with marriage.

A third common misconception is that the goals and values of lesbian and gay couples are different from those of heterosexual couples. In fact, research has found that the factors that influence relationship satisfaction, commitment, and stability are remarkably similar for both same-sex cohabiting couples and heterosexual married couples.

Far less research is available on the relationship experiences of people who identify as bisexual. If these individuals are in a same-sex relationship, they are likely to face the same prejudice and discrimination that members of lesbian and gay couples face. If they are in a heterosexual relationship, their experiences may be quite similar to those of people who identify as heterosexual unless they choose to come out as bisexual; in that case, they will likely face some of the same prejudice and discrimination that lesbian and gay individuals encounter.

Can lesbians and gay men be good parents?

Many lesbians and gay men are parents; others wish to be parents. In the 2000 U.S. Census, 33% of female same-sex couple households and 22% of male same-sex couple households reported at least one child under the age of 18 living in the home. Although comparable data are not available, many single lesbians and gay men are also parents, and many same-sex couples are part-time parents to children whose primary residence is elsewhere.

As the social visibility and legal status of lesbian and gay parents have increased, some people have raised concerns about the well-being of children in these families. Most of these questions are based on negative stereotypes about lesbians and gay men. The majority of research on this topic asks whether children raised by lesbian and gay parents are at a disadvantage when compared to children raised by heterosexual parents. The most common questions and answers to them are these:

Do children of lesbian and gay parents have more problems with sexual identity than do children of heterosexual parents?

For instance, do these children develop problems in gender identity and/or in gender role behavior? The answer from research is clear: sexual and gender identities (including gender identity, gender-role behavior, and sexual orientation) develop in much the same way among children of lesbian mothers as they do among children of heterosexual parents. Few studies are available regarding children of gay fathers.

Do children raised by lesbian or gay parents have problems in personal development in areas other than sexual identity?

For example, are the children of lesbian or gay parents more vulnerable to mental breakdown, do they have more behavior problems, or are they less psychologically healthy than other children? Again, studies of personality, self-concept, and behavior problems show few differences between children of lesbian mothers and children of heterosexual parents. Few studies are available regarding children of gay fathers.

Are children of lesbian and gay parents likely to have problems with social relationships?

For example, will they be teased or otherwise mistreated by their peers? Once more, evidence indicates that children of lesbian and gay parents have normal social relationships with their peers and adults. The picture that emerges from this research shows that children of gay and lesbian parents enjoy a social life that is typical of their age group in terms of involvement with peers, parents, family members, and friends.

Are these children more likely to be sexually abused by a parent or by a parent's friends or acquaintances?

There is no scientific support for fears about children of lesbian or gay parents being sexually abused by their parents or their parents' gay, lesbian, or bisexual friends or acquaintances.

In summary, social science has shown that the concerns often raised about children of lesbian and gay parents—concerns that are generally grounded in prejudice against and stereotypes about gay people—are unfounded. Overall, the research indicates that the children of lesbian and gay parents do not differ markedly from the children of heterosexual parents in their development, adjustment, or overall well-being.

What can people do to diminish prejudice and discrimination against lesbian, gay, and bisexual people?

Lesbian, gay, and bisexual people who want to help reduce prejudice and discrimination can be open about their sexual orientation, even as they take necessary precautions to be as safe as possible. They can examine their own belief systems for the presence of antigay stereotypes. They can make use of the lesbian, gay, and bisexual community—as well as supportive heterosexual people—for support.

Heterosexual people who wish to help reduce prejudice and discrimination can examine their own response to antigay stereotypes and prejudice. They can make a point of coming to know lesbian, gay, and bisexual people, and they can work with lesbian, gay, and bisexual individuals and communities to combat prejudice and discrimination. Heterosexual individuals are often in a good position to ask other heterosexual people to consider the prejudicial or discriminatory nature of their beliefs and actions. Heterosexual allies can encourage nondiscrimination policies that include sexual orientation. They can work to make coming out safe. When lesbians, gay men, and bisexual people feel free to make public their sexual orientation, heterosexuals are given an opportunity to have personal contact with openly gay people and to perceive them as individuals.

Studies of prejudice, including prejudice against gay people, consistently show that prejudice declines when members of the majority group interact with members of a minority group. In keeping with this general pattern, one of the most powerful influences on heterosexuals' acceptance of gay people is having personal contact with an openly gay person. Antigay attitudes are far less common among members of the population who have a close friend or family member who is lesbian or gay, especially if the gay person has directly come out to the heterosexual person.

Where can I find more information about homosexuality?

American Psychological Association
Lesbian, Gay, Bisexual, and Transgender Concerns Office
750 First Street, NE.
Washington, DC 20002
E-mail: lgbc@apa.org
Website: http://www.apa.org/pi/lgbc

Mental Health America
(formerly the National Mental Health Association)
2000 N. Beauregard Street, 6th Floor
Alexandria, VA 22311
Main Switchboard: (703) 684-7722
Toll-free: (800) 969-6MHA (6642)
TTY: (800) 433-5959
Fax: (703) 684-5968
Website: http://www.nmha.org/go/home

What Does Gay Mean? How to Talk with Kids about Sexual Orientation and Prejudice: An anti-bullying program designed to improve understanding and respect for youth who are gay/lesbian/bisexual/transgender (GLBT). Centered on an educational booklet called "What Does Gay Mean? How to Talk with Kids About Sexual Orientation and Prejudice," the program encourages parents and others to communicate and share values of respect with their children.

American Academy of Pediatrics (AAP)
Division of Child and Adolescent Health
141 Northwest Point Blvd.

Elk Grove Village, IL 60007
Office: (847) 228-5005
Fax: (847) 228-5097
Website: http://www.aap.org

Gay, Lesbian, and Bisexual Teens: Facts for Teens and Their Parents

Section 36.2

LGBT Depression

Major depression—or clinical depression—is a serious but common medical condition that affects LGBTs (lesbian, gay, bisexual, and transgender people) at a higher rate than the general population. A number of factors may contribute to this, from living in an often homophobic society to facing family rejection to being closeted in some or all aspects of life. If LGBTs experience higher rates of some mental disorders as several studies suggest (Mays & Cochran 2001), this may be fueled by discrimination.

Some of the symptoms of depression include:

• Persistent sad, anxious or "empty" feelings

• Feelings of guilt or hopelessness

• Markedly decreased interest in activities most of the day

• Decrease or increase in appetite and/or sleep

• Fatigue or loss of energy

(National Institute of Mental Health 2009)

Prevalence: Depression affects people of all ages and races. Most likely due to violence, discrimination, and isolation, members of the LGBT community experience higher rates of depression and suicidal thoughts than the general population. Possibly due to rejection from both gay and straight communities, bisexual women have been found to have significantly poorer mental health than either lesbians or heterosexual women. Studies show that the more confident women are in their sexual orientation, the less likely they are to experience depression.

Barriers to care: Heterosexist assumptions can adversely affect the quality of treatment, and fear of a negative experience keeps many LGBTs from seeking help. Organizations and individual therapists are not always LGBT friendly, and some therapists may not even recognize their own heterosexism. Staff can be judgmental toward LGBT sexuality, or be misinformed/uninformed about LGBT resources. LGBTs may experience discrimination against partners in favor of family of origin. Over 40% of lesbians recounted negative/mixed reactions from mental health professionals when they were open about sexuality (including instances of overt homophobia, discrimination, and perceived lack of empathy). (King & McKeown 2003).

Cultural and ethnic groups also have their own views of homosexuality and psychotherapy. African Americans have difficulty accepting LGBTs and are reluctant to seek psychiatric help. In Latino culture, Catholicism and family are central, while sex and women are hidden. Such cultural views make it more difficult for an individual to accept that they need to seek help.

LGBT Mental Health Resources

- GLBT National Hotline: 1-888-THE-GLNH (843-4564)

- Rainbow Youth Hotline: 1-877-LGBT-YTH (1-877-542-8984)

- LGBT Suicide Prevention Hotline: www.TheTrevorProject.org or 1-800-850-8078

- NAMI: www.nami.org or 1-800-950-NAMI (6264)

- Parents, Families and Friends of Lesbians and Gays: www.pflag.org

- Rainbow Heights Club: www.rainbowheights.org

- Association of Gay and Lesbian Psychiatrists: (215) 222-2800 www.aglp.org

- GayHealth.com: www.gayhealth.com

- National Foundation for Depressive Illness: www.depression.org

- Depression and Bipolar Support Alliance: (800) 826-3632 or www.dbsalliance.org

- American Foundation for Suicide Prevention: (888) 333-2377 or www.afsp.org

References

King, Michael & McKeown, Eamonn. (2003). LGB Report: Mental health and social wellbeing of gay men, lesbians and bisexuals in England and Wales. *Mind*, 5. http://www.pcsproud.org.uk/Summary findingsofLGBreport.pdf

Mays, V., & Cochran, S. (2001). Mental Health Correlates of Perceived Discrimination Among Lesbian, Gay, and Bisexual Adults in the United States. *American Journal of Public Health*, 91(11), 1869-1876. http://search.ebscohost.com/login.aspx?direct=true&db=a9h&AN=5461045 &site=ehost-live.

National Institute of Mental Health. (2009). Anxiety Disorders. U.S. Department of Health and Human Services. http://www.nimh.nih.gov/health/publications/anxiety-disorders/index.shtml

Chapter 37

Victims of Trauma and Disaster

Section 37.1

Common Reactions after Trauma

"Common Reactions after Trauma," U.S. Department of Veterans
Affairs (www.ptsd.va.gov), January 23, 2009.

After going through a trauma, survivors often say that their first
feeling is relief to be alive. This may be followed by stress, fear, and
anger. Trauma survivors may also find they are unable to stop thinking about what happened. Many survivors will show a high level of
arousal, which causes them to react strongly to sounds and sights
around them.

Most people have some kind of stress reaction after a trauma. Having such a reaction has nothing to do with personal weakness. Stress
reactions may last for several days or even a few weeks. For most
people, if symptoms occur, they will slowly decrease over time.

All kinds of trauma survivors commonly experience stress reactions.
This is true for veterans, children, and disaster rescue or relief workers. If you understand what is happening when you or someone you
know reacts to a traumatic event, you may be less fearful and better
able to handle things.

Reactions to a trauma may include the following:

- Feeling hopeless about the future

- Feeling detached or unconcerned about others

- Having trouble concentrating or making decisions

- Feeling jumpy and getting startled easily at sudden noises

- Feeling on guard and constantly alert

- Having disturbing dreams and memories or flashbacks

- Having work or school problems

You may also experience more physical reactions such as these:

- Stomach upset and trouble eating

- Trouble sleeping and feeling very tired

- Pounding heart, rapid breathing, feeling edgy
- Sweating
- Severe headache if thinking of the event
- Failure to engage in exercise, diet, safe sex, regular health care
- Excess smoking, alcohol, drugs, food
- Having your ongoing medical problems get worse

You may have more emotional troubles such as these:

- Feeling nervous, helpless, fearful, sad
- Feeling shocked, numb, and not able to feel love or joy
- Avoiding people, places, and things related to the event
- Being irritable or having outbursts of anger
- Becoming easily upset or agitated
- Blaming yourself or having negative views of oneself or the world
- Distrust of others, getting into conflicts, being over controlling
- Being withdrawn, feeling rejected or abandoned
- Loss of intimacy or feeling detached

Turn to your family and friends when you are ready to talk. They are your personal support system. Recovery is an ongoing gradual process. It doesn't happen through suddenly being "cured" and it doesn't mean that you will forget what happened. Most people will recover from trauma naturally. If your stress reactions are getting in the way of your relationships, work, or other important activities, you may want to talk to a counselor or your doctor. Good treatments are available.

Common Problems That Can Occur after a Trauma

Posttraumatic stress disorder (PTSD): PTSD is a condition that can develop after you have gone through a life-threatening event. If you have PTSD, you may have trouble keeping yourself from thinking over and over about what happened to you. You may try to avoid people and places that remind you of the trauma. You may feel numb. Lastly, if you have PTSD, you might find that you have trouble relaxing. You may startle easily and you may feel on guard most of the time.

Depression: Depression involves feeling down or sad more days than not. If you are depressed, you may lose interest in activities that used to be enjoyable or fun. You may feel low in energy and be overly tired. You may feel hopeless or in despair, and you may think that things will never get better. Depression is more likely when you have had losses such as the death of close friends. If you are depressed, at times you might think about hurting or killing yourself. For this reason, getting help for depression is very important.

Self-blame, guilt, and shame: Sometimes in trying to make sense of a traumatic event, you may blame yourself in some way. You may think you are responsible for bad things that happened, or for surviving when others didn't. You may feel guilty for what you did or did not do. Remember, we all tend to be our own worst critics. Most of the time, guilt, shame, or self-blame is not justified.

Suicidal thoughts: Trauma and personal loss can lead a depressed person to think about hurting or killing themselves. If you think someone you know may be feeling suicidal, you should directly ask them. You will NOT put the idea in their head. If someone is thinking about killing themselves, call the Suicide Prevention Lifeline 1-800-273-TALK (8255) (also available online at http://www.suicideprevention lifeline.org). You can also call a counselor, doctor, or 911.

Anger or aggressive behavior: Trauma can be connected with anger in many ways. After a trauma, you might think that what happened to you was unfair or unjust. You might not understand why the event happened and why it happened to you. These thoughts can result in intense anger. Although anger is a natural and healthy emotion, intense feelings of anger and aggressive behavior can cause problems with family, friends, or co-workers. If you become violent when angry, you just make the situation worse. Violence can lead to people being injured, and there may be legal consequences.

Alcohol/drug abuse: Drinking or "self-medicating" with drugs is a common, and unhealthy, way of coping with upsetting events. You may drink too much or use drugs to numb yourself and to try to deal with difficult thoughts, feelings, and memories related to the trauma. While using alcohol or drugs may offer a quick solution, it can actually lead to more problems. If someone close begins to lose control of drinking or drug use, you should try to get them to see a health care provider about managing their drinking or drug use.

Summing It All Up

Right after a trauma, almost every survivor will find him or herself unable to stop thinking about what happened. Stress reactions such as increased fear, nervousness, jumpiness, upsetting memories, and efforts to avoid reminders, will gradually decrease over time for most people.

Use your personal support systems, family, and friends, when you are ready to talk. Recovery is an ongoing gradual process. It doesn't happen through suddenly being "cured" and it doesn't mean that you will forget what happened. Most people will recover from trauma naturally over time. If your emotional reactions are getting in the way of your relationships, work, or other important activities, you may want to talk to a counselor or your doctor. Good treatments are available.

Section 37.2

Coping with Traumatic Events

"Coping with a Traumatic Event," Centers for Disease Control and Prevention (www.cdc.gov), February 20, 2009.

A Traumatic Event Turns Your World Upside Down

After surviving a disaster or act of violence, people may feel dazed or even numb. They may also feel sad, helpless, or anxious. In spite of the tragedy, some people just feel happy to be alive.

It is not unusual to have bad memories or dreams. You may avoid places or people that remind you of the disaster. You might have trouble sleeping, eating, or paying attention. Many people have short tempers and get angry easily.

These are all normal reactions to stress.

It Will Take Time Before You Start to Feel Better

You may have strong feelings right away. Or you may not notice a change until much later, after the crisis is over. Stress can change how you act with your friends and family. It will take time for you to feel better and for your life to return to normal. Give yourself time to heal.

These Steps May Help You Feel Better

A traumatic event disrupts your life. There is no simple fix to make things better right away. But there are actions that can help you, your family, and your community heal. Try these suggestions:

- Follow a normal routine as much as possible.

- Eat healthy meals. Be careful not to skip meals or to overeat.

- Exercise and stay active.

- Help other people in your community as a volunteer. Stay busy.

- Accept help from family, friends, co-workers, or clergy. Talk about your feelings with them.

- Limit your time around the sights and sounds of what happened. Don't dwell on TV, radio, or newspaper reports on the tragedy.

Sometimes the Stress Can Be Too Much to Handle Alone

- Ask for help if you are not able to take care of yourself or your children.

- Ask for help if you are not able to do your job.

- Ask for help if you use alcohol or drugs to get away from your problems.

- Ask for help if you feel sad or depressed for more than two weeks

- Ask for help if you think about suicide.

If you or someone you know is having trouble dealing with a tragedy, ask for help. Talk to a counselor, your doctor, or community organization, such as the National Suicide Prevention Lifeline (1-800-273-TALK).

Section 37.3

Disaster Survivors and Mental Health

"Disaster Mental Health Treatment," U.S. Department of
Veterans Affairs (www.ptsd.va.gov), July 2, 2010.

Disaster Mental Health Treatment

Disasters can cause a wide range of reactions in survivors. Research
has shown that right after a disaster, certain kinds of help can make
things easier for you. Most of those who are affected by disaster will
recover on their own given some time and help. Yet if a survivor is still
having trouble weeks after the disaster, he or she may need further
assistance.

After disaster, you are likely to do better if you feel—or are helped
to feel—safe, connected to others, and serene or calm. Those who are
hopeful and confident that they can cope with the results of a disaster
also tend to do better.

While group "debriefing" models have been used after disasters,
debriefing is not thought to be as useful as practical help, psychological first aid, and education.

Practical Help

A key to recovery from disasters is feeling that you have the resources with which to rebuild your life. The most basic resources include
food, safety, and shelter. Other important resources are family, community, school, and friends. In fact, having resources is so important
that many programs for disaster recovery focus on providing practical
help and building people's resources.

Psychological First Aid

Survivors in distress may benefit from psychological first aid. The
Psychological First Aid Field Operations Guide (PFA) (http://www
.ptsd.va.gov/professional/manuals/psych-first-aid.asp) teaches disaster
responders and others how to help those recovering from disaster. The

guide is based on the most important needs of survivors, such as safety, comfort, calming, and practical help. The guide also includes handouts to help survivors, with information on positive ways of coping, connecting with social supports, and links to needed services.

Education to Build Community Resilience

Resilience means being able to recover or bounce back after a disaster. One way to build resilience is education. Community members need to understand how disasters affect people. They need to know how to cope and use others for support, and how to get further help if needed.

Efforts to reach out and inform the community are sometimes provided by recovery workers, through the media, or on the internet. Education may focus on these topics:

- Reactions to disaster
- Building resilience and positive coping
- Providing support to each other
- Connecting to health and mental health care providers

Many types of healing practices also go into building community resilience. These practices involve communal, cultural, memorial, spiritual and religious healing practices. Training may be provided to local responders and healers, community leaders, and health providers. These workers are taught to make use of resources that are already in place or that occur naturally after disaster. Workers try to give survivors knowledge, attitudes, and skills that can be used to build the community. Part of the process also involves grieving the community's losses and making meaning of the disaster. Other goals include getting back to the normal rhythms and routines of life, and gaining a positive vision of the future, with renewed hope.

Crisis Counseling, Skill-Building, and Other Treatments

Programs and treatments exist for all levels of need after a disaster. One example is the Crisis Counseling Program (CCP). The Federal Emergency Management Agency (FEMA) supports CCPs for survivors of federally declared disasters. CCPs focus on both those affected by the disaster and the community as a whole. They provide survivors with practical help in coping with their current issues. They serve a full range of children, teens, parents or caretakers, families, and adults. CCPs also help businesses and neighborhoods. They focus not just on those at highest risk for problems, but also on providing resources to make the whole community stronger.

Skills in Psychological Recovery (SPR) [which is based in part on the Psychological First Aid Field Operations Guide (PFA)] is another model that can often be helpful. SPR works to teach all kinds of people skills that will help them be more resilient. SPR is given by trained and supervised crisis counselors. They work with you to help you develop skills, including the following:

- Problem-solving

- Planning more positive and meaningful activities

- Managing stress and reactions to the disaster

- Engaging in more helpful thinking

- Building healthy social connections

Some survivors may still be in distress after psychological first aid, crisis counseling, or SPR. For those in need of more intensive services, treatment may be needed for problems such as PTSD, anxiety, panic, depression, or guilt. Research supports cognitive behavioral therapy (CBT), a recommended treatment for trauma and PTSD.

Many standard treatments are being revised for use after disaster. An example of a trauma treatment tailored to disaster survivors is Cognitive Behavioral Treatment for Post-disaster Distress (CBT-PD). This is a 12-session program during which survivors learn about the following:

- Their symptoms

- A breathing technique to manage anxiety

- Engaging in pleasant activities

- Changing their ways of thinking to be more positive and helpful

This was used after Hurricane Katrina, and people improved even after only a few sessions of the treatment.

Summing It Up

Recovery programs after disaster span a wide range. The goals of these programs are to help both survivors and the community to recover. No matter where you are on the spectrum of disaster reactions, there should be a program to help you. With support, you can build your resources, resilience, skills, and mental health.

Chapter 38

Mental Health Issues among Minority and Immigrant Populations

Chapter Contents

Section 38.1

Mental Health Disparities among Minority Populations

Excerpted from "Mental Health 101," Office
of Minority Health (http://minorityhealth.hhs.gov),
July 8, 2008.

Disparities in Mental Health

Mental disorders constitute an immense burden on the U.S. population, with major depression now the leading cause of disability in the U.S., and schizophrenia, bipolar disorder (manic depressive disorder), and obsessive compulsive disorder ranked among the ten leading causes of disability. One person in four has been diagnosed with a mental disorder in the last 12 months and is consequently in need of services.

Minority populations are often over represented in our nation's most vulnerable populations: the poor, the uninsured, the homeless, and the incarcerated. They have little access and/or may under under-utilize mental health services. For those who do receive mental health interventions, the appropriateness and quality of those treatments remain in question. These unmet needs and provision of poor quality mental health services to minority populations is impacting the well being of our nation.

The United States population is composed of many diverse groups. Evidence indicates a persistent disparity in the health status of racial and ethnic minority populations, as compared with the overall health status of the U.S. population.

Over the next decade, the U.S. will continue to become more racially and ethnically diverse, increasing the demand for mental health services tailored to community needs. This will have significant consequences for the need and demand for providers of mental health services. Poverty, lack of adequate access to quality health services, few culturally and linguistically competent health providers and services, and lack of preventive health care are all factors that must be addressed.

A key finding of the Surgeon General's *Report on Mental Health: Culture, Race and Ethnicity* (2001) was that living in poverty has the most measurable effects on the rates of mental illness. Racial and ethnic minorities are overrepresented among the poor. People in the lowest socioeconomic positions are at least two to three times more likely than those in the highest positions to experience a mental disorder, and the overall rate of poverty among most racial and ethnic minority groups in the U.S. is much higher, than that of non-Hispanic whites. Racism and discrimination are highly stressful and can adversely affect health and mental health.

With advances in research, the causes and treatments for mental illness are better known today than ever before. According to recent reports, the great majority of mental illnesses are treatable. According to one National Institute of Mental Health study (2004), some have found that 80 percent of patients with depression can now recover. With treatment and recovery more reachable, everyone regardless of age, sex, religion, race, ethnicity, primary language or national origin should have the right and access to evidenced-based mental health services.

Addressing Stigma

Stigma continues to be a major barrier to seeking out care for mental health disorders. Many people are still confused between facts and myths. They don't understand what mental illnesses are and continue to believe that there is something shameful about them. In addition to shame, minorities often feel the legacy of racism and discrimination, leading to the distrust of health and mental health professionals. Feelings of stigma, discrimination, and mistrust of authorities preclude individuals in need from seeking out and receiving the help and treatments that can lead them to recovery.

Because the small numbers of minorities that do seek behavioral health care prefer seeking and receiving that care in primary care settings, it is in our best interest to nurture and further develop this entry point into treatment, and we must assure the presence of a sensitive workforce that is culturally and linguistically competent. As such, providers themselves will help to break down some of the barriers created by stigma, while providing needed care.

Mental Health Treatment

Although sensitivity to culture, race, gender, disability, poverty, and the need for consumer involvement are important considerations for care and treatment, barriers of access exist in the organization and financing of mental health services for adults.

Because of the lack of access to preventive care, early identification of mental illness and lack of quality interventions, the service needs of minorities may exceed those of whites. Poverty and lack of (or insufficient) medical insurance hampers access to care, often leading to more chronic mental health conditions. High concentrations of poverty in inner cities and the combination of isolation and poverty in rural and frontier areas pose additional challenges for residents of these areas.

In a report titled: "Health Centers' Role in Answering the Behavioral Health Needs of the Medically Underserved" (2004), the Health Resources and Services Administration (HRSA) reported that community health centers (CHC) are the primary care providers to 15 million medically underserved individuals. They have become critical sources of behavioral health services to those most vulnerable, particularly minority populations, the poor and the uninsured. According to the 2003 CHC Uniform Data System, health centers reported 2.1 million encounters for mental health conditions and 720,000 contacts for drug or alcohol dependence.

The Indian Health Service (IHS) is an integrated health care system that provides valuable mental health services to American Indians and Alaska Natives (AI/AN) through its Mental Health and Social Services program. This program is community oriented, clinical, and preventive—providing care to more than 1.6 million consumers, both urban and reservation-based. Nevertheless, the accessibility of mental health and substance abuse treatments continue to be a problem.

Mental Health and African Americans

- Poverty level affects mental health status. African Americans living below the poverty level, as compared to those over twice the poverty level, are four times more likely to report psychological distress.

- African Americans are 30% more likely to report having serious psychological distress than non-Hispanic whites.

- Non-Hispanic whites are more than twice as likely to receive antidepressant prescription treatments as are non-Hispanic blacks.

- The death rate from suicide for African American men was five times that for African American women, in 2005. However, the suicide rate for African Americans is generally lower than that of the non-Hispanic white population.

Mental Health and American Indians/Alaska Natives

- In 2006, suicide was the second leading cause of death for American Indian/Alaska Natives between the ages of 10 and 34.

- American Indian/Alaska Natives are almost three times as likely to experience feelings of sadness or hopelessness as compared to non-Hispanic whites.

- Violent deaths—unintentional injuries, homicide, and suicide—account for 75% of all mortality in the second decade of life for American Indian/Alaska Natives.

- While the overall death rate from suicide for American Indian/Alaska Natives is comparable to the white population, adolescent American Indian/Alaska Natives have death rates two to five times the rate for whites in the same age groups.

Mental Health and Asian Americans

- Suicide was the eighth leading cause of death for Asian Americans in 2005.

- Older Asian American women have the highest suicide rate of all women over age 65 in the United States. In 2005, the suicide rate for that group was 1.6 times greater than it was in the white population. The overall suicide rate for Asian Americans, however, is half that of the white population.

- Southeast Asian refugees are at risk for post-traumatic stress disorder (PTSD) associated with trauma experienced before and after immigration to the U.S. One study found that 70% of Southeast Asian refugees receiving mental health care were diagnosed with PTSD.

- For Asian Americans, the rate of serious psychological distress increases with lower levels of income, as it does in most other ethnic populations.

Mental Health and Hispanics

- Poverty level affects mental health status. Hispanics living below the poverty level, as compared to Hispanics over twice the poverty level, are twice as likely to report psychological distress.

- The death rate from suicide for Hispanic men is five times the rate for Hispanic women, in 2005. However, the suicide rate for Hispanics is half that of the non-Hispanic white population.

- Suicide attempts for Hispanic girls, grades 9–12, were 80% higher than for white girls in the same age group, in 2005.

- Non-Hispanic whites received mental health treatment three times more often than Hispanics, in 2005.

Section 38.2

Mental Health Needs of Immigrants

Who Are Immigrants?

Currently, 39.9 million people (12.9 percent of the population) living in the United States are foreign-born. As the foreign-born population has grown over the last few decades, so has the population of their children. Another 33 million individuals (11 percent) are native-born with at least one foreign-born parent. Today, one in five people living in the United States is a first-generation immigrant (born abroad to foreign-born parents) or a second-generation immigrant (born in the United States to a foreign-born parent or parents). All second-generation immigrants are U.S. citizens as mandated by the 14th Amendment. Thirty percent of young adults between the ages of 18 and 34 are first- or second-generation immigrants. Immigrant-origin children have become the fastest growing segment of the child population with one in three children under 18 projected to be the child of an immigrant by 2020.

Immigrants to the United States come from all over the world. During the previous great wave of migration, most new arrivals originated from Europe. But in the mid-1960s, immigrants began to contribute to the great diversification of our nation.

Since 1965, more than three-quarters of new immigrants arriving in the United States are "of color" with origins in Latin America, Asia, the Caribbean, and Africa. The largest group of immigrants comes from Latin America, a racially and ethnically complex region consisting of indigenous origin, white European origin, African origin, and mestizo (or mixed origin) populations. Asians account for 27.8 percent of the foreign born, and there has been a very rapid growth in immigration from Africa since 1960, from 35,355 to 1.4 million, with most of that growth occurring in the last decade.

The four states with the largest numbers of immigrants (California, Hawaii, New Mexico, and Texas) have already become "majority/minority" (less than 50 percent white) states. In the past two decades, a growing number of states with no previous immigrant population have seen very high rates of new migration. Southern states have experienced the most dramatic change in immigrant population compared to other states.

Immigrants arrive in the United States with varied levels of education but tend to be overrepresented at both the highest and lowest ends of the educational and skill continuum. They comprise a quarter of all U.S. physicians, 24 percent of the nation's science and engineering workers with a bachelor's degree, and 47 percent of scientists with doctorates. It is likely these percentages will be higher when the 2010 Census data are released.

At the other end of the spectrum, some immigrant adults have educational levels far below the average U.S. citizen. Some sectors of the U.S. economy rely heavily on "low-skilled" immigrants, including the agriculture, service, and construction industries. Approximately 75 percent of all hired farm workers and nearly all those involved in the production of fresh fruits and vegetables are either legal or undocumented immigrant adults.

An estimated 460 languages are currently spoken in homes in the United States. The National Center for Education Statistics estimates that between 1979 and 2008, the percentage of children who spoke a second language at home increased from nine percent to 21 percent. Of those individuals speaking a language other than English at home, 62 percent speak Spanish, 19 percent speak another Indo-European language, 15 percent speak an Asian or Pacific Island language, and the remaining four percent speak another language.

Immigrants also contribute to religious diversity. Religion is a fundamental part of life for most people throughout the world. Newly arrived immigrant adults and children who are feeling disoriented in their new land are particularly likely to turn to their religious communities in times of transition.

What Propels Migration?

Three factors have been identified as driving migration: reuniting with family members; searching for work; the need for humanitarian protection

Separated families often desire reunification, which may take years, especially when complicated by financial hurdles and immigration regulations. The longer the separation, the more complicated the family reunification and the greater the likelihood that children will report psychological symptoms.

Trends in the global economy stimulate migration because immigrants tend to follow where investments and jobs flow. Labor markets in global economies rely on foreign workers both in the highly paid knowledge-intensive sector as well as in the more labor-intensive sector. Economic difficulties in home countries along with higher wages in immigrant destinations lead large numbers of migrants to seek jobs outside their native countries.

Seeking humanitarian protection also contributes to U.S. immigration. By the first decade of the 21st century, there were approximately half a million refugees in the United States. The United States' stated immigration policy goal is to provide shelter to those fleeing their native countries because they face risk of persecution. Reasons for seeking humanitarian protection include wars, violence, and environmental disasters.

Dispelling the Myths

Although the number of immigrants in the United States is at an all-time high, the rate of immigration today is actually lower than during the last era of mass migration from 1880 to 1920, when European immigrants were arriving in America.

Contrary to popular belief, the number of undocumented immigrants is declining. The vast majority of immigrants in the United States are legal. In 1910, the rate of immigration reached a peak of 14.7 percent, while in 2009 the rate was 12.5 percent. After three decades of continuous growth, with a peak in unauthorized migration in 2000, the number has dropped by approximately one million during the last two years following the start of the recession in late 2007.

Economists have routinely debated the relative costs and benefits of immigration for the U.S. economy. Contrary to popular perceptions, undocumented immigrants are unable to access a host of services even though they regularly contribute to the federal system through taxes and social security payments automatically deducted from their wages.

There is, however, a general tension between federal governments and state governments when it comes to the economic consequences of immigration. The federal government keeps a large share of the taxes generated by immigrants, while local governments must bear many of the costs and provide the services immigrants consume, particularly for education.

Despite concerns about the immigrant population's inability or unwillingness to learn English, research finds a consistent pattern of language assimilation within a generation. Research suggests that immigrants today are highly motivated to learn English and do so more quickly than in previous generations. Compared to their U.S.-born peers, immigrant students have better attendance rates, more positive attitudes toward their teachers and school, higher feelings of being connected to their schools, and higher grades when controlling for parental education.

Resilience of the Population

Immigrants demonstrate a remarkable pattern of strengths. They have very high levels of engagement in the labor market, and the children of immigrants go on to out perform their parents. Although recently arrived immigrants often face many risks, including poverty, discrimination, taxing occupations, fewer years of schooling, and social isolation, they do better than expected on a wide range of outcomes compared with their counterparts remaining in the country of origin as well as second-generation immigrants.

What Is the Psychological Experience of Immigration?

Social Context of Reception

Socioecological model: Ecological approaches acknowledge that behavior does not occur in a vacuum but is affected by the larger culture and society, as well as the local community and its institutions. Thus, the social climate and receiving environment into which immigrants arrive help shape their experience in and adaptation to America. Also, today's immigrants may adopt American culture without losing the connection to their native culture, and thus enjoy the advantages of biculturalism.

Assimilation versus multiculturalism: The arrival of a new racially diverse wave of immigrants to the United States has highlighted the distinctions between assimilation (the melting pot) and multiculturalism (the salad bowl). Those in favor of cultural assimilation believe the best approach is for immigrants (and other minority groups) to rapidly blend into the dominant culture. They contend adopting the norms and rules of the dominant culture will eliminate ethnic differences and thus prejudice will be drastically reduced.

On the other hand, multicultural ideology holds that all cultural groups should have the opportunity to retain their basic cultural norms, values, traditions, and languages within a greater cultural framework. They believe that prejudice is reduced and self-esteem is enhanced through appreciation of group differences. In the end, the solution may involve preserving cultural distinctiveness while also developing a shared identity with those born in the United States.

The immigration debate, xenophobia, and discrimination: In the current anti-immigrant climate, xenophobia (hatred or fear of foreigners or strangers or of their politics or culture), and discrimination significantly impact the lives of immigrants. Many immigrants are discriminated against in employment, their neighborhoods, service agencies, and schools. Reasons include immigration status, skin color, language skills, and income and education levels. Immigrants are often negatively stereotyped and these stereotypes have negative consequences for well-being.

Neighborhoods/communities: Neighborhood relationships are particularly critical for new immigrants because many aspects of the new environment can be disorienting. Living in ethnic communities seems to protect immigrants from cultural isolation, which in turn, benefits their psychological adjustment. However, pressure to assimilate may be strong outside their ethnic group and lead to discrimination and its negative consequences.

New immigrants of color who settle in predominantly minority neighborhoods often have virtually no direct, regular, and intimate contact with middle-class white Americans. This in turn affects their opportunities to hear and use English, the quality of schools their children attend, and their access to desirable jobs. Concentrated poverty is associated with the lack of job opportunities, and youth in such neighborhoods are chronically under- or unemployed.

Acculturation and Adaptation

Acculturation and mental health: Acculturation is a multidimensional process that involves changes in many aspects of immigrants' lives, including language, cultural identity, attitudes and values, types of food and music preferred, media use, ethnic pride, ethnic social relations, cultural familiarity, and social customs.

Acculturation may occur in stages, with immigrants learning the new language first, followed by behavioral participation in the culture. While some settings, such as workplaces or schools, are predominantly culturally American, others, such as an immigrant's ethnic neighborhood and home environment, are predominantly of the heritage culture. From this perspective, acculturation to both cultures provides access to different kinds of resources that are useful in different settings, and in turn, hopefully linked to positive mental health outcomes.

But even immigrants who have lived in the United States for a long time and who appear to have adopted the American lifestyle may continue to maintain strong identification with, and hold the values of, their culture of origin. This has important implications for providing psychological services to this population. The process of integrating the social and cultural values, ideas, beliefs, and behavioral patterns of the culture of origin with those of the new culture can lead to acculturative stress if they conflict.

Acculturation gaps: Family acculturation gaps extend across a variety of parent-child relationships, and immigrant parents and children increasingly live in different cultural worlds. Because immigrant parents are immersed primarily in one cultural context and their children in another, they often know little of their children's lives outside the home. For immigrant children, it can be difficult to live with the expectations and demands of one culture in the home and another at school. Children may not turn to their parents with problems and concerns, believing their parents do not know the culture and its institutions well enough to provide them with good advice or assistance.

Social trust and civic engagement: Democratic societies require citizens to interact regularly with each other for political, economic, and social reasons. The current atmosphere of general social distrust in the United States coincides with, and is complicated by, the highest levels of immigration since the last great wave of migration from 1880 to 1920. For immigrants, involvement in U.S. society, politics, and communities represents successful integration into the life of the country.

A marker of whether new immigrants feel welcomed and accepted in this country is whether they are able to develop social trust and become involved in U.S. society, politics, and communities. While historically, civic engagement was defined as voting, definitions of civic engagement now include the following: attitudes toward political participation;

knowledge about government; commitment to society; activities that help those in need; collective action to fight for social justice.

Although nonnaturalized immigrant adults cannot vote, they can be involved in an array of civic projects. With citizenship and second-generation status come greater civic and political participation. Not speaking English blocks participation in some activities for the first generation. On the other hand, bilingual competencies can serve as tools for civic engagement among immigrant youth who become involved as culture brokers.

Trust and civic engagement do not occur in a vacuum. It remains to be seen how the general climate of distrust in the United States and the current crisis over immigration shape immigrant youths' civic trust and engagement. Research is needed on how the current political climate influences trust in the culture and future civic engagement.

Section 38.3

Children of Immigrants May Have a Higher Risk for Mental Disorders Than Their Parents

"U.S.-born Children of Immigrants May Have Higher Risk for Mental Disorders Than Parents," *Science Update*, National Institute of Mental Health (www.nimh.nih.gov), September 2009.

In the first studies to examine the effects of immigration and years of residence on the mental health of Caribbean Black, Latino, and Asian populations in the United States, researchers funded by the National Institute of Mental Health (NIMH) found that immigrants in general appear to have lower rates of mental disorders than their U.S.-born counterparts. A special section of the *American Journal of Public Health* published in January 2007 provides early findings from the National Survey of American Life (NSAL) and the National Latino and Asian American Study (NLAAS) on the prevalence of mental disorders and patterns of mental health service use among minority immigrants and later generations born in the U.S. It is also the first time that comparable studies of nationally representative samples of Caribbean Blacks, Latinos, and Asians have been published together in the same journal.

Overall, immigrants appear to have lower rates of mental disorders than second- or later-generation individuals, as seen in Table 38.1. However, within each group, risks for particular disorders may differ depending on ethnic subgroup, gender, English-language proficiency, years of living in the United States, and age at immigration. For example, Caribbean Black men in the United States had higher risks for mood and anxiety disorders in the past year than African American men. Caribbean Black women had lower past-year and lifetime risks for anxiety and substance abuse disorders compared with African American women. Among the Latino population in the United States, those who reported lower self-ratings of ability to speak, read, and write in English showed a reduced risk for substance use disorders and a lower overall risk for mental disorders. In contrast, Asian men who spoke English well were at lower risk for mental disorders over a lifetime; nativity was the most stable predictor of mental disorders in Asian women, with foreign-born women reporting fewer lifetime cases than U.S.-born women.

Patterns of mental health service use also varied among the different groups, but overall, U.S.-born children and grandchildren of immigrants showed greater service use than immigrants themselves. Among the diverse ethnic subgroups, the researchers also observed differences in patterns of service use according to a variety of ethnic- and immigration-related factors. For example, while Caribbean Blacks and African Americans showed similar mental health service use patterns overall, blacks from the Spanish-speaking Caribbean were more likely to report using specialty mental health services such as psychiatrists, psychologists, or mental health hotlines within the past year than African Americans or blacks of other Caribbean origins. Puerto Ricans reported significantly higher rates of overall mental health service use and specialty service use than all other Latino subgroups; however, foreign-born Latinos and those who spoke primarily Spanish, while much less likely to seek specialty services, used general medical services for mental health issues at comparable rates to other Latinos, suggesting lower recognition of psychiatric problems among these populations. While Asian Americans in general showed low rates of help-seeking, children of Asian immigrants, or second-generation individuals, showed more similar patterns of service use to immigrants than to third-generation individuals, who showed patterns comparable to the general population.

Table 38.1. Prevalence Rates of Mental Disorders among Different U.S. Population Groups

Population Group	Native Status	Lifetime Prevalence of Any Psychiatric Disorder	Past-Year Prevalence of Any Psychiatric Disorder
Caribbean Blacks	Foreign-Born	27.87	16.38
	U.S.-Born	30.54	14.79
Latinos	Foreign-Born	23.76	13.12
	U.S.-Born	36.77	18.57
Asians	Foreign-Born	15.16	8.00
	U.S.-Born	24.62	13.22
U.S. General Population*	All	46.4	26.2

* National Comorbidity Survey-Replication, 2005

Both the NSAL and NLAAS were part of the NIMH-supported Collaborative Psychiatric Epidemiological Survey (CPES) program, which also included the National Comorbidity Survey Replication. Together, these national surveys provide improved data on the mental health of racial and ethnic minorities living in the United States. The relative lack of this type of information in the past has created a barrier to service for immigrants and subsequent generations. Further research like the CPES studies that increases the understanding of mental health risks and service use among different population groups is critical for developing programs and services that meet the specific needs of these populations and may help reduce current health care disparities.

Chapter 39

The Link between Mental Health and Poverty

Mental ill-health and poverty are closely linked and inter-act in a complex negative cycle.

Studies over the last 20 years indicate a close interaction between factors associated with poverty and mental ill health:[1]

- Common mental disorders are about twice as frequent among the poor as among the rich.[2] For example, evidence indicates that depression is 1.5 to 2 times more prevalent among the low-income groups of a population.[8]

- People experiencing hunger or facing debts are more likely to suffer from common mental disorders.[3]

- Common mental disorders are also more prevalent for people living in poor and overcrowded housing.[4]

- Highest estimated prevalence of mental disorders can be found among people with the lowest levels of education or people who are unemployed.[5]

- In relation to severe mental disorders, and schizophrenia specifically, data show that:

"Breaking the Vicious Cycle Between Mental Ill-Health and Poverty," Mental Health Core to Development Information Sheet 1, 2007, http://www.who.int/mental_health/policy/development/1_Breakingviciouscycle_Infosheet.pdf. © 2007 World Health Organization. Reprinted with permission. Reviewed by David A. Cooke, MD, FACP, June 16, 2012.

- People with the lowest socioeconomic status (SES) have eight times more relative risk for schizophrenia than those of the highest SES;

- People with schizophrenia, in comparison with people without mental disorders, are four times more likely to be unemployed or partly employed;

- People with schizophrenia are one-third more likely not to have graduated from high school, and;

- Three times more likely to be divorced.[6]

Best evidence indicates that the relationship between mental ill-health and poverty is cyclical: poverty increases the risk of mental disorders and having a mental disorder increases the likelihoods of descending into poverty.

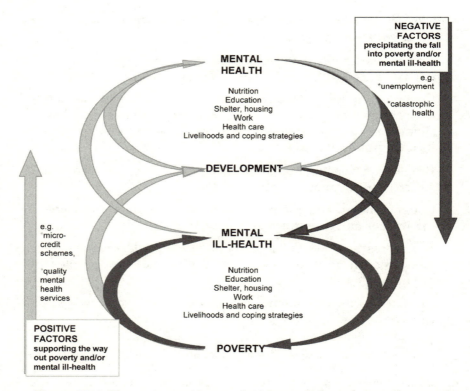

Figure 39.1. The cycles and factors linking mental health and development and mental ill-health and poverty.

- People living in poverty lack financial resources to maintain basic living standards, have fewer educational and employment opportunities, are exposed to adverse living environments, and are less able to access good quality health care.

- These stressful living conditions place people at higher risk of developing a mental disorder.

- People who develop a mental disorder may not be able to work because of their illness. Others, because of discrimination, may be systematically denied work opportunities or may lose their existing job.

- Lack of employment drives people deeper into poverty and people are unable to pay for the treatment that they need. In other cases a great deal of money is spent on ineffective and inappropriate mental health care, which means that people not only end up out of pocket but also fail to get better.

- Supportive community networks help to protect against the adverse effects of illness and poverty. But for people with mental disorders social support systems often disintegrate as the stigma and discrimination that they face leads to their marginalization, social exclusion, and human rights violations.

- All these factors further worsen their condition and perpetuate the negative cycle between poverty and mental ill health.

Most countries fail to devote sufficient resources to improving mental health.

Global data indicate that:

- Only 2% of national health budgets is dedicated to mental health.[7]

- 31% of countries have no specified mental health budget at all.[7]

- Although cheap and effective mental health treatments exist, it is estimated that 76 to 85% of people with serious mental disorders to not receive treatment in developing countries.[8]

- 69% of beds for mental health care are to be found in large psychiatric asylums which are associated with a wide range of human rights violations, instead of general hospitals in community settings.[7]

Mental health needs to be addressed in international and national health, development, or poverty reduction agendas.

In addition to being a burden in its own right, mental health is also co-morbid with other health problems, including both infectious and chronic diseases, and must therefore be addressed in order to achieve optimal health outcomes and to meet development goals.

The Millennium Development Goals (MDGs) [a set of eight goals adopted by members of the United Nations to improve conditions in poor countries] currently overlook mental health. But addressing mental issues will reinforce several of the MDGs:

- MDG 1: Eradicate extreme poverty: Providing treatment for people with mental disorders will enable them to get a job, reduce their health care costs, and help create the conditions necessary for them to rise out of poverty.[9]

- MDG 4: Reduce child mortality: Childhood failure to thrive is strongly associated with child mortality. Babies of depressed mothers are five times more likely to be underweight or stunted than babies of nondepressed mothers.[10] Addressing the mental health of women of childbearing age is therefore a crucial aspect of reducing child mortality.[9]

- MDG 5: Improve maternal health: Addressing depression in women of childbearing age is also an essential part of improving maternal health. A high number of women suffer from depression during pregnancy and after childbirth which can have a profound effect on their lives.[11] Indeed, today suicide is one of the leading causes of maternal death in developing countries. It is also possible that depression results in increased maternal mortality, through adversely affecting physical health as well as through suicide.[9]

- MDG 6: Combat HIV/AIDS, malaria, and other diseases: People living with infectious diseases such as HIV/AIDS are much more likely to suffer from depression.[9,12] According to published evidence, people with depression are less likely to adhere to medical treatment. Therefore, programs designed to combat HIV/AIDS must address mental health if health outcomes are to be improved.

People with mental disorders need to be targeted for poverty reduction and development programs to help bring them out of poverty and to promote development, e.g., through micro-credit schemes or employment programs.

References

1. Patel V. Poverty, inequality and mental health in developing countries. In *Poverty, Inequality and Health*, ed. D Leon & G Walt, Oxford, Oxford University Press, 2001: 247–262.

2. Patel V, Araya R, de Lima M, Ludermir A, Todd C. Women, poverty and common mental disorders in four restructuring societies. *Social Science and Medicine*, 1999, 49: 1461–1471.

3. Patel V, Araya R, de Lima M, Ludermir A, Todd C. Women, poverty and common mental disorders in four restructuring societies. *Social Science and Medicine*, 1999, 49: 1461-1471/The onset of common mental disorders in primary care attenders in Harare, Zimbabwe, *Psychological Medicine*, 1999, 29:97–104.

4. Araya R, Lewis G, Rojas G, Fritsch R. Education and income: which is more important for mental health? *J Epidemiol Community Health*. 2003 July; 57(7): 501–505.

5. WHO International Consortium of Psychiatric Epidemiology (2000). Cross-national comparisons of mental disorders. *Bulletin of the World Health Organization*, 78: 413-426.

6. Saraceno B., Barbui C., Poverty and Mental Illness. *Canadian Journal of Psychiatry* ,1997, 42(3): 285–290.

7. *Mental Health Atlas 2005*, Geneva, World Health Organization, 2005.

8. WHO World Mental Health Consortium, *JAMA*, June 2, 2004.

9. Miranda JJ and V Patel 2005: Achieving the Millennium Development Goals: Does Mental Health Play a Role. *PLoS Med* 2(10): e291. doi:10.1371/journal.pmed.0020291

10. Rahman A, Iqbal Z, Bunn J, Lovel H, Harrington R. Impact of maternal depression on infant nutritional status and illness: A cohort study, *Arch Gen Psychiatry*, 2004, 61: 946-952.

11. Eg. see Cooper PJ., Tomlinson M, Swartz L, et al., Post-partum depression and the mother-infant relationship in a South African peri-urban settlement. *British Journal of Psychiatry*, 1999, 175: 554-558.)

12. Unpublished WHO document. Lorenzo DR and Bertolote JM, Comorbidity and Mental Health. Geneva, World Health Organization, 2003.

Part Six

Mental Illness Co-Occurring with Other Disorders

Chapter 40

Caregivers and Mental Health

Chapter Contents

Section 40.1

Self-Care for Family Caregivers

Excerpted from "Taking Care of YOU: Self-Care for Family Caregivers,"
© 2008 Family Caregiver Alliance. Reprinted with permission. To view
the complete text of this article including a list of related organizations
providing information and assistance, visit www.caregiver.org.

First, Care for Yourself

On an airplane, an oxygen mask descends in front of you. What
do you do? As we all know, the first rule is to put on your own oxygen
mask before you assist anyone else. Only when we first help ourselves
can we effectively help others. Caring for yourself is one of the most
important—and one of the most often forgotten—things you can do as
a caregiver. When your needs are taken care of, the person you care
for will benefit, too.

Effects of Caregiving on Health and Well Being

We hear this often: "My husband is the person with Alzheimer's, but
now I'm the one in the hospital!" Such a situation is all too common.
Researchers know a lot about the effects of caregiving on health and
well being. For example, if you are a caregiving spouse between the
ages of 66 and 96 and are experiencing mental or emotional strain, you
have a risk of dying that is 63 percent higher than that of people your
age who are not caregivers. The combination of loss, prolonged stress,
the physical demands of caregiving, and the biological vulnerabilities
that come with age place you at risk for significant health problems
as well as an earlier death.

Older caregivers are not the only ones who put their health and well
being at risk. If you are a baby boomer who has assumed a caregiver
role for your parents while simultaneously juggling work and raising
adolescent children, you face an increased risk for depression, chronic
illness, and a possible decline in quality of life.

But despite these risks, family caregivers of any age are less likely
than noncaregivers to practice preventive healthcare and self-care

behavior. Regardless of age, sex, and race and ethnicity, caregivers report problems attending to their own health and well-being while managing caregiving responsibilities. They report:

- sleep deprivation;
- poor eating habits;
- failure to exercise;
- failure to stay in bed when ill;
- postponement of or failure to make medical appointments.

Family caregivers are also at increased risk for excessive use of alcohol, tobacco, and other drugs and for depression. Caregiving can be an emotional roller coaster. On the one hand, caring for your family member demonstrates love and commitment and can be a very rewarding personal experience. On the other hand, exhaustion, worry, inadequate resources, and continuous care demands are enormously stressful. Studies show that an estimated 46 percent to 59 percent of caregivers are clinically depressed.

Taking Responsibility for Your Own Care

You cannot stop the impact of a chronic or progressive illness or a debilitating injury on someone for whom you care. But there is a great deal that you can do to take responsibility for your personal well being and to get your own needs met.

Identifying Personal Barriers

Many times, attitudes and beliefs form personal barriers that stand in the way of caring for yourself. Not taking care of yourself may be a lifelong pattern, with taking care of others an easier option. However, as a family caregiver you must ask yourself, "What good will I be to the person I care for if I become ill? If I die?" Breaking old patterns and overcoming obstacles is not an easy proposition, but it can be done—regardless of your age or situation. The first task in removing personal barriers to self-care is to identify what is in your way. For example,

- Do you feel you have to prove that you are worthy of the care recipient's affection?

- Do you think you are being selfish if you put your needs first?

- Is it frightening to think of your own needs? What is the fear about?

- Do you have trouble asking for what you need? Do you feel inadequate if you ask for help? Why?

Sometimes caregivers have misconceptions that increase their stress and get in the way of good self-care. Here are some of the most commonly expressed:

- I am responsible for my parent's health.
- If I don't do it, no one will.
- If I do it right, I will get the love, attention, and respect I deserve.

"I never do anything right," or "There's no way I could find the time to exercise" are examples of negative "self-talk," another possible barrier that can cause unnecessary anxiety. Instead, try positive statements: "I'm good at giving John a bath." "I can exercise for 15 minutes a day." Remember, your mind believes what you tell it.

Because we base our behavior on our thoughts and beliefs, attitudes and misconceptions like those noted above can cause caregivers to continually attempt to do what cannot be done, to control what cannot be controlled. The result is feelings of continued failure and frustration and, often, an inclination to ignore your own needs. Ask yourself what might be getting in your way and keeping you from taking care of yourself.

Moving Forward

Once you've started to identify any personal barriers to good self-care, you can begin to change your behavior, moving forward one small step at a time. Following are some effective tools for self-care that can start you on your way.

Tool #1: Reducing Personal Stress

How we perceive and respond to an event is a significant factor in how we adjust and cope with it. The stress you feel is not only the result of your caregiving situation but also the result of your perception of it—whether you see the glass as half-full or half-empty. It is important to remember that you are not alone in your experiences.

Your level of stress is influenced by many factors, including the following:

- Whether your caregiving is voluntary. If you feel you had no choice in taking on the responsibilities, the chances are greater that you will experience strain, distress, and resentment.

- Your relationship with the care recipient. Sometimes people care for another with the hope of healing a relationship. If healing does not occur, you may feel regret and discouragement.

- Your coping abilities. How you coped with stress in the past predicts how you will cope now. Identify your current coping strengths so that you can build on them.

- Your caregiving situation. Some caregiving situations are more stressful than others. For example, caring for a person with dementia is often more stressful than caring for someone with a physical limitation.

- Whether support is available.

Steps to Managing Stress

1. **Recognize warning signs early.** These might include irritability, sleep problems, and forgetfulness. Know your own warning signs, and act to make changes. Don't wait until you are overwhelmed.

2. **Identify sources of stress.** Ask yourself, "What is causing stress for me?" Sources of stress might be too much to do, family disagreements, feelings of inadequacy, inability to say no.

3. **Identify what you can and cannot change.** Remember, we can only change ourselves; we cannot change another person. When you try to change things over which you have no control, you will only increase your sense of frustration. Ask yourself, "What do I have some control over? What can I change?" Even a small change can make a big difference. The challenge we face as caregivers is well expressed in words from the Serenity Prayer:

    > Grant me the serenity to
    > Accept the things I cannot change,
    > Courage to change the things I can,
    > And the wisdom to know the difference.

4. **Take action.** Taking some action to reduce stress gives us back a sense of control. Stress reducers can be simple activities like walking and other forms of exercise, gardening, meditation, having coffee with a friend. Identify some stress reducers that work for you.

Tool #2: Setting Goals

Setting goals or deciding what you would like to accomplish in the next three to six months is an important tool for taking care of yourself. Here are some sample goals you might set:

- Take a break from caregiving.

- Get help with caregiving tasks like bathing and preparing meals.

- Feel more healthy.

Goals are generally too big to work on all at once. We are more likely to reach a goal if we break it down into smaller action steps. Once you've set a goal, ask yourself, "What steps do I take to reach my goal?" Make an action plan by deciding which step you will take first, and when. Then get started!

Example: Goal and Action Steps

Goal: Feel more healthy.

Possible Action Steps

1. Make an appointment for a physical check-up.

2. Take a half-hour break once during the week.

3. Walk three times a week for 10 minutes.

Tool #3: Seeking Solutions

Seeking solutions to difficult situations is, of course, one of the most important tools in caregiving. Once you've identified a problem, taking action to solve it can change the situation and also change your attitude to a more positive one, giving you more confidence in your abilities.

Steps for Seeking Solutions

1. **Identify the problem.** Look at the situation with an open mind. The real problem might not be what first comes to mind. For example, you think that the problem is simply that you are tired all the time, when the more basic difficulty is your belief that "no one can care for John like I can." The problem? Thinking that you have to do everything yourself.

2. **List possible solutions.** One idea is to try a different perspective: "Even though someone else provides help to John in a different way than I do, it can be just as good." Ask a friend to help. Call Family Caregiver Alliance or the Eldercare Locator (see resource list at http://caregiver.org) and ask about agencies in your area that could help provide care.

3. **Select one solution from the list.** Then try it!

4. **Evaluate the results.** Ask yourself how well your choice worked.

5. **Try a second solution.** If your first idea didn't work, select another. But don't give up on the first; sometimes an idea just needs fine tuning.

6. **Use other resources.** Ask friends, family members and professionals for suggestions.

7. **If nothing seems to help, accept that the problem may not be solvable now.** You can revisit it at another time.

Note: All too often, we jump from step one to step seven and then feel defeated and stuck. Concentrate on keeping an open mind while listing and experimenting with possible solutions.

Tool #4: Communicating Constructively

Being able to communicate constructively is one of a caregiver's most important tools. When you communicate in ways that are clear, assertive and constructive, you will be heard and get the help and support you need. The information below shows basic guidelines for good communication.

Communication Guidelines

- **Use "I" messages rather than "you" messages.** Saying "I feel angry" rather than "You made me angry" enables you to express your feelings without blaming others or causing them to become defensive.

- **Respect the rights and feelings of others.** Do not say something that will violate another person's rights or intentionally hurt the person's feelings. Recognize that the other person has the right to express feelings.

- **Be clear and specific.** Speak directly to the person. Don't hint or hope the person will guess what you need. Other people are not mind readers. When you speak directly about what you need or feel, you are taking the risk that the other person might disagree or say no to your request, but that action also shows respect for the other person's opinion. When both parties speak directly, the chances of reaching understanding are greater.

- **Be a good listener.** Listening is the most important aspect of communication.

Tool #5: Asking for and Accepting Help

When people have asked if they can be of help to you, how often have you replied, "Thank you, but I'm fine." Many caregivers don't know how to marshal the goodwill of others and are reluctant to ask for help. You may not wish to "burden" others or admit that you can't handle everything yourself.

Be prepared with a mental list of ways that others could help you. For example, someone could take the person you care for on a 15-minute walk a couple of times a week. Your neighbor could pick up a few things for you at the grocery store. A relative could fill out some insurance papers. When you break down the jobs into very simple tasks, it is easier for people to help. And they do want to help. It is up to you to tell them how.

Help can come from community resources, family, friends, and professionals. Ask them. Don't wait until you are overwhelmed and exhausted or your health fails. Reaching out for help when you need it is a sign of personal strength.

Tips on How to Ask

- **Consider the person's special abilities and interests.** If you know a friend enjoys cooking but dislikes driving, your chances of getting help improve if you ask for help with meal preparation.

- **Resist asking the same person repeatedly.** Do you keep asking the same person because she has trouble saying no?

- **Pick the best time to make a request.** Timing is important. A person who is tired and stressed might not be available to help out. Wait for a better time.

- **Prepare a list of things that need doing.** The list might include errands, yard work, a visit with your loved one. Let the "helper" choose what she would like to do.

- **Be prepared for hesitance or refusal.** It can be upsetting for the caregiver when a person is unable or unwilling to help. But in the long run, it would do more harm to the relationship if the person helps only because he doesn't want to upset you. To the person who seems hesitant, simply say, "Why don't you think about it." Try not to take it personally when a request is turned down. The person is turning down the task, not you. Try not to let a refusal prevent you from asking for help again. The person who refused today may be happy to help at another time.

- **Avoid weakening your request.** "It's only a thought, but would you consider staying with Grandma while I went to church?" This request sounds like it's not very important to you. Use "I" statements to make specific requests: "I would like to go to church on Sunday. Would you stay with Grandma from 9 a.m. until noon?"

Tool #6: Talking to the Physician

In addition to taking on the household chores, shopping, transportation, and personal care, 37 percent of caregivers also administer medications, injections, and medical treatment to the person for whom they care. Some 77 percent of those caregivers report the need to ask for advice about the medications and medical treatments. The person they usually turn to is their physician.

But while caregivers will discuss their loved one's care with the physician, caregivers seldom talk about their own health, which is equally important. Building a partnership with a physician that addresses the health needs of the care recipient and the caregiver is crucial. The responsibility of this partnership ideally is shared between you the caregiver, the physician, and other healthcare staff. However, it will often fall to you to be assertive, using good communication skills, to ensure that everyone's needs are met—including your own.

Tips on Communicating with Your Physician

- **Prepare questions ahead of time.** Make a list of your most important concerns and problems. Issues you might want to discuss with the physician are changes in symptoms, medications, or general health of the care recipient, your own comfort in your caregiving situation, or specific help you need to provide care.

- **Enlist the help of the nurse.** Many caregiving questions relate more to nursing than to medicine. In particular, the nurse can answer questions about various tests and examinations, preparing for surgical procedures, providing personal care, and managing medications at home.

- **Make sure your appointment meets your needs.** For example, the first appointment in the morning or after lunch and the last appointment in the day are the best times to reduce your waiting time or accommodate numerous questions. When you schedule your appointment, be sure you convey clearly the reasons for your visit so that enough time is allowed.

- **Call ahead.** Before the appointment, check to see if the doctor is on schedule. Remind the receptionist of special needs when you arrive at the office.

- **Take someone with you.** A companion can ask questions you feel uncomfortable asking and can help you remember what the physician and nurse said.

- **Use assertive communication and "I" messages.** Enlist the medical care team as partners in care. Present what you need, what your concerns are, and how the doctor and/or nurse can help. Use specific, clear "I" statements like the following: "I need to know more about the diagnosis; I will feel better prepared for the future if I know what's in store for me." Or "I am feeling rundown. I'd like to make an appointment for myself and my husband next week."

Tool #7: Starting to Exercise

You may be reluctant to start exercising, even though you've heard it's one of the healthiest things you can do. Perhaps you think that physical exercise might harm you or that it is only for people who are young and able to do things like jogging. Fortunately, research suggests that you can maintain or at least partly restore endurance, balance, strength, and flexibility through everyday physical activities like walking and gardening. Even household chores can improve your health. The key is to increase your physical activity by exercising and using your own muscle power.

Exercise promotes better sleep, reduces tension and depression, and increases energy and alertness. If finding time for exercise is a problem, incorporate it into your daily activity. Perhaps the care recipient can walk or do stretching exercise with you. If necessary, do frequent short exercises instead of those that require large blocks of time. Find activities you enjoy.

Walking, one of the best and easiest exercises, is a great way to get started. Besides its physical benefits, walking helps to reduce psychological tension. Walking 20 minutes a day, three times a week, is very beneficial. If you can't get away for that long, try to walk for as long as you can on however many days you can. Work walking into your life. Walk around the mall, to the store or a nearby park. Walk around the block with a friend.

Tool #8: Learning from Our Emotions

It is a strength to recognize when your emotions are controlling you (instead of you controlling your emotions). Our emotions are messages we need to listen to. They exist for a reason. However negative or painful, our feelings are useful tools for understanding what is happening to us.

Even feelings such as guilt, anger, and resentment contain important messages. Learn from them, then take appropriate action.

For example, when you cannot enjoy activities you previously enjoyed, and your emotional pain over-shadows all pleasure, it is time to seek treatment for depression—especially if you are having thoughts of suicide. Speaking with your physician is the first step. (Please refer Caregiving and Depression below.)

Caregiving often involves a range of emotions. Some feelings are more comfortable than others. When you find that your emotions are intense, they might mean the following:

- That you need to make a change in your caregiving situation.
- That you are grieving a loss.
- That you are experiencing increased stress.
- That you need to be assertive and ask for what you need.

Summing Up

Remember, it is not selfish to focus on your own needs and desires when you are a caregiver—it's an important part of the job. You are responsible for your own self-care. Focus on the following self-care practices:

- Learn and use stress-reduction techniques.
- Attend to your own healthcare needs.
- Get proper rest and nutrition.

- Exercise regularly.

- Take time off without feeling guilty.

- Participate in pleasant, nurturing activities.

- Seek and accept the support of others.

- Seek supportive counseling when you need it, or talk to a trusted counselor or friend.

- Identify and acknowledge your feelings.

- Change the negative ways you view situations.

- Set goals.

It's up to you!

Credits

1. Shultz, Richard and Beach, Scott (1999). Caregiving as a Risk for Mortality: The Caregiver Health Effects Study. *JAMA,* December 15, 1999, Vol. 282, No. 23.

Thanks: A special thank you the Powerful Tools for Caregivers program for permission to use information from *The Caregiver Helpbook* and their "Powerful Tools for Caregivers Class Leader Tips Manual." *The Caregiver Helpbook*, written by Vicki Schmall, Ph.D., Marilyn Cleland, R.N. and Marilynn Sturdevant, RN, MSW, LCSW, (2000) is highly recommended reading for caregivers. The book can be ordered directly from Powerful Tools for Caregivers, 4110 SE Hawthorne Blvd., #703, Portland, OR 97214, (503) 719-6980, http://www.powerfultools forcaregivers.org.

Section 40.2

Caregiving and Depression

Introduction

Could the sadness, loneliness, or anger you feel today be a warning sign of depression? It's possible. It is not unusual for caregivers to develop mild or more serious depression as a result of the constant demands they face in providing care.

Caregiving does not cause depression, nor will everyone who provides care experience the negative feelings that go with depression. But in an effort to provide the best possible care for a family member or friend, caregivers often sacrifice their own physical and emotional needs and the emotional and physical experiences involved with providing care can strain even the most capable person. The resulting feelings of anger, anxiety, sadness, isolation, exhaustion—and then guilt for having these feelings—can exact a heavy toll.

Everyone has negative feelings that come and go over time, but when these feelings become more intense and leave caregivers totally drained of energy, crying frequently, or easily angered by their loved one or other people, it may well be a warning sign of depression. Concerns about depression arise when the sadness and crying don't go away or when those negative feelings are unrelenting.

Unfortunately, feelings of depression are often seen as a sign of weakness rather than a sign that something is out of balance. Comments such as "snap out of it" or "it's all in your head" are not helpful, and reflect a belief that mental health concerns are not real. Ignoring or denying your feelings will not make them go away.

Early attention to symptoms of depression through exercise, a healthy diet, positive support of family and friends, or consultation with a trained health or mental health professional may help to prevent the development of a more serious depression over time.

Symptoms of Depression

People experience depression in different ways. Some may feel a general low-level sadness for months, while others suffer a more sudden and intense negative change in their outlook. The type and degree of symptoms vary by individual and can change over time. Consider these common symptoms of depression. Have you experienced any of the following for longer than two weeks?

- A change in eating habits resulting in unwanted weight gain or loss
- A change in sleep patterns—too much sleep or not enough
- Feeling tired all the time
- A loss of interest in people and/or activities that once brought you pleasure
- Becoming easily agitated or angered
- Feeling that nothing you do is good enough
- Thoughts of death or suicide, or attempting suicide
- Ongoing physical symptoms that do not respond to treatment, such as headaches, digestive disorders, and chronic pain.

Special Caregiver Concerns

What do lack of sleep, dementia, and whether you are male or female have in common? Each can contribute in its own way to a caregiver's increased risk for depression.

Dementia and Care

Researchers have found that a person who provides care for someone with dementia is twice as likely to suffer from depression as a person providing care for someone without dementia. The more severe the case of dementia such as that caused by Alzheimer's disease, the more likely the caregiver is to experience depression. It is critical for caregivers, especially in these situations, to receive consistent and dependable support.

- **Caring for a person with dementia can be all consuming.** It is different from other types of caregiving. Not only do caregivers spend significantly more hours per week providing care, they report more employment problems, personal stress, mental and physical health problems, less time to do the things they enjoy, less time to spend with other family members, and more family conflict than nondementia caregivers. As stressful as the deterioration of a loved one's mental and physical abilities may be for the caregiver, dealing with dementia-related behavior is an even bigger contributor to developing symptoms of depression. Dementia-related symptoms such as wandering, agitation, hoarding, and embarrassing conduct makes every day challenging and makes it harder for a caregiver to get rest or assistance in providing care.

- **Women experience depression at a higher rate than men.** Women, primarily wives and daughters, provide the majority of caregiving. In the United States, approximately 12 million women experience clinical depression each year, at approximately twice the rate of men. A National Mental Health Association survey on the public's attitude and beliefs about clinical depression found that more than one-half of women surveyed still believe it is "normal" for a woman to be depressed during menopause.

The study also found that many women do not seek treatment for depression because they are embarrassed or in denial about being depressed. In fact, 41% of women surveyed cited embarrassment or shame as barriers to treatment.

- **Men who are caregivers deal with depression differently.** Men are less likely to admit to depression and doctors are less likely to diagnose depression in men. Men will more often "self treat" their depressive symptoms of anger, irritability, or powerlessness with alcohol or overwork. Although male caregivers tend to be more willing than female caregivers to hire outside help for assistance with home care duties, they tend to have fewer friends to confide in or positive activities outside the home. The assumption that depressive symptoms are a sign of weakness can make it especially difficult for men to seek help.

- **Lack of sleep contributes to depression.** While sleep needs vary, most people need eight hours a day. Loss of sleep as a result of caring for a loved one can lead to serious depression. The important thing to remember is that even though you may not be able to get your loved one to rest throughout the night, you can arrange to get much needed sleep. Hiring a respite worker to be with your loved one while you take a nap or finding a care center or scheduling a stay over with another family member for a few nights are ways to keep your caregiving commitment while getting the sleep you need.

- **Depression can persist after placement in a care facility.**
  Making the decision to move a loved one to a care center is very
  stressful. While many caregivers are finally able to catch up on
  much needed rest, loneliness, guilt, and monitoring the care a
  loved one receives in this new location can add new stress. Many
  caregivers feel depressed at the time of placement and some continue to feel depressed for a long time after.

People assume that once caregiving is over, the stress from providing hands-on care will go away. Yet, researchers found that even three
years after the death of a spouse with dementia, some former caregivers continued to experience depression and loneliness. In an effort to
return their life to normal, former caregivers may need to seek out
help for depression as well.

What to Do If You Think You Have Depression

Depression deserves to be treated with the same attention afforded
any other illness, such as diabetes or high blood pressure. If you feel
uncomfortable using the term depression, tell the professional that
you are "feeling blue" or "feeling down." The professional will get the
message. The important thing is to seek help.

Those with chronic illnesses also may suffer from depression. If you
suspect this is the case with your loved one, look for an opportunity to
share your concern with him or her. If they are reluctant to talk about
it with you, encourage a trusted friend to talk with them, or consider
leaving a message for their doctor regarding your concern prior to
their next appointment.

How Is Depression Treated?

The first step to getting the best treatment for depression is to meet
with a mental health professional such as a psychiatrist, psychologist,
or social worker. At the same time, schedule a physical exam with your
doctor. Certain medications, as well as some medical conditions such as
viral infection, can cause the same symptoms as depression, and can be
evaluated by your physician during an exam. The exam should include
lab tests and an interview that tests for mental status to determine if
speech, memory, or thought patterns have been affected.

Although it's not unusual for a physician to prescribe antidepressant medication, medication alone may not be the most effective treatment for depression. The guidance of a mental health professional

throughout your treatment is strongly recommended. The therapist or counselor will listen to your concerns, screen you for symptoms of depression, and assist you in setting up an appropriate course of treatment.

One way to find a professional is to ask a friend for the name of someone they know and trust. You may also find someone by asking your minister or rabbi, your doctor, or, if you are employed, you may check your employer's health insurance provider list or EAP program. In addition, national organizations can provide contact information for mental health professionals in your community. (See the FCA fact sheet "Finding a Professional in your Area" available online at http://caregiver.org)

It is important to trust and feel comfortable with the professional you see. It is not uncommon to request a free introductory phone or in-person meeting to help determine if the professional is the right match for your particular needs and style. It is appropriate to clarify what the cost will be, how much your insurance will pay and how many scheduled sessions you should expect to have with the mental health therapist. Any treatment should be evaluated regularly to ensure that it continues to contribute towards your improved health and growth.

Strategies to Help Yourself

Depressive disorders can make one feel exhausted, helpless, and hopeless. Such negative thoughts and feelings make some people feel like giving up. It is important to realize that these negative views are part of the depression and may not accurately reflect the situation. The National Institute of Mental Health offers the following recommendations for dealing with depression:

- Set realistic goals in light of the depression and assume a reasonable amount of responsibility.

- Break large tasks into small ones, set some priorities, and do what you can as you can.

- Try to be with other people and to confide in someone; it is usually better than being alone and secretive.

- Participate in activities that may make you feel better, such as mild exercise, going to a movie or ballgame, or attending a religious, social, or community event.

- Expect your mood to improve gradually, not immediately. Feeling better takes time.

- It is advisable to postpone important decisions until the depression has lifted. Before deciding to make a significant transition—change jobs, get married or divorced—discuss it with others who know you well and have a more objective view of your situation.

- People rarely "snap out of" a depression. But they can feel a little better day-by-day.

- Remember, positive thinking will replace the negative thinking that is part of the depression. The negative thinking will be reduced as your depression responds to treatment.

- Let your family and friends help you.

Direct assistance in providing care for your loved one, such as respite care relief, as well as positive feedback from others, positive self-talk, and recreational activities are linked to lower levels of depression. Look for classes and support groups available through caregiver support organizations to help you learn or practice effective problem-solving and coping strategies needed for caregiving. For your health and the health of those around you, take some time to care for yourself.

Chapter 41

Cancer and Mental Health

Chapter Contents

Section 41.1

Psychological Stress and Cancer

Excerpted from "Psychological Stress and Cancer: Questions and Answers," National Cancer Institute (www.cancer.gov), April 29, 2008.

The complex relationship between physical and psychological health is not well understood. Scientists know that psychological stress can affect the immune system, the body's defense against infection and disease (including cancer); however, it is not yet known whether stress increases a person's susceptibility to disease.

What is psychological stress?

Psychological stress refers to the emotional and physiological reactions experienced when an individual confronts a situation in which the demands go beyond their coping resources. Examples of stressful situations are marital problems, death of a loved one, abuse, health problems, and financial crises.

How does stress affect the body?

The body responds to stress by releasing stress hormones, such as epinephrine (also called adrenaline) and cortisol (also called hydrocortisone). The body produces these stress hormones to help a person react to a situation with more speed and strength. Stress hormones increase blood pressure, heart rate, and blood sugar levels. Small amounts of stress are believed to be beneficial, but chronic (persisting or progressing over a long period of time) high levels of stress are thought to be harmful.

Stress that is chronic can increase the risk of obesity, heart disease, depression, and various other illnesses. Stress also can lead to unhealthy behaviors, such as overeating, smoking, or abusing drugs or alcohol, that may affect cancer risk.

Can stress increase a person's risk of developing cancer?

Studies done over the past 30 years that examined the relationship between psychological factors, including stress, and cancer risk have produced conflicting results. Although the results of some studies have indicated a link between various psychological factors and an increased risk of developing cancer, a direct cause-and-effect relationship has not been proven.

Some studies have indicated an indirect relationship between stress and certain types of virus-related tumors. Evidence from both animal and human studies suggests that chronic stress weakens a person's immune system, which in turn may affect the incidence of virus-associated cancers, such as Kaposi sarcoma and some lymphomas.

More recent research with animal models (animals with a disease that is similar to or the same as a disease in humans) suggests that the body's neuroendocrine response (release of hormones into the blood in response to stimulation of the nervous system) can directly alter important processes in cells that help protect against the formation of cancer, such as DNA repair and the regulation of cell growth.

How does stress affect people who have cancer?

Studies have indicated that stress can affect tumor growth and spread, but the precise biological mechanisms underlying these effects are not well understood. Scientists have suggested that the effects of stress on the immune system may in turn affect the growth of some tumors. However, recent research using animal models indicates that the body's release of stress hormones can affect cancer cell functions directly.

A review of studies that evaluated psychological factors and outcome in cancer patients suggests an association between certain psychological factors, such as feeling helpless or suppressing negative emotions, and the growth or spread of cancer, although this relationship was not consistently seen in all studies. In general, stronger relationships have been found between psychological factors and cancer growth and spread than between psychological factors and cancer development.

Section 41.2

Depression in Cancer Patients

Excerpted from PDQ® Cancer Information Summary. National Cancer
Institute; Bethesda, MD. Depression (PDQ): Patient Version. Updated
08/2011. Available at: http://cancer.gov. Accessed November 24, 2011.

Overview

Depression is a disabling illness that affects about 15% to 25% of
cancer patients. It affects men and women with cancer equally. People
who face a diagnosis of cancer will experience different levels of stress
and emotional upset. Important issues in the life of any person with
cancer may include fear of death, interruption of life plans, changes in
body image and self-esteem, changes in social role and lifestyle, and
money and legal concerns. Everyone who is diagnosed with cancer will
react to these issues in different ways and may not experience serious
depression or anxiety.

Sadness and grief are normal reactions to the crises faced during cancer, and will be experienced at times by all people. Because
sadness is common, it is important to distinguish between normal
levels of sadness and depression. An important part of cancer care is
the recognition of depression that needs to be treated. Some people
may have more trouble adjusting to the diagnosis of cancer than
others may. Major depression is not simply sadness or a blue mood.
Major depression affects about 25% of patients and has common
symptoms that can be diagnosed and treated. Symptoms of depression that are noticed when a patient is diagnosed with cancer may
be a sign that the patient had a depression problem before the
diagnosis of cancer.

Cancer and Depression Risk Factors

Some people with cancer may have a higher risk for developing depression. The cause of depression is not known, but the risk factors for
developing depression are known. Risk factors may be cancer-related
and noncancer-related.

Cancer-related risk factors include depression at the time of cancer diagnosis, poorly controlled pain, an advanced stage of cancer, increased physical impairment or pain, pancreatic cancer, being unmarried and having head and neck cancer, and treatment with some anticancer drugs.

Noncancer-related risk factors include history of depression, lack of family support, other life events that cause stress, family history of depression or suicide, previous suicide attempts, history of alcoholism or drug abuse, and having many illnesses at the same time that produce symptoms of depression (such as stroke or heart attack).

The most common type of depression in people with cancer is called reactive depression. This shows up as feeling moody and being unable to perform usual activities. The symptoms last longer and are more pronounced than a normal and expected reaction but do not meet the criteria for major depression. When these symptoms greatly interfere with a person's daily activities, such as work, school, shopping, or caring for a household, they should be treated in the same way that major depression is treated (such as crisis intervention, counseling, and medication, especially with drugs that can quickly relieve distressing symptoms). Basing the diagnosis on just these symptoms can be a problem in a person with advanced cancer since the illness may be causing decreased functioning. It is important to identify the difference between fatigue and depression since they can be assessed and treated separately. In more advanced illness, focusing on despair, guilty thoughts, and a total lack of enjoyment of life is helpful in diagnosing depression.

Medical factors may also cause symptoms of depression in patients with cancer. Medication usually helps this type of depression more effectively than counseling, especially if the medical factors cannot be changed (for example, dosages of the medications that are causing the depression cannot be changed or stopped). Some medical causes of depression in patients with cancer include uncontrolled pain; abnormal levels of calcium, sodium, or potassium in the blood; anemia; vitamin B 12 or folate deficiency; fever; and abnormal levels of thyroid hormone or steroids in the blood.

Depression and Drug Interactions

Patients with cancer may be treated with a number of drugs throughout their care. Some drugs do not mix safely with certain other drugs, foods, herbals, and nutritional supplements. Certain combinations may reduce or change how drugs work or cause life-threatening side effects. It is important that the patient's healthcare providers be told about all the drugs, herbals, and nutritional supplements the patient is taking, including drugs taken in patches on the skin. This can help prevent unwanted reactions.

Treatment with Psychotherapy

Several psychiatric therapies have been found to be helpful in the treatment of depression related to cancer. Most therapy programs for depression are given in four to 30 hours and are offered in both individual and group settings. They may include sessions about cancer education or relaxation skills. These therapies are often used in combination and include crisis intervention, psychotherapy, and thought/behavior techniques. Patients explore methods of lowering distress, improving coping and problem-solving skills; enlisting support; reshaping negative and self-defeating thoughts; and developing a close personal bond with an understanding health care provider. Talking with a clergy member may also be helpful for some people.

Specific goals of these therapies include the following:

- Assist people diagnosed with cancer and their families by answering questions about the illness and its treatment, explaining information, correcting misunderstandings, giving reassurance about the situation, and exploring with the patient how the diagnosis relates to previous experiences with cancer.

- Assist with problem solving, improve the patient's coping skills, and help the patient and family to develop additional coping skills. Explore other areas of stress, such as family role and lifestyle changes, and encourage family members to support and share concern with each other.

- Ensure that the patient and family understand that support will continue when the focus of treatment changes from trying to cure the cancer to relieving symptoms. The health care team will treat symptoms to help the patient control pain and remain comfortable, and will help the patient and his or her family members maintain dignity.

Cancer support groups may also be helpful in treating depression in patients with cancer, especially adolescents. Support groups have been shown to improve mood, encourage the development of coping skills, improve quality of life, and improve immune response. Support groups can be found through the wellness community, the American

Cancer Society, and many community resources, including the social work departments in medical centers and hospitals.

Recent studies of psychotherapy in patients with cancer, including training in problem solving, have shown that it helps decrease feelings of depression.

Suicidal Patients with Cancer

The incidence of suicide in cancer patients may be as much as 10 times higher than the rate of suicide in the general population. One study has shown that the risk of suicide in patients with cancer is highest in the first months after diagnosis, and that this risk decreases significantly over decades. Passive suicidal thoughts are fairly common in patients with cancer. The relationships between suicidal tendency and the desire for hastened death, requests for physician-assisted suicide, and/or euthanasia are complicated and poorly understood. Men with cancer are at an increased risk of suicide compared with the general population, with more than twice the risk. Overdosing with painkillers and sedatives is the most common method of suicide by patients with cancer, with most cancer suicides occurring at home. The occurrence of suicide is higher in patients with oral, pharyngeal, and lung cancers, and in HIV-positive patients with Kaposi sarcoma. The actual incidence of suicide in cancer patients is probably underestimated, since there may be reluctance to report these deaths as suicides.

General risk factors for suicide in a person with cancer include a history of mental problems, especially those associated with impulsive behavior (such as borderline personality disorders), a family history of suicide, a history of suicide attempts, depression, substance abuse, the recent death of a friend or spouse, or having little social support.

Cancer-specific risk factors for suicide include a diagnosis of oral, throat, or lung cancer (often associated with heavy alcohol and tobacco use); advanced stage of disease and poor prognosis; confusion /delirium; poorly controlled pain; physical impairments such as loss of mobility, loss of bowel and bladder control, amputation, loss of eyesight or hearing, paralysis, inability to eat or swallow; tiredness; and exhaustion.

Patients who are suicidal require careful evaluation. The risk of suicide increases if the patient reports thoughts of suicide and has a plan to carry it out. Risk continues to increase if the plan is "lethal," that is, the plan is likely to cause death. A lethal suicide plan is more likely to be carried out if the way chosen to cause death is available to the person, the attempt cannot be stopped once it is started, and help is unavailable. When a person with cancer reports thoughts of death, it is important to determine whether the underlying cause is depression or a desire to control unbearable symptoms. Prompt identification and treatment of major depression is important in decreasing the risk for suicide. Risk factors, especially hopelessness (which is a better predictor for suicide than depression) should be carefully determined. The assessment of hopelessness is not easy in the person who has advanced cancer with no hope of a cure. It is important to determine the basic reasons for hopelessness, which may be related to cancer symptoms, fears of painful death, or feelings of abandonment.

Talking about suicide will not cause the patient to attempt suicide; it actually shows that this is a concern and permits the patient to describe his or her feelings and fears, providing a sense of control. A crisis intervention-oriented treatment approach should be used which involves the patient's support system. Contributing symptoms, such as pain, should be aggressively controlled and depression, psychosis, anxiety, and underlying causes of delirium should be treated. These problems are usually treated in a medical hospital or at home. Although not usually necessary, a suicidal patient with cancer may need to be hospitalized in a psychiatric unit.

The goal of treatment of suicidal patients is to attempt to prevent suicide that is caused by desperation due to poorly controlled symptoms. Patients close to the end of life may not be able to stay awake without a great amount of emotional or physical pain. This often leads to thoughts of suicide or requests for aid in dying. Such patients may need sedation to ease their distress.

Other treatment considerations include using medications that work quickly to alleviate distress (such as antianxiety medication or stimulants) while waiting for the antidepressant medication to work; limiting the quantities of medications that are lethal in overdose; having frequent contact with a health care professional who can closely observe the patient; avoiding long periods of time when the patient is alone; making sure the patient has available support; and determining the patient's mental and emotional response at each crisis point during the cancer experience.

Pain and symptom treatment should not be sacrificed simply to avoid the possibility that a patient will attempt suicide. Patients often have a method to commit suicide available to them. Incomplete pain and symptom treatment might actually worsen a patient's suicide risk.

Frequent contact with the health professional can help limit the amount of lethal drugs available to the patient and family. Infusion devices that limit patient access to medications can also be used at home or in the hospital. These are programmable, portable pumps with coded access and a locked cartridge containing the medication. These pumps are very useful in controlling pain and other symptoms. Some pumps can give multiple drug infusions, and some can be programmed over the phone. The devices are available through home care agencies, but are very expensive. Some of the expense may be covered by insurance.

Assisted Dying, Euthanasia, and Decisions Regarding End of Life

Respecting and promoting patient control has been one of the driving forces behind the hospice movement and right-to-die issues that range from honoring living wills to promoting euthanasia (mercy killing). These issues can create a conflict between a patient's desire for control and a physician's duty to promote health. These are issues of law, ethics, medicine, and philosophy. Some physicians may favor strong pain control and approve of the right of patients to refuse life support, but do not favor euthanasia or assisted suicide. Often patients who ask for physician-assisted suicide can be treated by increasing the patient's comfort and relieving symptoms, thereby reducing the patient's need for drastic measures. Patients with the desire to die should be carefully evaluated and treated for depression.

Palliative Sedation

The decision whether to sedate a patient at the end of life is difficult and involves many factors. The goal of palliative sedation is not to shorten life but to make the end of life more comfortable. Palliative sedation may be considered in order to relieve uncontrolled physical suffering, depression, or anxiety. Certain drugs are given to sedate the patient and may be combined with treatment for pain and agitation. Palliative sedation may be temporary, as in patients with delirium or trouble breathing.

A patient's thoughts and feelings about end-of-life sedation may depend greatly on his or her own culture and beliefs. Some patients who are nearing the end of life may want to be sedated. Other patients may wish to have no procedures, including sedation, just before death. It is important for the patient to tell family members and health care providers of his or her wishes about sedation at the end of life. When patients make their wishes about sedation known ahead of time, doctors and family members can be sure they are doing what the patient would want.

Considerations for Depression in Children

Most children cope with the emotions related to cancer and not only adjust well, but show positive emotional growth and development. A small number of children, however, develop psychological problems including depression, anxiety, sleeping problems, relationship problems, and are uncooperative about treatment. A mental health specialist should treat these children.

Children with severe late effects of cancer have more symptoms of depression. Anxiety usually occurs in younger patients, while depression is more common in older children. Most cancer survivors are generally able to adapt and adjust successfully to cancer and its treatment; however, a small number of cancer survivors have difficulty adjusting.

Individual and group counseling are usually used as the first treatment for a child with depression, and are directed at helping the child to master his or her difficulties and develop in the best way possible. Play therapy may be used as a way to explore the younger child's view of him- or herself, the disease, and treatment. From the beginning of treatment, a child needs help to understand, at his or her developmental level, the diagnosis of cancer and the treatment involved. A doctor may prescribe medications, such as antidepressants, for children.

Section 41.3

Cognitive Disorders and Delirium in Advanced Cancer

PDQ® Cancer Information Summary. National Cancer Institute; Bethesda, MD. Cognitive Disorders and Delirium (PDQ): Patient Version. Updated 08/2011. Available at: http://cancer.gov. Accessed November 24, 2011.

Overview

Cognitive disorders and delirium are conditions in which the patient experiences a confused mental state and changes in behavior. People who have cognitive disorders or delirium may fall in and out of consciousness and may have problems with attention, thinking, awareness, emotion, memory, muscle control, and sleeping and waking.

Delirium occurs frequently in patients with cancer, especially in patients with advanced cancer. Delirium usually occurs suddenly and the patient's symptoms may come and go during the day. This condition can be treated and is often temporary, even in people with advanced illness. In the last 24 to 48 hours of life, however, delirium may be permanent due to problems such as organ failure.

Causes of Cognitive Disorders and Delirium

Cognitive disorders and delirium may be complications of cancer and cancer treatment, especially in people with advanced cancer.

In patients with cancer, cognitive disorders and delirium may be due to the direct effects that cancer has on the brain, such as the pressure of a growing tumor. Cognitive disorders and delirium may also be caused by indirect effects of cancer or its treatment, including the following:

- Organ failure

- Electrolyte imbalances: Electrolytes are important minerals (including salt, potassium, calcium, and phosphorous) that are needed to keep the heart, kidneys, nerves, and muscles working correctly.

- Infection

- Symptoms caused by the cancer but that occur apart from the local or distant spread of the tumor (paraneoplastic syndromes), such as inflammation of the brain.

- Medication side effects: Patients with cancer usually take many medications. Some drugs have side effects that include delirium and confusion. The effects of these drugs usually go away after the drug is stopped.

- Withdrawal from drugs that depress (slow down) the central nervous system (brain and spinal cord).

Risk factors for delirium include having a serious disease and having more than one disease. Other conditions besides having cancer may place a patient at risk for developing delirium, including advanced cancer or other serious illness, having more than one disease, older age, previous mental disorder (such as dementia), low levels of albumin (protein) in the blood, infection, taking medications that affect the mind or behavior, and taking high doses of pain medication.

Early identification of risk factors may help prevent the onset of delirium or may reduce the length of time it takes to correct it.

Effects of Cognitive Disorders and Delirium

Cognitive disorders and delirium can be upsetting to the family and caregivers, and may be dangerous to the patient if judgment is affected. These conditions can cause the patient to act unpredictably and sometimes violently. Even a quiet or calm patient can suddenly experience a change in mood or become agitated, requiring increased care. The safety of the patient, family, and caregivers is most important.

Patients with cognitive disorders or delirium are more likely to fall, be incontinent (unable to control bladder and/or bowels), and become dehydrated (drink too little water to maintain health). They often require a longer hospital stay than patients without cognitive disorders or delirium.

The confused mental state of these patients may hinder their communication with family members and the health care providers. Assessment of the patient's symptoms becomes difficult and the patient may be unable to make decisions regarding care. Agitation in these patients may be mistaken as an expression of pain. Conflict can arise among the patient, family, and staff concerning the level of pain medication needed.

Diagnosis of Cognitive Disorders and Delirium

A patient who suddenly becomes agitated or uncooperative, experiences personality or behavior changes, has impaired thinking, decreased attention span, or intense, unusual anxiety or depression, may be experiencing cognitive disorders or delirium. Patients who develop these symptoms need to be assessed completely.

Early symptoms of delirium are similar to symptoms of anxiety, anger, depression, and dementia. Delirium that causes the patient to be very inactive may appear to be depression. Delirium and dementia are difficult to tell apart, since both may cause disorientation and impair memory, thinking, and judgment. Dementia may be caused by a number of medical conditions, including Alzheimer disease. Some differences in the symptoms of delirium and dementia include the following:

- Patients with delirium often go in and out of consciousness. Patients who have dementia usually remain alert.

- Delirium may occur suddenly. Dementia appears gradually and gets worse over time.

- Sleeping and waking problems are more common with delirium than with dementia.

In elderly patients who have cancer, dementia is often present along with delirium, making diagnosis difficult. The diagnosis is more likely dementia if symptoms continue after treatment for delirium is given.

In patients aged 65 or older who have survived cancer for more than five years, the risk for cognitive disorders and dementia is increased, apart from the risk for delirium. Regular screening of the patient and monitoring of the patient's symptoms can help in the diagnosis of delirium.

Treatment of Delirium

Deciding if, when, and how to treat a person with delirium depends on the setting, how advanced the cancer is, the wishes of the patient and family, and how the delirium symptoms are affecting the patient. Monitoring alone may be all that is necessary for patients who are not dangerous to themselves. In other cases, symptoms may be treated or causes of the delirium may be identified and treated.

Treatment of the Symptoms of Delirium by Changing the Patient's Surroundings

Controlling the patient's surroundings may help reduce mild symptoms of delirium. Changes—such as putting the patient in a quiet, well-lit room with familiar objects, placing a clock or calendar where the patient can see it, reducing noise, having family present, and limiting changes in caregivers—may be effective.

To prevent a patient from harming himself or herself or others, physical restraints also may be necessary.

Treatment of the Causes of Delirium

The standard approach to managing delirium is to find and treat the causes. Symptoms may be treated at the same time. Identifying the causes of delirium will include a physical examination to check general signs of health, including checking for signs of disease. A medical history of the patient's past illnesses and treatments will also be taken. In a terminally ill delirious patient being cared for at home, the doctor may do a limited assessment to determine the cause or may treat just the symptoms.

Treatment may include stopping or reducing medications that cause delirium, giving fluids into the bloodstream to correct dehydration, giving drugs to correct hypercalcemia (too much calcium in the blood), and giving antibiotics for infections.

Treatment of the Symptoms of Delirium with Medication

Drugs called antipsychotics may be used to treat the symptoms of delirium. Drugs that sedate (calm) the patient may also be used, especially if the patient is near death. All of these drugs have side effects and the patient will be monitored closely by a doctor. The decision to use drugs that sedate the patient will be made in cooperation with family members after efforts have been made to reverse the delirium.

Delirium, Sedation, and End-of-Life Issues

The decision to use drugs to sedate the patient who is near death and has symptoms of delirium, pain, and difficult breathing presents ethical and legal issues for both the doctor and the family. When the symptoms of delirium are not relieved with standard treatment approaches and the patient is experiencing severe distress and suffering, the doctor may discuss the option to give drugs that will sedate the patient. This decision is guided by the following principles:

- Health care professionals who have experience in palliative care make repeated assessments of the patient's response to treatments. The family is always included.

- The need to use drugs that sedate the patient is evaluated by a multidisciplinary team of health care professionals.

- Temporary sedation should be considered.

- A multidisciplinary team of health care professionals will work with the family to ensure that the family's views are assessed and understood. The family may need support from the health care team and mental health professionals while palliative sedation is used.

Chapter 42

Codependency and Mental Health

Minding Your Mental Health

Codependency is used to describe the person who becomes the caretaker of an addicted or troubled individual. The individual can be addicted to alcohol, drugs, or gambling. Or, he or she can be troubled by a physical or emotional illness. Codependents can be this individual's partner, lover, child, parent, brother, sister, co-worker, or friend. Codependents do these things:

- *Enable* or allow the person to continue his or her self-destructive or troubled behavior

- *Rescue* the person who has gotten into trouble from things, such as an arrest, accident, being absent or late for work

- *Make excuses* for the person's behavior

- *Deny* that the person has a problem

Typical Roles That Codependents Play

- **Rescuer:** Saves the person from unpleasant situations, for example, putting an alcoholic to bed after he/she passes out

- **Caretaker:** Takes care of all household and financial chores which hold the family together

"Mental Health: Codependency," U.S. Navy (www.nehc.med.navy.mil), February 25, 2009.

- **Joiner:** Rationalizes that the person's behavior is normal by simply allowing it to take place or by taking part in the same behavior as the addicted or troubled individual

- **Hero:** Becomes the "super person" to preserve the family image

- **Complainer:** Blames the person and makes him or her the scapegoat for all problems

- **Adjuster:** Withdraws from the family and acts like he/she doesn't care

Most codependents do not realize they have a co-dependent problem. They focus more energy on another's actions and needs than on their own. They think they are actually helping the troubled person, but they are not.

Questions to Ask

Do you do three or more of the following? If yes, see a counselor. If not, see Self-Help below.

- Think more about another person's behavior and problems than about your own life

- Feel anxious about the addicted or troubled person's behavior and constantly check on them to try to catch them in their bad behavior

- Worry that if you stop trying to control the other person, that he or she will fall apart

- Blame yourself for this person's problems

- Cover up or rescue this person when they are caught in a lie or other embarrassing situation related to their addiction or other problem

- Deny that this person has a real problem with drugs, alcohol, etc. and become angry and/or defensive when others suggest there is an addiction or other substance abuse problem

You may not be truly codependent, but you should become aware of how your behavior may be enabling an addicted or troubled individual.

Self-Help

Most codependents are not in touch with their co-dependency and may need help to see it. The following self-help tips are general suggestions. For many people, these are not easy to do without the help of a counselor.

- Read books on codependency. You can find these in the library and bookstores. You may find you identify with what you read and gain understanding.

- Focus on these three C's:
  - You did not Cause the other person's problem.
  - You can't Control the other person.
  - You can't Cure the problem.

- Don't lie, make excuses, or cover up for the abuser's drinking, drug, or other problem. Admit to yourself that this way of living is not normal and that the abuser or troubled person has a problem that needs professional help.

- Refuse to come to the person's aid. Every time you bail the abuser out of trouble, you reinforce their helplessness and your hopelessness.

- If you or your children are being physically, verbally, or sexually abused, do not allow it to continue. Seek the help of shelters for victims of domestic violence.

- Know that there are many support groups which help codependents. Examples are self-help groups for family and friends of substance abusers, such as Al-Anon, Alateen, and Children of Alcoholics Foundation (COAF). Other self-help and support groups are offered through community health education programs.

- Continue your normal family routines, for example, include the drinker when he/she is sober.

- Focus on your own feelings, desires, and needs. Begin to do what is good for your own well-being.

- Allow children to express their feelings. Show them how by expressing your own.

- Set limits on what you will and won't do. Be firm and stick to these limits.

- Engage in new experiences and interests. Find diversion from your loved one's problem.

- Take responsibility for yourself and others in the family to live a better life whether your loved one recovers or not.

What You Can Do for a Friend or Relative

Persons who are codependent may not realize they have a problem, deny they have a problem, and/or refuse to get help. If you think someone you know is codependent, the following tips can help you help them:

- Let them know that you are concerned for their well-being and health.

- Encourage them to seek professional help and/or join a support group.

Chapter 43

Diabetes and Mental Health

Depression

- People with diabetes are at greater risk for depression.
- Poor diabetes control can cause symptoms that look like depression.
- If physical causes are ruled out, you may be referred to a specialist for mental health treatment, including psychotherapy and antidepressant medication.

Feeling down once in a while is normal. But some people feel a sadness that just won't go away. Life seems hopeless. Feeling this way most of the day for two weeks or more is a sign of serious depression.

Does Diabetes Cause Depression?

At any given time, most people with diabetes do not have depression. But studies show that people with diabetes have a greater risk of depression than people without diabetes. There are no easy answers about why this is true.

The stress of daily diabetes management can build. You may feel alone or set apart from your friends and family because of all this extra work.

If you face diabetes complications such as nerve damage, or if you are having trouble keeping your blood sugar levels where you'd like, you may feel like you're losing control of your diabetes. Even tension between you and your doctor may make you feel frustrated and sad.

Just like denial, depression can get you into a vicious cycle. It can block good diabetes self-care. If you are depressed and have no energy, chances are you will find such tasks as regular blood sugar testing too much. If you feel so anxious that you can't think straight, it will be hard to keep up with a good diet. You may not feel like eating at all. Of course, this will affect your blood sugar levels.

Spotting Depression

Spotting depression is the first step. Getting help is the second. If you have been feeling really sad, blue, or down in the dumps, check for these symptoms:

- **Loss of pleasure:** You no longer take interest in doing things you used to enjoy.

- **Change in sleep patterns:** You have trouble falling asleep, you wake often during the night, or you want to sleep more than usual, including during the day.

- **Early to rise:** You wake up earlier than usual and cannot to get back to sleep.

- **Change in appetite:** You eat more or less than you used to, resulting in a quick weight gain or weight loss.

- **Trouble concentrating:** You can't watch a TV program or read an article because other thoughts or feelings get in the way.

- **Loss of energy:** You feel tired all the time.

- **Nervousness:** You always feel so anxious you can't sit still.

- **Guilt:** You feel you "never do anything right" and worry that you are a burden to others.

- **Morning sadness:** You feel worse in the morning than you do the rest of the day.

- **Suicidal thoughts:** You feel you want to die or are thinking about ways to hurt yourself.

If you have three or more of these symptoms, or if you have just one or two but have been feeling bad for two weeks or more, it's time to get help.

Getting Help

If you are feeling symptoms of depression, don't keep them to your-self. First, talk them over with your doctor. There may a physical cause for your depression.

Poor control of diabetes can cause symptoms that look like depres-sion. During the day, high or low blood sugar may make you feel tired or anxious. Low blood sugar levels can also lead to hunger and eating too much. If you have low blood sugar at night, it could disturb your sleep. If you have high blood sugar at night, you may get up often to urinate and then feel tired during the day.

Other physical causes of depression can include the following:

- Alcohol or drug abuse

- Thyroid problems

- Side effects from some medications

Do not stop taking a medication without telling your doctor. Your doctor will be able to help you discover if a physical problem is at the root of your sad feelings.

Mental Health Treatment

If you and your doctor rule out physical causes, your doctor will most likely refer you to a specialist. You might talk with a psychia-trist, psychologist, psychiatric nurse, licensed clinical social worker, or professional counselor. In fact, your doctor may already work with mental health professionals on a diabetes treatment team.

All of these mental health professionals can guide you through the rough waters of depression. In general, there are two types of treatment:

- Psychotherapy or counseling

- Antidepressant medication

Psychotherapy

Psychotherapy with a well-trained therapist can help you look at the problems that bring on depression. It can also help you find ways

587

to relieve the problem. Therapy can be short term or long term. You should be sure you feel at ease with the therapist you choose.

Medication

If medication is advised, you will need to consult with a psychiatrist (a medical doctor with special training in diagnosing and treating mental or emotional disorders). Psychiatrists are the only mental health professionals who can prescribe medication and treat physical causes of depression.

If you opt for trying an antidepressant drug, talk to the psychiatrist and your primary care provider about side effects, including how it might affect your blood sugar levels. Make sure that the doctors will consult about your care when needed. Many people do well with a combination of medication and psychotherapy.

If you have symptoms of depression, don't wait too long to get help. If your health care provider cannot refer you to a mental health professional, contact your local psychiatric society or psychiatry department of a medical school, or the local branch of organizations for psychiatric social workers, psychologists, or mental health counselors. Your local American Diabetes Association may also be a good resource for counselors who have worked with people with diabetes.

Chapter 44

Epilepsy and Mental Health

Depression and anxiety disorders are very common in people with epilepsy. The altered brain activity that causes epileptic seizures can lead to depressive moods and the stress of living with a chronic condition can worsen feelings of depression and anxiety. As a consequence, epilepsy may be more difficult to manage as depression is sometimes known to make seizures more frequent[1] and can take away the motivation to manage epilepsy effectively.

Fortunately, once diagnosed, depression and anxiety disorders can be safely and effectively treated at the same time as epilepsy. Treatments for mental health conditions can greatly improve quality of life and can reduce the frequency and impact of seizures.[2] This chapter looks at the relationship between epilepsy, depression, and anxiety disorders, and gives advice on how to manage these conditions if they occur.

What Is Epilepsy?

Epilepsy is a common neurological (brain) condition characterized by disruptions in regular brain activity known as seizures. Epilepsy affects around one percent of the population.[3] Although epilepsy is more

Excerpted from "Depression and Anxiety Disorders People with Epilepsy" (Fact Sheet 47), reprinted with permission from BeyondBlue: The National Depression Initiative, www.beyondblue.org.au. © 2010 Beyond Blue Ltd. All rights reserved. The complete text of this factsheet including additional references and resources is available online at www.beyondblue.org.au.

likely to be diagnosed in childhood or senior years, it is not confined to any age group, sex or race.

There are many types of seizures. These are commonly grouped as:[4]

- **Partial seizures:** Causing strange sensations, twitching, or changes in mood and behavior

- **Generalized seizures:** Causing unconsciousness, stiffness, and jerking of the muscles.

Frequent seizures may cause difficulties at school or the workplace, as well as sometimes hindering the development of new friendships and relationships. Fortunately, epilepsy can be managed with antiepileptic medications and more than 70 percent of people become seizure-free with treatment.[3] With sensible management of diet, alcohol intake, and seizure triggers, it is possible to lead a full and active life.

What Are the Links Between Depression, Anxiety Disorders, and Epilepsy?

Research shows there are strong links between depression, anxiety disorders, and epilepsy—around half of all adults with epilepsy experience depression[5] and around one in five experiences generalized anxiety disorder (GAD).[2] The rate of anxiety is similar to that for people with other chronic illnesses such as asthma or diabetes. It seems that, as for these conditions, the stress of living with epilepsy increases the risk of anxiety disorders.[5]

It's a slightly different story for depression. People with epilepsy experience depression at two to three times the rate of the general population[2] and are more likely to experience depression than people with other chronic conditions.[6] This means that while these depressive feelings can be partly due to the stress of living with a chronic condition, they are mainly caused by the same abnormal brain activity that normally occurs with seizures.[2]

The connections between epilepsy, depression, and anxiety disorders are complex.

- **Depression may exist before the diagnosis of epilepsy:** People with a history of depression are four to six times more likely to develop epilepsy.[7] This is because the genetic or biological factors that cause both epilepsy and depression[2] sometimes express themselves as unexplained feelings of sadness before the first recognizable seizure.[5] If untreated, this makes the onset of epilepsy more likely, particularly when symptoms of depression, such as sleep deprivation and alcohol misuse, can further increase the chance of a seizure occurring.[1]

- **Depressive symptoms may be directly caused by seizures:** These brain disruptions may have little or no physical symptoms, but can lead to unexplained feelings of sadness, guilt, or an inability to take pleasure in any activity.[8] Some people may only have depressive feelings prior to, or after, seizure, while for others it is ongoing. Seizures may also cause serious thoughts of suicide, regardless of whether or not the person feels negatively about his/her life.[7]

- **Depression or anxiety may develop soon after a diagnosis of epilepsy:** Being diagnosed with a chronic condition is a negative life event, like loss, separation, or trauma, which can result in feelings such as denial, anger, grief, and lowered self-esteem. These are all a normal part of adapting to changes in lifestyle and the way you view yourself and your life. However, for some people these feelings do not pass with time and can lead to the development of depression.

- **Depression or an anxiety disorder may develop as a consequence of living with epilepsy:** Over time, the impact of epilepsy on health,[9] work,[10] relationships[11] and overall quality of life,[6] as well as the social stigma attached to seizures,[12,13] can lead to social isolation, lowered self-esteem, and depression, particularly in those with epilepsy for more than five years.[14]

Regardless of whether depression or anxiety disorders come before or after epilepsy, both conditions can severely affect quality of life and can do so even more than the seizures themselves.[13] These conditions together can also create a vicious cycle—just as poorly controlled seizures increase the risk of depression, untreated depression makes seizures more frequent[1] and more severe.[7]

An important thing to remember is that if you do experience depression or an anxiety disorder, effective treatments are available and recovery is possible. Epilepsy management becomes easier as depression lifts and treatments that tackle depression, such as psychological therapy, also reduce the frequency of seizures.[2]

What Is Depression?

Depression is more than just sadness or a low mood—it's a serious illness that can have severe effects on both physical and mental health.

People with depression find it hard to function every day and may be reluctant to participate in activities they once enjoyed. Being aware of the signs of depression and seeking help if you think you may need it are important because effective treatments are available.

Signs of Depression

People may be experiencing depression if, for more than two weeks, they have been behaving in a way that is out of character. Common behaviors associated with depression include:

- moodiness that is out of character;
- increased irritability and frustration;
- finding it hard to accept minor personal criticism;
- spending less time with friends and family;
- loss of interest in pleasurable activities (such as eating, sex, exercise);
- being awake throughout the night;
- increased alcohol and/or drug use;
- staying home from work;
- increased physical health complaints such as fatigue or pain;
- being reckless or taking unnecessary risks;
- slowing down of thoughts or actions.

Everyone experiences some or all of these symptoms from time to time, but when symptoms are severe and lasting, it's time to seek professional help.

What Is Anxiety?

Most people feel anxious sometimes, but for some people, anxious feelings are overwhelming and cannot be brought under control easily. An anxiety disorder is a serious condition that makes it hard for the person to cope from day to day. There are many types of anxiety disorders, each with a range of symptoms. Living with epilepsy is one of many things—such as a family history of mental health problems, stressful life events, personality factors—that may trigger anxiety. Combined with a chronic physical illness, lost educational or employment opportunities, financial worries, and the constant fear of seizures can lead to the development of an anxiety disorder.

Signs of Anxiety

A person may be experiencing an anxiety disorder if, for some time, worry and fear have got in the way of other parts of life—like how things are at work or in relationships. An anxiety disorder will usually be far more intense than normal anxiety and go on for weeks, months or even longer. An anxiety disorder can be expressed in different ways such as uncontrollable worry, intense fear (phobias or panic attacks), or upsetting dreams or flashbacks of a traumatic event.

Like depression, there are effective treatments available for anxiety disorders.

Helpful Tips for Managing Anxiety and Depression

If you have epilepsy and you suspect you may be experiencing depression or an anxiety disorder—and/or you have a diagnosis—the following tips may be helpful:

- Speak to your doctor about your concerns and discuss treatment options.
- Accept help, support, and encouragement from family and friends.
- Avoid feeling isolated by becoming involved in support groups and social activities.
- Exercise regularly.
- Eat healthily and include a wide variety of nutritious foods.
- Achieve and maintain a healthy weight.
- Get enough sleep.
- Allow yourself time to relax and reduce your stress.
- Go to your doctor for regular check-ups.

What Are the Treatments for Anxiety and Depression?

Managing depression and anxiety disorders can greatly improve people's well-being and quality of life as well as their epilepsy and their attitude towards it.[7] There is a range of effective treatments for people with epilepsy who experience an anxiety disorder or depression.

Different types of depression and anxiety disorders require different types of treatments. These may range from physical exercise for preventing and treating mild depression, through to psychological treatments for anxiety disorders and depression, and a combination of psychological and drug treatments for more severe levels of depression and anxiety disorders.

Whatever the reason for mental health problems, it is important to seek help as soon as possible. Depression and anxiety disorders are both common and treatable, and a doctor will be able to help you decide whether treatment is needed and what treatments are suitable.

- Psychological therapies may not only help with recovery, but can also help prevent a recurrence of depression or anxiety. These therapies help build skills in coping with stressful life circumstances.

- Cognitive behavior therapy (CBT) is one of the most researched psychological therapies and there is a lot of evidence to support its effectiveness in treating people for depression and anxiety disorders. It teaches people to think realistically about common difficulties, helping them to change their thought patterns and the way they react to certain situations.

- Interpersonal therapy (IPT) has also been researched and found to be effective for treatment of depression and some anxiety disorders. It helps people find new ways to get along with others and to resolve losses, changes and conflict in relationships.

- Antidepressant medication can play a role when people become severely depressed or when other treatments are ineffective. Some types of antidepressants can be helpful for the management of anxiety disorders. Deciding which antidepressants are best for a person can be complex. There is a range of factors that should be discussed with a doctor before starting antidepressants.

- Benzodiazepines are anti-anxiety and sedative drugs commonly used to help people cope with anxiety or insomnia. They are, however, addictive and so are only useful for a short period of time (two or three weeks) or if used intermittently.

It is important that any current medication for epilepsy, including over-the-counter preparations and herbal or natural remedies, is reviewed by a medical practitioner before starting a course of medication. Talk to the doctor or pharmacist to rule out the possibility of adverse interaction between any medications being taken.

In the past, some doctors feared antidepressant medications would cause problems for epilepsy treatment, but recent research has shown this is not true.[1,2] In fact, antidepressants can reduce the likelihood of seizures as well as treating depression.[2]

Antidepressant medication can take 14 to 21 days before it begins to work effectively. The prescribing health professional should discuss differences in effects and possible side-effects of medications. Stopping medication should only be done gradually, with a doctor's recommendation and under supervision.

Most people taking medication will also benefit from psychological therapies, which will reduce the likelihood of relapse after the person has stopped taking the medication. The Therapeutic Goods Administration (Australia's regulatory agency for medical drugs) and the manufacturers of antidepressants do not recommend antidepressants as a first-line treatment for depression in young people under the age of 18.

How to Get the Right Treatment

- **Be proactive:** As with physical health problems, the earlier you get help, the faster you can recover. That's why it is very important to get help at the first sign of any problems.

- **Be direct:** It's important to give the doctor or mental health professional the full picture. Writing down feelings or questions before your visit can help and makes it less likely you will forget to tell the doctor the important things. It may be useful to take a completed depression checklist along, such as those on the BeyondBlue website (www.beyondblue.org.au).

- **Be persistent:** Finding the right mental health professional is very important. If you don't feel comfortable with a doctor or other health professional, or suspect your mental health isn't being managed effectively, choose another doctor or get a second opinion.

- **Be prepared to follow the treatment plan:** For some people, it can take a while before they feel well again. It's important for your long-term recovery that you stick with treatment plans and let the doctor know when things aren't working or if you are experiencing side-effects.

Helpful Strategies

- If you have been recently diagnosed with epilepsy, be gentle on yourself. Think about how you have faced previous stressful situations in your life and what helped you cope (and what didn't). Get support from friends and family, and learn as much about epilepsy and its management as you can.

- Initially, most people find managing epilepsy a real challenge. Until seizures are controlled with medication, the possibility of seizures in public can be a real concern. You may find it helpful to contact other people with epilepsy so you can learn from them and share your experiences.

- Take a partner or carer with you when you go to the doctor. Not only can they help you remember what was discussed, ask questions, and give you support, but they may benefit from having a better understanding of epilepsy and its treatments.

- Remember that, like epilepsy, depression and anxiety disorders can be treated or managed. As having these conditions can affect the way you manage your epilepsy, it's important to seek help early—the sooner the better.

References

1. Jackson, M & Turkington, D. (2005) "Depression and Anxiety in Epilepsy." Journal of Neurology, Neurosurgery and Psychiatry 76: i45–i47.

2. Ekinci, O et al. (2008) "Depression and anxiety in children and adolescents with epilepsy: Prevalence, risk factors, and treatment." Epilepsy & Behavior 14: 8–18.

3. Epilepsy Action Australia (2008) Understanding Epilepsy. Available at: http://www.epilepsy.org.au/understanding_epilepsy.asp

4. Epilepsy Action Australia (2008) Epilepsy Explained. Available at: http://www.epilepsy.org.au/epilepsy_explained2.asp#1

5. Loney, J et al. (2008) "Anxiety and Depressive Symptoms in Children Presenting With a First Seizure." Pediatric Neurology 39(4): 236–240.

6. Thomson, E & Brennenstuhl, S. (2008) "The association between depression and epilepsy in a nationally representative sample." Epilepsia 50(5): 1051–1058.

7. Mazza, S. (2006) "Depression and suicide in epilepsy: fact or artefact?" Journal of the Neurological Sciences 260: 300–301.

8. Balabanov, A et al. (2004) "Unrecognized and Untreated: Preventing and Treating Depression in Patients With Epilepsy." *Psychiatric Times* 21(13): 23–32.

9. Yu, C et al. (2008) "Health behavior in teens with epilepsy: How do they compare with controls?" *Epilepsy & Behavior* 13: 90–95.

10. Baker, G. (2008) "Perceived impact of epilepsy in teenagers and young adults: An international survey." *Epilepsy & Behavior* 12: 395–401.

11. Devinsky, O. (2003) "Psychiatric comorbidity in patients with epilepsy: Implications for diagnosis and treatment." *Epilepsy & Behavior* 4: S2–S10.

12. Hamiwka, L et al. (2009) 'Are children with epilepsy at greater risk for bullying than their peers?' *Epilepsy & Behavior* 15: 500–505.

13. Boer, H et al. (2008) "The global burden and stigma of epilepsy." *Epilepsy & Behavior* 12: 540–546.

14. Mikhailov, S et al. (2004) "Depression as a Factor Affecting the Quality-of-Life Assessment in Patients with Epilepsy." *International Journal of Mental Health* 33(3): 63–68.

Chapter 45

Heart Disease and Mental Health

Mental Health and Heart Risk

What types of mental health problems can contribute to heart disease?

The mental health problems that can play a role in heart disease are usually broken down into two categories: emotional factors, including depression, anxiety, and hostility; and chronic stressors, including low social support, the strain of being a caregiver, and work stress.

How common are mental health problems for people with heart disease?

A large survey showed that 2.8% of otherwise healthy people experienced psychological distress symptoms that fall short of a diagnosis for mental illness. By comparison, 10% of women with heart failure, 6.4% for those who had had a heart attack, and 4.1% of people with other types of heart disease experienced psychological distress. In this survey, women were more likely than men to show signs of psychological distress (67.2% vs. 32.8%).

From "Mental Health and Heart Risk," "Mental Health and Heart Risk: Anxiety," and "Stress and Heart Risk." Reprinted with permission from www .hearthealthywomen.org, © 2012. All rights reserved. The complete text of these documents, including references, is available online at http://www.hearthealthy women.org/am-i-at-risk/stress-mentalhealth/mental-health.html, /mh2.html, and /mh5.html.

Women are also more prone to depression than men after a heart attack or bypass surgery. A study of more than 93,000 women found that having any sort of serious heart-related event such as a heart attack or stroke or a major procedure to treat heart disease (e.g., bypass surgery) makes a person much more likely to suffer from depression. Your doctor can recommend ways to deal with any mental health problems you may be having.

What is depression?

A person is considered to be clinically depressed if they have a depressed mood and a lack of interest in activities that used to be enjoyable, lasting for at least 2 weeks, and accompanied by at least one of the following: changes in appetite, sleep disturbance, fatigue, agitation, feelings of guilt or worthlessness, problems concentrating, and suicidal thoughts.

Symptoms of Depression

Source: National Institute of Mental Health

- Persistent sad, anxious, or empty mood
- Feelings of hopelessness, pessimism
- Feelings of guilt, worthlessness, helplessness
- Loss of interest or pleasure in hobbies and activities that were once enjoyed, including sex
- Decreased energy, fatigue, being "slowed down"
- Difficulty concentrating, remembering, making decisions
- Insomnia, waking up early, or oversleeping
- Loss of appetite and weight loss, or overeating and weight gain
- Thoughts of death or suicide; suicide attempts
- Restlessness, irritability
- Persistent physical symptoms that do not respond to treatment, such as headaches, digestive disorders, and chronic pain

How common is depression?

According to the National Institute for Mental Health, about 18.8 million Americans (9.5% of the population) 18 years and older suffer from depression in a given year; nearly twice as many women (12%) as men (6.6%) suffer from depression each year.

An even greater number of women have depressive symptoms that are not severe enough to be classified as clinical depression. In the Women's Health Initiative Study (WHI) of more than 93,000 post-menopausal women without clinical depression, depressive symptoms were reported by nearly 16% of women. Hispanic and American-Indian Alaskan-Native women had the highest rates of depressive symptoms while Asian-Pacific Islanders had the lowest rates.

How common is depression for people with heart disease?

A national survey found that for people age 15 to 54 years, about 5% will suffer from depression. The rate of depression among people with heart disease was about three times higher (15%).

How does depression affect my risk of heart disease?

Depression affects heart health in many ways, though more research is needed to understand exactly how. Depression can alter your heart's ability to beat properly; it can increase the buildup of fatty plaques in your blood vessels; and it has been linked to eating and exercise habits.

A study of nearly 63,000 women in the Nurse's Health Study found that women who experienced the symptoms of depression were 50% more likely to die of heart disease than women who did not, even after other heart disease risk factors were taken into account. Depression also increases the chance of having another heart attack in people who have already had one. The more depressed you are, the higher your risk of having heart troubles.

Mental Health and Heart Risk—Anxiety

What is anxiety?

Anxiety is a state of fear, worry, or uneasiness, sometimes about future events. Anxiety may also occur in certain situations, as is the case with social anxiety. It may also take the form of panic attacks. Phobic anxiety is a condition where a specific phobia causes a person to have anxiety. A phobia is a fear that is irrational or excessive.

Accompanying the fear is a strong desire to avoid what you fear and, in some cases, an inability to function at normal tasks in your job or social settings. Examples of phobias include fear of enclosed spaces, fear of heights, or fear of being out in public.

601

How common is anxiety for people with heart disease?

Approximately 19.1 million Americans age 18 to 54 have an anxiety disorder (13.3% of the total population). Women are more likely than men to have an anxiety disorder, and about twice as many women than men suffer from panic disorder, post traumatic stress disorder, generalized anxiety, agoraphobia (fear of open spaces), as well as other phobias.

Symptoms of Anxiety

Source: National Institute of Mental Health

- Unable to relax or concentrate
- Easily startled
- Fatigue
- Headaches
- Muscle tension and muscle aches
- Trembling or twitching
- Irritability
- Sweating or hot flashes
- Feeling lightheaded or out of breath
- Nauseous
- Going to the bathroom frequently
- Trouble falling or staying asleep

How does anxiety affect my risk of heart disease?

General anxiety has been linked to heart disease risk in only a few studies. However, having a phobia has been strongly linked to poor heart health in men but not in women. Three studies of nearly 35,000 men have shown a strong link between phobic anxiety and death from heart disease. However, one large study of more than 72,000 women did not conclusively find a link between this kind of anxiety and heart disease-related deaths. Women are more likely than men to suffer anxiety from their phobias, and this condition is often linked to depression.

Anxiety affects the way the heart beats, making it less able to adjust to increases in heart rate. Anxiety has been linked to an increased risk of sudden cardiac death—a sudden, unexplained failure of the heart, often with little or no warning—but not the risk of heart attacks.

Stress and Heart Risk

What is stress?

Stress is a mentally or emotionally disruptive condition that occurs in response to outside influences. It is usually characterized by a faster heart rate, a rise in blood pressure, tensing of the muscles, irritability, and depression.

Can stress affect my risk of heart disease?

Yes. However, when researchers talk about the effects of stress, they speak specifically to the kinds of events that trigger this response. Many of these triggers are short term, such as experiencing a death in the family or surviving a car crash. However, stressors that are likely to affect your risk of heart disease are more long term. They are often called chronic stressors. Chronic stressors include those discussed below.

Lack of social support: Social support is the friendship, encouragement, and companionship that family and friends provide. People with fewer connections to friends and family have a higher risk of heart disease and heart attack. In a review of 15 studies that examined the effects of social factors on heart disease, having a relatively small network of family and friends increased a person's risk of having heart disease 2- to 3-fold over time, compared with people who have larger social support groups.

In a study of over 500 women who likely had heart disease, those who had larger, more supportive social networks had fewer risk factors including lower blood sugar levels, lower rates of smoking, and lower rates of high blood pressure and diabetes, and were slimmer than those with smaller social circles.

While living alone has been shown to increase the risk of heart disease in men, the same has not been seen in women because women are more likely than men to develop close friendships outside of marriage.

Poverty: Not earning much money increases the risk of heart attacks in both healthy people and those with heart disease. This may be due, in part, to both the stress of poverty and reduced access to healthcare. Poverty has also been linked to poorer health habits, higher rates of heart disease risk factors, increased levels of high-risk behaviors such as smoking and drinking alcohol, and other psychosocial risk factors such as chronic stress. Researchers also think that much of the risk associated with smaller social circles could be explained by income level. A large, all-female study showed that women with the fewest social ties were much more likely to have an annual income below $20,000 and a low income level was significantly associated with an increased risk of death. Your income level is also related to the type of work you do, which may influence your stress level.

Work-related stress: The relationship between work stress and heart disease is still up for discussion. Data from a study of more than 3,000 people (44% were women) show that over 10 years, women in high-powered jobs with high degrees of authority and control had almost three times the risk of developing heart disease than women in high-demand jobs who had little control over the work they do, such as factory workers. This is different than the findings in men, where those with lots of control over their work are less likely to have heart disease than those with busy jobs but little control. In another large study of over 10,000 people, being stressed at work was significantly related to heart disease risk in men and women, regardless of job type.

In a study of more than 1,300 women, having a "high pressure deadline at work" made both men and woman six times more likely to have a heart attack within the next 24 hours. A change in financial circumstances tripled a woman's risk of heart attack. Women were also three times more likely to experience a heart attack if they had recently taken on more responsibilities at work, particularly if they were unhappy about these new responsibilities.

However, the Nurses' Health Study of more than 35,000 women found that job strain was not related to an increased risk of heart disease. Women in this study were between the ages of 46 and 71 and were followed for an average of four years. Though they were all registered nurses, they performed different jobs, some of which were more stressful than others. After adjusting for other risk factors including age and smoking, women in high-strain jobs did not have a higher incidence of heart disease compared with those in low-strain jobs, and neither women in active or passive jobs showed an increased risk of heart disease.

Marital stress: Marital stress may be a greater risk for women who already have some form of heart disease than for those with healthy hearts. One all-female report found that severe stress in a marriage or live-in relationship can triple a woman's risk of a second heart attack or angina. Marital stress may also affect risk factors. Women in the Pittsburgh Healthy Women Study who were either dissatisfied with their marriage, were divorced, or widowed were significantly more likely to develop metabolic syndrome after nearly 12 years. Single women, however, showed no significant difference from happily married women.

Caregiver stress: Caring for people who are elderly, ill, or disabled is burdensome and stressful for many families and may lead to depression. Studies have shown that female caregivers are less likely to take care of their own health, and their blood pressure tends to rise when they are in the presence of the person they care for.

In the Nurses' Health Study, of more than 54,000 women, those who cared for a disabled or ill spouse for nine hours or more per week were about twice as likely to develop heart disease in the next four years. However, caring for disabled or ill parents, children, or friends did not significantly increase a woman's risk. Other results from the Nurses' Health Study also showed that being under strain from caregiving could increase your risk of death from any cause.

Caring for a family member or spouse isn't always bad for your health. The risks are not due to the act of caregiving alone, but occur only when the act is viewed as stressful.

How can depression or stress be treated?

There are many things you can do to combat depression and stress. Finding social support either from friends and family or through a support group can be helpful. Managing your stress can also help treat depression.

There are also several different types of treatments available for women who are under a lot of stress—the key is to find the method that is right for you. Many women find that relaxation exercises and meditation help alleviate stress. Relaxation exercises involve the flexing and releasing of major muscle groups. Breathing exercises also help to reduce stress. Exercise has also been shown to be a very effective way of reducing stress because it reduces the amount of stress hormones that your body releases. Many cardiac rehabilitation programs also teach stress management techniques.

If you can't lower stress or depression by yourself, you may want professional help. Licensed therapists, psychologists, marriage and family therapists, pastoral counselors, clinical social workers, and psychiatrists offer short-term psychotherapy. A psychiatrist may also help a person overcome their depression. Talk to your doctor. There are medications that he or she can prescribe to help treat depression called selective serotonin reuptake inhibitors such as Zoloft and Paxil. Though these medications do have serious side effects, most studies show that they are safe and effective for people with heart disease. Your doctor can help you weigh the risks and benefits of using these medications.

Chapter 46

Human Immunodeficiency Virus (HIV) and Mental Health

Overview

If you are diagnosed with HIV, your physical health is not the only issue you have to deal with. Along with the physical illness are mental health conditions that may come up, such as depression and anxiety. Mental health refers to the overall well-being of a person, including a person's mood, emotions, and behavior.

Many people are surprised when they learn that they have been infected with HIV. Some people feel overwhelmed by the changes that they will need to make in their lives. It is normal to have strong reactions when you find out you are HIV positive, including feelings such as fear, anger, and a sense of being overwhelmed. Often people feel helpless, sad, and anxious about the illness.

Some things to keep in mind about your feelings:

- No matter what you are feeling, you have a right to feel that way.

- There are no "wrong" or "right" feelings; feelings just are.

- Feelings come and go.

- You have choices about how you respond to your feelings.

"Coping with HIV/AIDS: Mental Health" August 3, 2011. Reprinted with permission from http://hivinsite.ucsf.edu, a project of the University of California San Francisco Center for HIV Information. © 2011 Regents of the University of California. All rights reserved.

There are many things you can do to deal with the emotional aspects of having HIV. What follows are some of the most common feelings associated with a diagnosis of HIV and suggestions on how to cope with these feelings. You may experience some, all, or none of these feelings, and you may experience them at different times.

Denial

People who find out that they are HIV positive often deal with the news by denying that it is true. You may believe that the HIV test was not accurate or that there was a mix-up with the result, even after confirmatory testing shows that it is a true positive. This is a natural and normal first reaction.

At first, this denial may even be helpful, because it can give you time to get used to the idea of infection. However, if not dealt with, denial can be dangerous; you may fail to take certain precautions or reach out for the necessary help and medical support.

It is important that you talk out your feelings with your doctor, a therapist, or someone you trust. It is important to do this so that you can begin to receive the care and support you need.

Anger

Anger is another common and natural feeling related to being diagnosed with HIV. Many people are upset about how they got the virus or angry that they didn't know they had the virus.

Ways to deal with feelings of anger include the following:

- Talk about your feelings with others, such as people in a support group, or with a counselor, friend, or social worker.

- Try to get some exercise—like gardening, walking, or dancing—to relieve some of the tension and angry feelings you may be experiencing.

- Avoid situations—involving certain people, places, and events—that cause you to feel angry or stressed out. Using drugs or alcohol when you feel angry can be dangerous for you and lead to conflict or violence that might otherwise have been avoidable.

Sadness or Depression

It is also normal to feel sad when you learn you have HIV. If, over time, you find that the sadness doesn't go away or is getting worse, talk with your doctor or someone else you trust. You may be depressed.

Symptoms of depression can include the following, especially if they last for more than two weeks:

- Feeling sad, anxious, irritable, or hopeless
- Gaining or losing weight
- Sleeping more or less than usual
- Moving slower than usual or finding it hard to sit still
- Losing interest in the things you usually enjoy
- Feeling tired all the time
- Feeling worthless or guilty
- Having a hard time concentrating
- Thinking about death or giving up
- Persistent loss of libido or interest in sex

To deal with these symptoms, you may want to:

- Talk with your doctor about treatments for depression, such as therapy or medicines
- Get involved with a support group
- Spend time with supportive people, such as family members and friends

If your mood swings or depression get very severe, or if you ever think about suicide, call your doctor right away. Your doctor can help you.

Finding the right treatment for depression takes time; so does recovery. If you think you may be depressed, don't lose hope. Instead, talk to your health care provider and seek help for depression.

Fear and Anxiety

Fear and anxiety may be caused by not knowing what to expect after you've been diagnosed with HIV, or by not knowing how others will treat you if they find out you have HIV. You also may be afraid of telling people—friends, family members, and others—that you are HIV positive.

Fear can make your heart beat faster or make it hard for you to sleep. Anxiety also can make you feel nervous or agitated. Fear and anxiety might make you sweat, feel dizzy, or feel short of breath.

Ways to control your feelings of fear and anxiety include the following:

- Learn as much as you can about HIV. HIV infection is now a very treatable disease and most HIV-infected people can live long, healthy lives if they seek medical care and take good care of themselves. Current HIV medications can be very well tolerated and in general do not lead to the body changes that were seen with older treatments.

- Have your questions answered by your doctor.

- Talk with your friends, family members, and health care providers.

- Join a support group.

- Help others who are in the same situation, such as by volunteering at an HIV service organization. This may empower you and lessen your feelings of fear.

- Talk to your doctor about medicines for anxiety if the feelings don't lessen with time or if they get worse.

Stress

If you are HIV infected, you and your loved ones constantly have to deal with stress. Stress is unique and personal to each of us. When stress does occur, it is important to recognize the fact and deal with it. Some ways to handle stress are discussed below. As you gain more understanding about how stress affects you, you will come up with your own ideas for coping with stress.

- Try physical activity. When you are nervous, angry, or upset, try exercise or some other kind of physical activity. Walking, yoga, and gardening are just some of the activities you might try to release your tension.

- Take care of yourself. Be sure you get enough rest and eat well. If you are irritable from lack of sleep or if you are not eating right, you will have less energy to deal with stressful situations. If stress keeps you from sleeping, you should ask your doctor for help.

- Talk about it. It helps to talk to someone about your concerns and worries. You can talk to a friend, family member, counselor, or health care provider.

- Let it out. A good cry can bring relief to your anxiety, and it might even prevent a headache or other physical problem. Taking some deep breaths also releases tension.

AIDS Dementia

HIV/AIDS and some medications for treating HIV may affect your brain. When HIV itself infects the brain, it can cause a condition known as AIDS dementia complex (ADC). Symptoms can include the following:

- Forgetfulness
- Confusion
- Difficulty paying attention
- Slurred speech
- Sudden shifts in mood or behavior
- Muscle weakness
- Clumsiness

If you think you may have ADC:

- Don't be afraid to tell your doctor that you think something is wrong. These symptoms can be subtle in the beginning, and telling your care providers about your concerns can help them to diagnose and treat you early.

- Keep a notepad with you and write down details about your symptoms whenever they occur. This information can help your doctor to help you.

- Build as much support as possible, including friends, family, and health care providers. Although it's possible to treat ADC successfully, it may take a while for some symptoms to go away.

Coping Tips

It is completely normal to have an emotional reaction upon learning that you are infected with HIV, such as anxiety, anger, or depression. These feelings do not last forever. As noted above, there are many things that you can do to help take care of your emotional needs. Here are just a few ideas:

- Talk about your feelings with your doctor, friends, family members, or other supportive people.

- Try to find activities that relieve your stress, such as exercise or hobbies.

- Try to get enough sleep each night to help you feel rested.

611

- Learn relaxation methods such as meditation, yoga, or deep breathing.

- Limit the amount of caffeine, nicotine, alcohol, and recreational drugs you use.

- Eat small, healthy meals throughout the day.

- Join a support group.

There are many kinds of support groups that provide a place where you can talk about your feelings, help others, and get the latest information about HIV/AIDS. Check with your health care provider for a listing of local support groups.

More specific ways to care for your emotional well-being include various forms of therapy and medication. Used alone or in combination, these may be helpful in dealing with the feelings you are experiencing. Therapy can help you better express your feelings and find ways to cope with your emotions. Medicines that may be able to help with anxiety and depression are also available.

You should always talk with your doctor about your options. There are many ways to care for your emotional health, but treatments must be carefully chosen by your physician based on your specific circumstances and needs.

The most important thing to remember is that you are not alone; there are support systems in place to help you, including doctors, psychiatrists, family members, friends, support groups, and other services.

Resources

- AIDS.org: Telling Others You Are HIV Positive (http://www.aids.org/factSheets/204-Telling-Others-You-are-HIV-Positive.html). Issues and guidelines about telling family members, friends, and others that you are HIV positive.

- American Academy of Family Physicians: HIV: Coping With the Diagnosis (http://www.familydoctor.org/038.xml). Q and A about coping with fear, legal issues, and other information.

- The Body: Mental Health (http://www.thebody.com/mental.html). Articles and links on depression, anxiety, stress, relationships, and other mental health issues.

- The Body: AIDS Hotlines and Organizations (http://www.thebody.com/hotlines.html). A comprehensive listing of HIV/AIDS hotlines and organizations, including a state-by-state breakout of HIV/AIDS organizations and support groups.

- Centers for Disease Control and Prevention's Caring for Someone with AIDS at Home: Providing Emotional Support (http://www.cdc.gov/hiv/resources/brochures/careathome/care5.htm). Information for caregivers and loved ones on providing emotional support.

- HIV InSite Links: Hotlines (http://hivinsite.ucsf.edu/InSite?page=li-01-04)

- HIV InSite Links: Mental Health (http://hivinsite.ucsf.edu/InSite?page=li-04-20). Links to organizations and other resources dealing with depression, anxiety, stress and other mental health issues.

- Pets Are Wonderful Support (PAWS) (http://www.pawssf.org). A non-profit organization that focuses on pets as a way to improve the mental health and well-being of people with HIV/AIDS. Includes information on health issues and international list of organizations.

Chapter 47

Pain and Mental Health

Chapter Contents

Section 47.1

When Pain Accompanies Depression

The two-way connection between depression and pain has been known since the days of Hippocrates. Gastrointestinal problems, headache, and other less specific aches and pains are common features of depression. Conversely, depression frequently sets in when individuals are battling persistent pain. Studies have also documented that as an individual's number of physical complaints increases, so does the likelihood that depression may occur.

Paying Attention to Pain

Pain can serve as an early indicator of many things—including depression. When pain persists after depression is diagnosed and its emotional symptoms have been treated, it can also alert a healthcare provider that a patient is at risk for a recurrence of depression. In addition to pointing to the possible presence of depression, persistent pain can also signal another physical problem that needs further medical evaluation.

Because of the significant link between depression and physical pain, it's important to identify and address pain while diagnosing and treating depression. Ironically, pain can make it more difficult to diagnose depression. In general, both patients and doctors may be more comfortable discussing physical symptoms than emotional concerns. As a result, addressing physical ailments may take precedence over probing more deeply for the possibility that pain is signaling the presence of depression.

What Is Chronic Pain?

Physical hurt is an unavoidable part of life. It is expected that irritability, agitation, and stress will accompany pain. Normally, as pain subsides, so do these responses. But chronic pain is pain that lasts much longer than would be expected from a specific injury or physical problem. When pain becomes chronic, the body reacts in many ways. Decreased energy, muscle pain, or weakness, and difficulty performing both physically and mentally can occur. Chronic pain can bring about neurochemical changes in the body, which can increase sensitivity to pain and cause an individual to experience pain in parts of the body that do not normally hurt.

This type of pain can interfere with sleep, which can then lead to daytime fatigue and lowered productivity. Ongoing pain can also make it difficult to interact with other people, resulting in the impairment of social interactions, relationships, sexual activity, and even the possible loss of jobs and income. Life with chronic pain can be extremely challenging, leading to feelings of irritability and even hopelessness when it seems there is no relief in sight. It's no surprise that this type of pain is so frequently associated with depression.

Understanding the Link between Depression and Pain

Depression and chronic pain share some of the same neurotransmitters—brain chemicals that act as messengers traveling between nerves—as well as some of the same nerve pathways, and depression and pain can interact in a vicious cycle. Depression magnifies pain, changing the brain's sensitivity to painful stimuli and reducing a person's coping skills. And the constant stress of experiencing chronic pain can lead to a cascade of other medical problems linked with depression, making it still more difficult to break the cycle.

Breaking the Cycle

Because chronic pain and depression are so intertwined, they are best treated together. The good news is that effective tools and lifestyle changes exist to both relieve the symptoms of depression and help manage chronic pain.

Specifically, medication is commonly employed to fight both depression and pain, since they share some of the same neurotransmitters. Antidepressants have also been shown to be effective in reducing an individual's sensitivity to pain, as well as improving sleep and overall quality of life. Psychotherapy and a number of different self-care strategies including relaxation techniques are also beneficial.

Each individual's experience with depression is different, and each calls for a unique treatment plan. You and your healthcare provider must work together to develop the plan that's right for you. If you are facing both depression and chronic pain, it is important that your treatment plan addresses every aspect of your life impacted by depression and/or pain. Visit "Know Your Treatment Options" (http://www .depressiontoolkit.org/treatmentoptions/default.asp) for information about the many tools you and your healthcare provider can consider, including medication and psychotherapy. In addition, visit "Take Care of Yourself" (http://www.depressiontoolkit.org/takecare/default.asp) for even more lifestyle tools and ideas you can incorporate into your plan, including exercise, stress management, and healthy sleep and eating habits.

Section 47.2

Anxiety and Chronic Pain

"Chronic Pain," © 2012 Anxiety and Depression Association of America (www.adaa.org); reprinted with permission.

Muscle tension, body soreness, headaches. For people with anxiety disorders, pain like this may be all too familiar.

Pain can be a common symptom—and sometimes a good indicator—of an anxiety disorder, particularly generalized anxiety disorder (GAD).

Beyond everyday aches and pains, some people will also suffer a diagnosed chronic pain disease such as arthritis or fibromyalgia. And a co-occurring chronic pain disease can make functioning even more difficult for someone with an anxiety disorder.

But people can manage anxiety disorders and chronic pain to lead full and productive lives.

Chronic Pain and Anxiety Disorders

Many chronic pain disorders are common in people with anxiety disorders.

Arthritis is a wide-ranging term that describes a group of more than 100 medical conditions that affect the musculoskeletal system, specifically the joints.

Symptoms include pain, stiffness, inflammation, and damage to joint cartilage and surrounding structures. Damage can lead to joint weakness, instability, and deformities that can interfere with basic daily tasks. Systemic forms of arthritis can affect the whole body and can cause damage to virtually any bodily organ or system.

Anxiety, depression, and other mood disorders are common among people who have arthritis, and very often in younger arthritis sufferers.

Fibromyalgia is a chronic medical condition that causes widespread muscle pain and fatigue.

Migraine is severe pain felt on one or both sides of the head, normally occurring around the temples or behind one eye or ear.

Back pain is more common in people with anxiety and mood disorders than those without them. Illness, accidents, and infections are among the causes of back pain.

Symptoms include persistent aches or stiffness anywhere along the spine; sharp, localized pain in the neck, upper back, or lower back, especially after lifting heavy objects or engaging in strenuous activity; and chronic ache in the middle or lower back, especially after sitting or standing for extended periods.

Complications

An anxiety disorder along with chronic pain can be difficult to treat. Those who suffer from chronic pain and have an anxiety disorder may have a lower tolerance for pain. People with an anxiety disorder may be more sensitive to medication side effects or be more fearful of side effects—and they may also be more fearful of pain—than someone who experiences pain without anxiety.

Treatment

Many treatments for anxiety disorders may also improve chronic pain symptoms.

Medications: Some people with an anxiety disorder and chronic pain may be able to take one medication for the symptoms of both conditions, such as treating fibromyalgia with a selective serotonin reuptake inhibitor (SSRI). Some anxiolytics, tricyclic antidepressants, and monoamine oxidase inhibitors (MAOIs) are effective for headache pain.

Therapy: Cognitive-behavior therapy (CBT) is used to treat anxiety disorders as well as chronic pain conditions. It is one type of effective therapy.

Relaxation: Relaxation techniques help people develop the ability to cope more effectively with the stresses that contribute to anxiety and pain. Common techniques include breathing retraining, progressive muscle relaxation, and exercise.

Complementary and alternative medicine: Yoga, acupuncture, and massage are among the complementary and alternative techniques that relieve the symptoms of anxiety disorders as well as chronic pain.

Lifestyle

Many lifestyle changes that improve the symptoms of an anxiety disorder also help the symptoms of chronic pain.

Exercise: Regular exercise strengthens muscles, reduces stiffness, improves flexibility, and boosts mood and self-esteem. Always check with your doctors before beginning an exercise regimen.

Sleep: A good night's sleep is key for anxiety disorders and chronic pain conditions. Symptoms of both types of conditions often become worse without enough sleep.

Consistent sleep and wake times, a good sleep environment (comfortable room temperature, no TV or other distractions), and avoiding caffeine late in the day and at night can help promote restful sleep.

Nutrition: People with anxiety should limit or avoid caffeine and alcohol, which can trigger panic attacks and worsen anxiety symptoms. According to the National Fibromyalgia Association, certain foods aggravate some musculoskeletal conditions, including dairy products, gluten (found in wheat, oats, barley, and rye), corn, sugar, and members of the nightshade family (potatoes, tomatoes, eggplant, peppers, and tobacco).

Those who experience can pain reduce their intake of tea, coffee, alcohol, red meat, and acid-forming foods. A health professional can provide more guidance about healthful foods and which to avoid.

Section 47.3

Psychological Factors of Chronic Back Pain

The Mind-Body Issue

Traditionally, we have thought of pain as a signal transmitted from the periphery to the brain—such as when a finger touches a hot plate. This understanding of pain serves well for very brief acute pain; however, it is only a small part of the story when pain is longer lasting.

Just as there are nerve tracts that carry pain signals upward to the brain, there are also tracts coming down from the brain that regulate the sensitivity of the spinal cord and thus determine how much pain we perceive. These tracts can amplify pain—making a trivial stimulation seem terrible—and can block it, which probably explains why quarterbacks and combat soldiers can carry out remarkable activities, and only after some time realize that they've been injured.

Additionally, there are genetic differences in the responses to stimulation. For example, a metal disc heated to exactly 120° and placed on the forearm will be experienced by some as barely uncomfortable (pain of 1/10) and by others as excruciating (pain of 9/10). Functional brain imaging at the time of the experiment confirms that those who report severe pain actually have greater activation of several areas in the brain that process pain, while those who feel little pain have little brain activation. Thus we conclude that, unless other factors interfere, pain is whatever the patient tells us it is.

Is It Mental?

Psychological factors rarely seem to be an important cause of prolonged pain, but they invariably affect it—for better or for worse.

Attention and vigilance account for much of the psychological modulation of pain. Pain that the brain thinks is important will be amplified, and those that it thinks are of no consequence will be lessened. (Just as a mother in a noisy New York apartment sleeps soundly as ambulances and car horns sound through the night, but awakens instantly when her baby whimpers.)

Mood profoundly affects pain, and even something as simple as reading a short story that is either funny or tragic changes people's thresholds and tolerance to experimental pain.

Research over the last 35 years has demonstrated that pain, as well as numerous other factors, changes the central nervous system in ways that lead to prolonged pain, even when the illness or injury that initiated it has healed. In fact, most chronic pain is more attributable to sensitization of the nervous system than to problems in the body parts that hurt.

These findings help to explain why people with normal-looking feet can have constant burning, why perfectly healthy people have headaches, and why the majority of people with chronic back pain have no findings on exam or imaging to account for it.

In the past, it was often assumed that when people had serious complaints of pain in healthy body parts, that their pain was imagined, psychologically induced, or exaggerated. We now know that this was a misjudgment on the part of medical providers.

What You Think Governs What You Do

Behavior, however, is another matter, and here psychological and environmental reinforcers play a prominent role in determining function. So we see people with very severe health problems and very severe pain who have well preserved work, play, and socialization, while we see others with far less pathology whose lives appear to have stopped.

In addition to such obvious factors as anxiety, stress, and depression, there are others that impact function. One is the person's intellectual understanding of their health—the person who believes that activity endangers their spinal fusion may become an unnecessary invalid, while a more confident person with the same medical condition may be golfing.

A person's confidence in his/her own strength and abilities is also important. Those who feel competent tend to function better and have better quality of life than those who lack self confidence.

Catastrophic Thinking

Catastrophizing, the tendency to assume that the worst that can happen is true, has been shown to promote pain and dysfunction. In the case of back pain, a person whose thoughts tend to run in the direction of, "This is horrible, there's no way I can stand it, I'm damaged for the rest of my life," will likely suffer more (and have less fun) than one who thinks, "the majority of people have back pain, and I'm getting more than my share of it, but I know there will be days that are better and days that are worse."

Who's Got the Power?

People who believe that their future depends on others—surgeons, spouses, Workers' Compensation insurers, foremen, etc,—tend to be more depressed, more functionally impaired, and in worse pain than those who recognize that they are in charge of their own lives.

Learn to Live with It

These may be the most feared words that a person with chronic pain can hear, with the implication that the rest of your life is going to be about enduring suffering. Fortunately that is not the case. Those who learn to live with pain do have to accept that there is so far no cure for most chronic pains, but most go on to have joyous and productive lives in which they feel a blessing and not a burden to their loved ones.

It's not easy or automatic, and we don't come with instruction manuals telling us how to do it. These may be useful hints:

Acceptance

In order to do what we can, we need to stop trying to do what we can't. At some point, it's time to stop looking for diagnoses and cures, and to decide to make the best life possible out of an unfortunate situation. Acceptance does not mean giving up; it means taking charge and having the fullest life possible, despite the pain.

Fitness

There may be nothing more important for reducing pain and increasing function than maintaining physical fitness. It clearly improves not only pain, but the anxiety and depression that often accompany it. Yes, it hurts at first. Yes, it would feel better at first to take a pain pill and go to bed. But over the long term, the fitter you are, the better you'll feel—and the more you'll be able to do with those who love you. You do need advice for this, though. The wrong exercises can increase many pains, and most patients require a slow and gradual increase in activities in order to avoid overdoing and crashing.

Fitness means weight management as well. Many studies show that obesity is associated with chronic pain. Weight loss is difficult, but with commercial weight loss programs that provide food guidance along with ongoing support, one can lose weight and keep it off without ever going hungry.

Stress Reduction

Stress is a funny thing. It can be good or bad. And if you have constant pain, you may want most of all to be comfortable. On the other hand, you've probably had more fun in roller coasters than in your favorite recliner, so you don't want to always take it easy.

Relaxation training, yoga, guided imagery, self-hypnosis, and biofeedback training all harness the individual's ability to learn to regulate the body's "fight or flight" response that tends to increase pain.

Cognitive therapy can help, especially if your beliefs about life, yourself, other people, or your health situation have become liabilities, interfering with your quality of life more than helping it.

Staying Active

One of the fathers of pain psychology noted that patients who have something better to do don't seem to hurt as much. The converse of this is the aphorism that if your life is empty, pain will fill it up.

Indeed, most patients find that when they're preoccupied with their grandchildren, or involved in some activity that consumes them, they are much less aware of the pain.

Medical advice to "let pain be your guide" is great for acute pain, but it is toxic for chronic pain. Seek clear answers from your physician as to whether you are at risk for harm to your body (as distinguished from hurt), and then let life be your guide.

Interpersonal Support

During acute pain, most have loved ones who are sympathetic and helpful. As the pain becomes chronic it seems that whatever they do is wrong. If they note that there isn't much physical disease going on and wonder if you're exaggerating the pain, it tends to lead to depression, anger, and decreased function. If they baby you, wait on you, and/or begin to make decisions for you, it tends to lead to regression, helplessness, and then depression. If friends get tired of hearing about the pain and drift away, it leads to loneliness and resentment.

It seems that the best response for those who love you is to accept that the pain is real, that they can't take it away, and that you aren't sick and don't need to be treated like a child. It helps if they give attention in the form of an invitation to the movies or a picnic rather than in the form of caretaking. It is important that loved ones ensure that your pain does not govern their lives.

Mutual Help

There may be nothing lonelier in life than living with chronic pain. It feels as though no one can really understand. Not true.

There are several organizations of people with chronic pain that provide education and support. The American Chronic Pain Association (www.theacpa.org) provides a great deal of education to patients and families about pain, how to deal with it, and various treatments for it. Many cities have ACPA groups in which people provide mutual help and support. And they definitely understand your pain—they have it too.

References

- National Pain Foundation. Living with Pain. www.nationalpain foundation.org/ Accessed 12/13/2011

- National Institute of Neurological Disorders & Stroke. NINDS Chronic Pain Information Page. www.ninds.nih.gov/ Accessed 12/13/2011

- American Psychological Association. Psychology Help Center: Coping with Chronic Pain. www.apa.org/ Accessed 12/13/2011

Chapter 48

Parkinson Disease and Mental Health

Depression not only affects your brain and behavior—it affects your entire body. Depression has been linked with other health problems, including Parkinson disease. Dealing with more than one health problem at a time can be difficult, so proper treatment is important.

What is depression?

Major depressive disorder, or depression, is a serious mental illness. Depression interferes with your daily life and routine and reduces your quality of life. About 6.7 percent of U.S. adults ages 18 and older have depression.

Signs and Symptoms of Depression

- Ongoing sad, anxious, or empty feelings
- Feeling hopeless
- Feeling guilty, worthless, or helpless
- Feeling irritable or restless
- Loss of interest in activities or hobbies once enjoyable, including sex
- Feeling tired all the time

"Depression and Parkinson's Disease," National Institute of Mental Health (www.nimh.nih.gov), 2011.

- Difficulty concentrating, remembering details, or making decisions

- Difficulty falling asleep or staying asleep, a condition called insomnia, or sleeping all the time

- Overeating or loss of appetite

- Thoughts of death and suicide or suicide attempts

- Ongoing aches and pains, headaches, cramps, or digestive problems that do not ease with treatment.

What is Parkinson disease?

Parkinson disease is a chronic disorder that worsens over time and results in the loss of brain cells that produce dopamine, a chemical messenger that controls movement. Parkinson disease usually affects people over age 50. These are the main symptoms of Parkinson disease:

- Tremor, or shaking, in the hands, arms, legs, jaw, and face

- Rigidity, or stiffness, of the arms, legs, and torso

- Slowness of movement

- Impaired balance and coordination

Parkinson can also affect thinking and emotions. At present, there is no way to predict or prevent Parkinson disease.

How are depression and Parkinson disease linked?

For people with depression and Parkinson disease, each illness can make symptoms of the other worse. For example, people with both illnesses tend to have more movement problems and greater levels of anxiety than those who have just depression or Parkinson disease. Compared with people who are depressed but do not have Parkinson, people who have both illnesses may have lower rates of sadness and guilt, but greater problems with concentration. One recent brain imaging study also suggests that people with Parkinson disease may have an unusually high number of reuptake pumps for the brain chemical messenger serotonin. Serotonin helps regulate mood, but overactive pumps reduce serotonin levels, possibly leading to depressive symptoms in some people with Parkinson disease.

How is depression treated in people who have Parkinson disease?

Depression is diagnosed and treated by a health care provider. Treating depression can help you manage your Parkinson disease treatment and improve your overall health. Recovery from depression takes time but treatments are effective.

At present, the most common treatments for depression include the following:

- Cognitive behavioral therapy (CBT), a type of psychotherapy, or talk therapy, that helps people change negative thinking styles and behaviors that may contribute to their depression

- Selective serotonin reuptake inhibitor (SSRI), a type of antidepressant medication that includes citalopram (Celexa), sertraline (Zoloft), and fluoxetine (Prozac)

- Serotonin and norepinephrine reuptake inhibitor (SNRI), a type of antidepressant medication similar to SSRI that includes venlafaxine (Effexor) and duloxetine (Cymbalta).

While currently available depression treatments, particularly SSRIs, are generally well tolerated and safe for people with Parkinson disease, talk with your health care provider about side effects, possible drug interactions, and other treatment options. For the latest information on medications, visit the U.S. Food and Drug Administration website (www.fda.gov). Not everyone responds to treatment the same way. Medications can take several weeks to work, may need to be combined with ongoing talk therapy, or may need to be changed or adjusted to minimize side effects and achieve the best results.

A variety of medications can provide dramatic relief from the symptoms of Parkinson disease. However, no current medication can stop the progression of the disease, and in many cases, medications lose their benefit over time. In such cases, the doctor may recommend deep brain stimulation, a surgery that places a battery-operated medical device called a neurostimulator—similar to a heart pacemaker—to deliver electrical stimulation to areas in the brain that control movement. Some doctors recommend physical therapy or muscle-strengthening exercises to improve movement and balance and make it easier to continue doing daily tasks, such as getting dressed and bathing. Although usually associated with treating severe or treatment-resistant depression, electroconvulsive therapy may improve Parkinson disease symptoms in some people.

Chapter 49

Sleep Disorders and Mental Health

Chapter Contents

Section 49.1

Depression and Sleep

Feeling sad every now and then is a fundamental part of the human experience, especially during difficult or trying times. In contrast, persistent feelings of sadness, anxiety, hopelessness, and disinterest in things that were once enjoyed are symptoms of depression, an illness that affects at least 20 million Americans. Depression is not something that a person can ignore or simply will away. Rather, it is a serious disorder that affects the way a person eats, sleeps, feels, and thinks. The cause of depression is not known, but it can be effectively controlled with treatment.

The relationship between sleep and depressive illness is complex—depression may cause sleep problems and sleep problems may cause or contribute to depressive disorders. For some people, symptoms of depression occur before the onset of sleep problems. For others, sleep problems appear first. Sleep problems and depression may also share risk factors and biological features and the two conditions may respond to some of the same treatment strategies. Sleep problems are also associated with more severe depressive illness.

Insomnia is very common among depressed patients. Evidence suggests that people with insomnia have a ten-fold risk of developing depression compared with those who sleep well. Depressed individuals may suffer from a range of insomnia symptoms, including difficulty falling asleep (sleep onset insomnia), difficulty staying asleep (sleep maintenance insomnia), unrefreshing sleep, and daytime sleepiness. However, research suggests that the risk of developing depression is highest among people with both sleep onset and sleep maintenance insomnia.

Obstructive sleep apnea (OSA) is also linked with depression. In a study of 18,980 people in Europe conducted by Stanford researcher Maurice Ohayon, MD, PhD, people with depression were found to be five times more likely to suffer from sleep-disordered breathing (OSA is the most common form of sleep disordered breathing). The good news is that treating OSA with continuous positive airway pressure (CPAP) may improve depression; a 2007 study of OSA patients who used CPAP for one year showed that improvements in symptoms of depression were significant and lasting.

In many cases, because symptoms of depression overlap with symptoms of sleep disorders, there is a risk of misdiagnosis. For example, depressed mood can be a sign of insomnia, OSA, or narcolepsy. Restless legs syndrome (RLS), a neurological condition that causes discomfort in the legs and sleep problems, is also associated with depression. According to the Restless Legs Syndrome Foundation, approximately 40% of people with RLS complain of symptoms that would indicate depression if assessed without consideration of a sleep disorder.

Many children and adolescents with depression suffer from sleep problems such as insomnia or hypersomnia (excessive sleepiness) or both. According to recent research, children with depression who suffer from both insomnia and hypersomnia are more likely to have severe and longer-lasting depression. They are also more likely to suffer from weight loss, impaired movement, and anhedonia (an inability to feel pleasure). Additionally, the National Sleep Foundation's 2006 Sleep in America poll, which focused on children aged 11 to 17, found a strong association between negative mood and sleep problems. Among adolescents who reported being unhappy, 73% reported not sleeping enough at night.

Depression affects all types of people from all over the world, but certain people are more likely than others to develop depression, including women and older adults. Among older adults, higher rates of depression and sleep problems may be explained in part by higher rates of physical illness. Among women, motherhood and hormonal changes throughout the life cycle (menstruation, menopause) may contribute to higher rates of depression. Among women and older adults, higher rates of depression may also be explained by higher rates of insomnia in these groups.

Seasonal affective disorder (SAD), also known as "winter depression," is one type of depression. SAD is believed to be influenced by the changing patterns of light and darkness that occur with the approach of winter. Circadian rhythms are regulated by the body's internal clock and by exposure to sunshine. When the days get shorter in autumn, circadian rhythms may become desynchronized and trigger depression. For most people with SAD, depressive symptoms resolve in springtime with increasing hours of daylight when the days lengthen out.

Living with depression can be extremely difficult. Depression not only affects the way a person feels and thinks but research suggests that it is also associated with serious chronic health problems such as heart disease. If you are experiencing symptoms of depression, it is very important to seek treatment as soon as possible.

Symptoms

Symptoms of depression vary from person to person. The following is a list of the most common symptoms. Some depression patients have only one of these, while others may have some, most or all:

- Feelings of hopelessness, helplessness and sadness
- Thoughts of death or suicide
- Loss of interest in things that were once pleasurable
- Concentration problems
- Forgetfulness
- Loss of libido
- Changes in weight and appetite
- Daytime sleepiness
- Loss of energy
- Insomnia

Depression may also be accompanied by anxiety, low self-esteem, and physical symptoms such as back pain, headaches, and gastrointestinal problems. Sleep problems such as insomnia and daytime sleepiness are often among the most debilitating features of depression.

Depressive illness may take different forms, including major depressive disorder (MDD), dysthymia, and bipolar disorder. MDD refers to an impaired ability to eat, sleep, work, think, enjoy activities, and feel pleasure. Dysthymia is a mild yet more persistent form of depression. Another form of depressive illness is bipolar disorder (manic depressive illness), which is characterized by extreme highs and lows. During high phases, bipolar patients may be energetic, talkative, and joyful. During lows, they experience symptoms of depression.

Treatment

Treatment for depression typically involves a combination of psychotherapy (including cognitive-behavioral therapy) and/or pharmacological (drug) treatment. Each of these therapies may be used to treat both depression and insomnia and treatment for sleep problems is often an integral part of depression therapy.

Treatment for depression may be complicated by sleep disorders. For example, patients with both OSA and depression should avoid sedating antidepressant medications due to their potential to suppress breathing and worsen OSA. Before beginning therapy for depression, talk to your physician about any sleep symptoms you are experiencing. In some cases, effectively treating the sleep problem may be enough to alleviate the symptoms of depression.

Cognitive behavioral therapy (CBT) is a behavioral approach to treating depression that is increasingly popular due to its effectiveness and lack of side effects. The essential features of CBT for depression include cognitive restructuring, a technique that targets the thoughts that lead to depressive feelings, and behavioral activation, which targets behavior that may perpetuate depression. CBT may be used to treat insomnia and depression at the same time.

There are a number of different medications used to treat insomnia, and your physician will work with you to determine which is best for you. Some of the most common drug treatments for depression are:

- **Selective serotonin reuptake inhibitors (SSRIs):** SSRIs effectively improve mood in many patients, but they may also cause or worsen insomnia.

- **Tricyclic antidepressants:** Tricyclic antidepressants are typically sedating, but they may also carry serious side effects such as high blood pressure.

- **Mood stabilizing anticonvulsants and lithium:** These drugs are commonly used to treat bipolar disorder.

In addition to the above treatment options, patients who suffer from SAD may benefit from bright light therapy. Light therapy may involve exposure to natural light (light from the sun) or treatment with a light box. Light therapy is considered safe, but little evidence exists to support its effectiveness at treating SAD or other forms of depression. Consult your physician before beginning any form of light therapy, as exposure to the sun or bright light may cause negative effects.

Some individuals show significant improvements in depression symptoms following a night of partial or complete sleep deprivation, leading physicians to consider using sleep deprivation as an intervention. However, such improvements are unreliable and are reversed after a night of normal sleep, making sleep deprivation an impractical therapeutic choice for depression. Moreover, sleep deprivation carries the potential for serious side effects such as extreme sleepiness, cognitive impairment, and an increased risk of injury or traffic accidents.

In preparation for a visit to a health professional for depression evaluation and treatment, it is helpful to keep track of your mood and to use a sleep diary for a period of two weeks. Sharing this information with your therapist will help guide treatment and the correct diagnosis.

Treating clinical depression may take time. Depression medications often take weeks to take full effect and some individuals may need to try a variety of drugs before finding the one that suits them best. Keep in mind that you should not stop taking a depression medication because your symptoms improve as this may cause symptoms to recur or other ill effects. Always consult your health care provider before making any changes to your depression therapy or any medication regimen.

Addressing sleep symptoms are of critical importance to recovery from depression. Be sure to discuss any sleep problems that persist as mood improves. Such problems may signal the presence of an underlying sleep disorder.

Coping

Depression can be stressful and exhausting. It can also make you feel helpless and hopeless. In addition to treatment with a medical or mental health professional, here are some tips for helping you cope with depression on a daily basis:

- Keep a regular sleep/wake schedule
- Get into bright light soon after waking in the morning
- Get some form of exercise every day
- Avoid afternoon naps if you have nighttime insomnia
- Limit caffeine and alcohol
- Ask loved ones for help—you should not face depression alone

Section 49.2

Disordered
Sleep and Anxiety

Many of us toss and turn or watch the clock when we can't sleep for a night or two. But for some, a restless night is routine.

More than 40 million Americans suffer from chronic, long-term sleep disorders, and an additional 20 million report sleeping problems occasionally, according to the National Institutes of Health.

Stress and anxiety may cause sleeping problems or make existing problems worse. And having an anxiety disorder exacerbates the problem.

Sleep disorders are characterized by abnormal sleep patterns that interfere with physical, mental, and emotional functioning. Stress or anxiety can cause a serious night without sleep, as do a variety of other problems.

Insomnia is the clinical term for people who have trouble falling asleep, difficulty staying asleep, waking too early in the morning, or waking up feeling unrefreshed.

Other common sleep disorders include sleep apnea (loud snoring caused by an obstructed airway), sleepwalking, and narcolepsy (falling asleep spontaneously). Restless leg syndrome and bruxism (grinding of the teeth while sleeping) are conditions that also may contribute to sleep disorders.

Anxiety Disorder or Sleep Disorder: Which Comes First?

Either one. Anxiety causes sleeping problems, and new research suggests sleep deprivation can cause an anxiety disorder.

Research also shows that some form of sleep disruption is present in nearly all psychiatric disorders. Studies also show that people with chronic insomnia are at high risk of developing an anxiety disorder.

Health Risks

The risks of inadequate sleep extend way beyond tiredness. Sleeplessness can lead to poor performance at work or school, increased risk of injury, and health problems.

In addition to anxiety and mood disorders, those with sleep disorders are risk for heart disease, heart failure, irregular heartbeat, heart attack, high blood pressure, stroke, diabetes, and obesity.

Treatment

If you suspect you have a sleep disorder, visit a primary care physician, mental health professional, or sleep disorders clinic. Treatment options include sleep medicine and cognitive-behavior therapy, which teaches how to identify and modify behaviors that perpetuate sleeping problems.

Treatment options for an anxiety disorder also include cognitive-behavior therapy, as well as relaxation techniques, and medication. Your doctor or therapist may recommend one or a combination of these treatments.

Reduce Anxiety, Sleep Soundly

To reduce anxiety and stress:

- **Meditate:** Focus on your breath—breathe in and out slowly and deeply—and visualize a serene environment such as a deserted beach or grassy hill.

- **Exercise:** Regular exercise is good for your physical and mental health. It provides an outlet for frustrations and releases mood-enhancing endorphins. Yoga can be particularly effective at reducing anxiety and stress.

- **Prioritize your to-do list:** Spend your time and energy on the tasks that are truly important, and break up large projects into smaller, more easily managed tasks. Delegate when you can.

- **Play music:** Soft, calming music can lower your blood pressure and relax your mind and body.

- **Get an adequate amount of sleep:** Sleeping recharges your brain and improves your focus, concentration, and mood.

- **Direct stress and anxiety elsewhere:** Lend a hand to a relative or neighbor, or volunteer in your community. Helping others will take your mind off of your own anxiety and fears.

- **Talk to someone:** Let friends and family know how they can help, and consider seeing a doctor or therapist.

To sleep more soundly:

- Make getting a good night's sleep a priority. Block out seven to nine hours for a full night of uninterrupted sleep, and try to wake up at the same time every day, including weekends.

- Establish a regular, relaxing bedtime routine. Avoid stimulants like coffee, chocolate, and nicotine before going to sleep, and never watch TV, use the computer, or pay bills before going to bed. Read a book, listen to soft music, or meditate instead.

- Make sure your bedroom is cool, dark, and quiet. Consider using a fan to drown out excess noise, and make sure your mattress and pillows are comfortable.

- Use your bedroom as a bedroom—not for watching TV or doing work—and get into bed only when you are tired. If you don't fall asleep within 15 minutes, go to another room and do something relaxing.

- Regular exercise will help you sleep better, but limit your workouts to mornings and afternoons.

- Avoid looking at the clock. This can make you anxious in the middle of the night. Turn the clock away from you.

- Talk to your doctor if you still have problems falling asleep. You may need a prescription or herbal sleep remedy.

Chapter 50

Stroke and Mental Health

Recovery after Stroke: Coping with Emotions

Dealing with a flood of emotions can be hard for stroke survivors. Some emotions are normal responses to the changes in your life after stroke. Others are common but should not be considered a normal part of stroke recovery. If you suffer from depression, anxiety or emotions that are not in line with the occasion, seek help.

Dealing with Depression

Grieving for what you have lost is good for you. But when sadness turns to depression, it's time to act. Depression can take hold right after a stroke, during rehabilitation (rehab) or after you go home. It can be—but not always—caused by brain damage from the stroke. Mild or major, it is the most common emotional problem faced by survivors.

Depression symptoms include:

- Feeling sad or "empty" most of the time

- Loss of interest or pleasure in ordinary activities

- Fatigue or feeling "slowed down"

- Sudden trouble sleeping or oversleeping

- Sudden loss of appetite or weight gain

"Recovery After Stroke: Coping with Emotions," © 2009 National Stroke Association (www.stroke.org). All rights reserved. Reprinted with permission.

- Being unable to concentrate, remember or make decisions like you used to

- Feeling worthless or helpless

- Feelings of guilt

- Ongoing thoughts of death or suicide, suicide planning or attempts

- A sudden change in how easily you are annoyed

- Crying all the time

Some useful tips:

- Make the most of rehab; the more you recover, the better you will feel

- Spend time with family and friends

- Maintain your quality of life by staying active and doing things you enjoy

- Seek help soon after you note symptoms

Your treatment may include counseling, medicine or both.

Having Extreme Anxiety

Anxiety is an overwhelming sense of worry or fear. It can include increased sweating or heart rate. Among stroke survivors, feelings of anxiety are common. Often, stroke survivors suffer from both depression and anxiety at the same time.

Anxiety can affect rehab progress, daily living, relationships, and quality of life. So, be sure to seek help right away.

Anxiety symptoms include:

- Ongoing worrying, fear, restlessness and irritability that don't seem to let up

- Low energy

- Poor concentration

- Muscle tension

- Feeling panicky and out of breath

- Scary rapid heart beat

- Shaking

- Headache

- Feeling sick to your stomach

Again, treatment may include counseling, medicine or both.

Uncontrolled Emotions

Do you find yourself laughing or crying at all the wrong times? If so, you may suffer from pseudobulbar affect (PBA). Also called emotional incontinence or pathologic lability, PBA is a common medical problem among stroke survivors. It can cause you to laugh at a funeral or cry at a comedy club. It can even make you cry uncontrollably for little or no reason. For this, it is often confused with depression. But, PBA is not depression.

People with PBA are unable to control their emotional expressions the way they used to. When this happens in social settings, they feel embarrassed, frustrated and angry. They also sense that others are uneasy. They may avoid work, public places and family get-togethers. This can lead to feelings of fear, shame and isolation.

There is no treatment approved by the Federal Drug Administration (FDA) for PBA, though antidepressant drugs can help.

These things may help you cope with PBA:

- Be open about it. Warn people that you cannot always control your emotions. Explain that the emotions you show on the outside don't always reflect how you feel on the inside.

- Distract yourself. If you feel an outburst coming on, focus on something boring or unrelated. Try counting the number of items on a shelf.

- Note the posture you take when crying. When you think you are about to cry, change your posture.

- Breathe in and out slowly until you are in control.

- Relax your forehead, shoulders and other muscles that tense up when crying.

What Can Help

- Ask your doctor about emotional changes and symptoms early on.

- Ask your family to stimulate your interest in people and social activities.

- Stay as active as possible and stay involved in your hobbies.

- Set goals and measure accomplishment.

- Plan daily activities to provide structure and sense of purpose.

- Stay involved with people, thoughts and activities that you enjoy.

- Get information on stroke recovery from National Stroke Association. Visit www.stroke.org or call 1-800-STROKES (1-800-787-6537).

- Contact your local stroke association.

- Join a stroke support group. Other survivors will understand your issues, and offer support and ideas to help you manage your emotions.

- Speak openly and honestly to your caregivers about your emotional changes. They'll be glad you did, and together you can work out a solution.

Professionals Who Can Help

- Psychologists, psychiatrists and other mental health professionals experienced with stroke-related emotional disorders.

Remember

Rehabilitation is a lifetime commitment and an important part of recovering from a stroke. Through rehabilitation, you relearn basic skills such as talking, eating, dressing and walking. Rehabilitation can also improve your strength, flexibility and endurance. The goal is to regain as much independence as possible.

Remember to ask your doctor, "Where am I on my stroke recovery journey?"

Part Seven

Additional Help and Information

Chapter 51

A Glossary of Mental Health Terms

accrued deficits: The delays or lack of development in emotional, social, academic, or behavioral skills that a child or adolescent experiences because of untreated mental illness. The mental illness keeps the individual from developing these life skills at the usual stage of life. An individual may never fully make up for these deficiencies.[1]

action potential: Transmission of signal from the cell body to the synaptic terminal at the end of the cell's axon. When the action potential reaches the end of the axon the neuron releases chemical (neurotransmitters) or electrical signals.[2]

acute: Refers to a disease or condition that has a rapid onset, marked intensity, and short duration.[1]

addiction: A chronic, relapsing disease characterized by compulsive drug seeking and use and by long-lasting changes in the brain.[3]

amygdala: The brain's "fear hub," which helps activate the fight-or-flight response and is also involved in emotions and memory.[2]

anterior cingulate cortex: Brain component involved in attention, emotional responses, and many other functions.[2]

Terms marked [1] are excerpted from *The Science of Mental Illness*, Copyright © 2005 by BSCS. All rights reserved. Reprinted with permission. Terms marked [2] are excerpted from "Brain Basics," National Institute of Mental Health, November 2, 2011. Terms marked [3] are excerpted from "Research Reports: Comorbidity: Addiction and Other Mental Illnesses," National Institute on Drug Abuse, September 2010.

antidepressant: A medication used to treat depression.[1]

antisocial personality disorder: A disorder characterized by antisocial behaviors that involve pervasive disregard for and violation of the rights, feelings, and safety of others. These behaviors begin in early childhood (conduct disorder) or the early teenage years and continue into adulthood.[3]

anxiety disorder: Any of a group of illnesses that fill people's lives with overwhelming anxieties and fears that are chronic and unremitting. Anxiety disorders include panic disorder, obsessive-compulsive disorder, post-traumatic stress disorder, phobias, and generalized anxiety disorder.[1]

anxiety: An abnormal sense of fear, nervousness, and apprehension about something that might happen in the future.[1]

attention deficit hyperactivity disorder (ADHD): A mental illness characterized by an impaired ability to regulate activity level (hyperactivity), attend to tasks (inattention), and inhibit behavior (impulsivity). For a diagnosis of ADHD, the behaviors must appear before an individual reaches age seven, continue for at least six months, be more frequent than in other children of the same age, and cause impairment in at least two areas of life (school, home, work, or social function).[1]

autism: A developmental brain disorder that typically affects a person's ability to communicate, engage in social interactions, and respond appropriately to the environment. Some people with autism have few problems with learning and speech, and are able to function well in society. Others may be significantly impaired or have serious language delays. Autism makes some people seem closed off and shut down; others seem locked into repetitive behaviors and rigid patterns of thinking.[1]

axon: The long, fiber-like part of a neuron by which the cell carries information to target cells.[1]

bipolar disorder: A depressive disorder in which a person alternates between episodes of major depression and mania (periods of abnormally and persistently elevated mood). Also referred to as manic-depression.[1]

cell body: Contains the nucleus and cytoplasm of a cell.[2]

cell membrane: The boundary separating the inside contents of a cell from its surrounding environment.[2]

cerebrum: The upper part of the brain that consists of the left and right hemispheres.[1]

chronic: Refers to a disease or condition that persists over a long period of time.[1]

cognition: Conscious mental activity that informs a person about his or her environment. Cognitive actions include perceiving, thinking, reasoning, judging, problem solving, and remembering.[1]

comorbidity: The occurrence of two disorders or illnesses in the same person, either at the same time (co-occurring comorbid conditions) or with a time difference between the initial occurrence of one and the initial occurrence of the other (sequentially comorbid conditions).[3]

conduct disorder: A personality disorder of children and adolescents involving persistent antisocial behavior. Individuals with conduct disorder frequently participate in activities such as stealing, lying, truancy, vandalism, and substance abuse.[1]

cytoplasm: The substance filling a cell, containing all the chemicals and parts needed for the cell to work properly.[2]

delusion: A false belief that persists even when a person has evidence that the belief is not true.[1]

dendrite: The specialized fibers that extend from a neuron's cell body and receive messages from other neurons.[1]

depression (depressive disorders): A group of diseases including major depressive disorder (commonly referred to as depression), dysthymia, and bipolar disorder (manic-depression). See bipolar disorder, dysthymia, and major depressive disorder.[1]

Diagnostic and Statistical Manual of Mental Disorders, 4th Edition (DSM-IV): A book published by the American Psychiatric Association that gives general descriptions and characteristic symptoms of different mental illnesses. Physicians and other mental health professionals use the *DSM-IV* to confirm diagnoses for mental illnesses. [1] [Note: *DSM-V* is expected to be released in 2013.]

DNA: The "recipe of life," containing inherited genetic information that helps to define physical and some behavioral traits.[2]

dopamine: A neurotransmitter mainly involved in controlling movement, managing the release of various hormones, and aiding the flow of information to the front of the brain.[2]

dysthymia: A depressive disorder that is less severe than major depressive disorder but is more persistent. In children and adolescents, dysthymia lasts for an average of four years.[1]

electroconvulsive therapy (ECT): A treatment for severe depression that is usually used only when people do not respond to medications and psychotherapy. ECT involves passing a low-voltage electric current through the brain. The person is under anesthesia at the time of treatment. ECT is not commonly used in children and adolescents.[1]

electroencephalography (EEG): A method of recording the electrical activity in the brain through electrodes attached to the scalp.[1]

epigenetics: The study of how environmental factors like diet, stress, and post-natal care can change gene expression (when genes turn on or off)—without altering DNA sequence.[2]

frontal lobe: One of the four divisions of each cerebral hemisphere. The frontal lobe is important for controlling movement and associating the functions of other cortical areas.[1]

gene: A segment of DNA that codes to make proteins and other important body chemicals.[2]

glutamate: The most common neurotransmitter in a person's body, which increases neuronal activity, is involved in early brain development, and may also assist in learning and memory.[2]

gray matter: The portion of brain tissue that is dark in color. The gray matter consists primarily of nerve cell bodies, dendrites, and axon endings.[1]

hallucination: The perception of something, such as a sound or visual image, that is not actually present other than in the mind.[1]

hippocampus: A portion of the brain involved in creating and filing new memories.[2]

hypothalamus: The part of the brain that controls several body functions, including feeding, breathing, drinking, temperature, and the release of many hormones.[1]

hypothalamic-pituitary-adrenal (HPA) axis: A brain-body circuit which plays a critical role in the body's response to stress.[2]

impulse: An electrical communication signal sent between neurons by which neurons communicate with each other.[2]

magnetic resonance imaging (MRI): An imaging technique that uses magnetic fields to take pictures of the structure of the brain.[1]

major depressive disorder: A depressive disorder commonly referred to as depression. Depression is more than simply being sad; to be diagnosed with depression, a person must have five or more characteristic symptoms nearly every day for a two-week period.[1]

mania: Feelings of intense mental and physical hyperactivity, elevated mood, and agitation.[1]

manic-depression: *See* bipolar disorder.[1]

mental illness: A health condition that changes a person's thinking, feelings, or behavior (or all three) and that causes the person distress and difficulty in functioning.[1]

mental retardation: A condition in which a person has an IQ that is below average and that affects an individual's learning, behavior, and development. This condition is present from birth.[1]

mutation: A change in the code for a gene, which may be harmless or even helpful, but sometimes give rise to disabilities or diseases.[2]

myelin: A fatty material that surrounds and insulates the axons of some neurons.[1]

neural circuit: A network of neurons and their interconnections.[2]

neuron (nerve cell): A unique type of cell found in the brain and body that processes and transmits information.[1]

neurosis: A term no longer used medically as a diagnosis for a relatively mild mental or emotional disorder that may involve anxiety or phobias but does not involve losing touch with reality.[1]

neurotransmission: The process that occurs when a neuron releases neurotransmitters that relay a signal to another neuron across the synapse.[1]

neurotransmitter: A chemical produced by neurons that carries messages to other neurons.[1]

nucleus: A structure within a cell that contains DNA and information the cell needs for growing, staying alive, and making new neurons.[2]

obsessive-compulsive disorder (OCD): An anxiety disorder in which a person experiences recurrent unwanted thoughts or rituals that the individual cannot control. A person who has OCD may be plagued by persistent, unwelcome thoughts or images or by the urgent need to engage in certain rituals, such as hand washing or checking.[1]

oppositional defiant disorder: A disruptive pattern of behavior of children and adolescents that is characterized by defiant, disobedient, and hostile behaviors directed toward adults in positions of authority. The behavior pattern must persist for at least six months.[1]

panic disorder: An anxiety disorder in which people have feelings of terror, rapid heart beat, and rapid breathing that strike suddenly and repeatedly with no warning. A person who has panic disorder cannot predict when an attack will occur and may develop intense anxiety between episodes, worrying when and where the next one will strike.[1]

phobia: An intense fear of something that poses little or no actual danger. Examples of phobias include fear of closed-in places, heights, escalators, tunnels, highway driving, water, flying, dogs, and injuries involving blood.[1]

pituitary gland: An endocrine organ closely linked with the hypothalamus. The pituitary secretes a number of hormones that regulate the activity of other endocrine organs in the human body.[1]

positron emission tomography (PET): An imaging technique for measuring brain function in living subjects by detecting the location and concentration of small amounts of radioactive chemicals.[1]

positron: A positively charged particle that has the same mass and spin as—but the opposite charge of—an electron.[1]

postsynaptic neuron: The neuron that receives messages from other neurons.[1]

post-traumatic stress disorder (PTSD): A disorder that develops after exposure to a highly stressful event (for example, wartime combat, physical violence, or natural disaster). Symptoms include sleeping difficulties, hypervigilance, avoiding reminders of the event, and re-experiencing the trauma through flashbacks or recurrent nightmares.[3]

prefrontal cortex: A highly developed area at the front of the brain that, in humans, plays a role in executive functions such as judgment, decision making and problem solving, as well as emotional control and memory.[2]

presynaptic neuron: The neuron that sends messages to other neurons by releasing neurotransmitters into the synapse.[1]

psychiatrist: A medical doctor (M.D.) who specializes in treating mental diseases. A psychiatrist evaluates a person's mental health along with his or her physical health and can prescribe medications.[1]

psychiatry: The branch of medicine that deals with identifying, studying, and treating mental, emotional, and behavioral disorders.[1]

psychologist: A mental health professional who has received specialized training in the study of the mind and emotions. A psychologist usually has an advanced degree such as a Ph.D.[1]

psychosis: A serious mental disorder in which a person loses contact with reality and experiences hallucinations or delusions.[1]

psychotherapy: A treatment method for mental illness in which a mental health professional (psychiatrist, psychologist, counselor) and a patient discuss problems and feelings to find solutions. Psychotherapy can help individuals change their thought or behavior patterns or understand how past experiences affect current behaviors.[1]

receptor: A molecule that recognizes specific chemicals, including neurotransmitters and hormones, and transmits the message into the cell on which the receptor resides.[1]

relapse: The reoccurrence of symptoms of a disease.[1]

reuptake pump: The large molecule that carries neurotransmitter molecules back into the presynaptic neuron from which they were released. Also referred to as a transporter.[1]

risk factor: Something that increases a person's risk or susceptibility to harm.[1]

schizophrenia: A chronic, severe, and disabling brain disease. People with schizophrenia often suffer terrifying symptoms such as hearing internal voices or believing that other people are reading their minds, controlling their thoughts, or plotting to harm them. These symptoms may leave them fearful and withdrawn. Their speech and behavior can be so disorganized that they may be incomprehensible or frightening to others.[1]

selective serotonin reuptake inhibitors (SSRIs): A group of medications used to treat depression. These medications cause an increase in the amount of the neurotransmitter serotonin in the brain.[1]

self-medication: The use of a substance to lessen the negative effects of stress, anxiety, or other mental disorders (or side effects of their pharmacotherapy). Self-medication may lead to addiction and other drug- or alcohol-related problems.[3]

serotonin: A neurotransmitter that regulates many functions, including mood, appetite, and sensory perception.[1]

single photon emission computed tomography (SPECT): A brain imaging process that measures the emission of single photons of a given energy from radioactive tracers in the human body.[1]

St. John's wort: An herb sometimes used to treat mild cases of depression. Although the popular media have reported successes using St. John's wort, it is not a recommended treatment. The scientific evidence for its effectiveness and safety is not conclusive.[1]

stigma: A negative stereotype about a group of people.[1]

symptom: Something that indicates the presence of a disease.[1]

synapse: The site where presynaptic and postsynaptic neurons communicate with each other.[1]

synaptic space: The intercellular space between a presynaptic and postsynaptic neuron. Also referred to as the synaptic cleft.[1]

syndrome: A group of symptoms or signs that are characteristic of a disease. In this module, the word syndrome is used as a synonym for illness.[1]

transporter: A large protein on the cell membrane of axon terminals. It removes neurotransmitter molecules from the synaptic space by carrying them back into the axon terminal that released them. Also referred to as the reuptake pump.[1]

ventricle: One of the cavities or spaces in the brain that are filled with cerebrospinal fluid.[1]

vesicle: A membranous sac within an axon terminal that stores and releases neurotransmitters.[1]

Chapter 52

Crisis Hotlines and Helplines

Important Information about Suicide

Are you thinking of suicide? If yes, please do the following:

- Dial: 911

- Dial: 800-273-TALK (8255)

- Check yourself into the emergency room.

- Tell someone who can help you find help right away.

- Stay away from things that might hurt you.

Remember: Most people can be treated with a combination of antidepressant medication and talk therapy. Talk to a health professional for guidance.

No Insurance?

- Go to the nearest hospital emergency room.

- Look in your local Yellow Pages under Mental Health and/or Suicide Prevention and then call the mental health organizations/

Excerpted from "Mental Health: Preventing Suicide" and "Mental Health: Help Hotlines" Office on Women's Health (www.womenshealth.gov), March 29, 2010. Additional information compiled from various sources deemed reliable. All contact information was verified and updated in June 2012. Inclusion does not imply endorsement, and there is no implication association with omission.

crisis phone lines that are listed. There may be clinics or counseling centers in your area operating on a sliding or no-fee scale.

- Some pharmaceutical companies have "Free Medication Programs" for those who qualify. Visit the National Alliance for the Mentally Ill website at http://www.nami.org for more information.

Helplines and Hotlines

Below is a list of toll-free national helplines and hotlines that provide anonymous, confidential information to callers. They can answer questions and help you in times of need.

AIDS Alliance for Children, Youth and Families
Toll-Free: 888-917-AIDS (888-917-2437)

Alcohol and Drug Helpline
Toll-Free: 800-821-HELP (800-821-4357)

American Foundation for Suicide Prevention
Toll-Free: 888-333-AFSP (888-333-2377)

Boys Town National Hotline
Crisis hotline that helps parents and children cope
with stress and anxiety.
Toll-Free: 800-448-3000

Center for Substance Abuse Treatment
Toll-Free: 800-729-6686

Childhelp National Child Abuse Hotline
Toll-Free: 800-4-A-CHILD (800-422-4453)

Covenant House
Helping homeless youth in the United States and Canada.
Toll-Free: 800-999-9999
Toll-Free TTY: 800-999-9915

Depression and Bipolar Support Alliance
Toll-Free: 800-826-3632

Hopeline
Toll-Free: 800-442-HOPE (800-442-4673)

Kristin Brooks Hope Center
Toll-Free: 800-442-HOPE (800-442-4673)

Mental Health America
For a referral to specific mental health service or support program in your community.
Toll-Free: 800-969-NMHA (800-969-6642)

National Alcoholism and Substance Abuse Information Center
Toll-Free: 800-662-HELP (800-662-4357)
Toll-Free: 800-784-6776

National Alliance on Mental Illness (NAMI)
Toll-Free: 800-950-NAMI (800-950-6264)

National Domestic Violence Hotline
Toll-Free: 800-799-SAFE (800-799-7233)

National Eating Disorders Association Information and Referral Helpline
Toll-Free: 800-931-2237

National Mental Health Information Center
Toll-Free: 800-789-2647
Toll-Free TDD: 866-889-2647

National Organization for Victim Assistance
Toll-Free: 800-TRY-NOVA (800-879-6682) (Victims/Survivors only)

National Runaway Switchboard
Toll-Free: 800-RUNAWAY (800-786-2929)

National Sexual Assault Hotline
Toll-Free: 800-656-HOPE (800-656-4673)

National Suicide Prevention Hotline
Toll-Free: 800-273-TALK (800-273-8255)

Postpartum Support International
Toll-Free: 800-994-4PPD (800-994-4773)

Postpartum Depression (PPD) Moms
Toll-Free: 800-PPD-MOMS (800-773-6667)

S.A.F.E. Alternatives
Toll-Free: 800-DONTCUT (800-366-8288)

Suicide Prevention Crisis Center
Toll-Free: 877-7-CRISIS (877-727-4747)

Trevor Project

Suicide prevention helpline for lesbian, gay, bisexual, transgender, and questioning youth.
Toll-Free: 866-4U-TREVOR (866-488-7386)

Chapter 53

Mental Health Organizations

Alzheimer's Association
225 North Michigan Avenue
Floor 17
Chicago, IL 60601-7633
Toll-Free: 800-272-3900
(Helpline)
Toll-Free TDD: 866-403-3073
(Helpline)
Phone: 312-335-8700
TDD: 312-335-5886
Toll-Free Fax: 866-699-1246
Website: www.alz.org
E-mail: info@alz.org

American Academy of Child and Adolescent Psychiatry
3615 Wisconsin Avenue, NW
Washington, DC 20016-3007
Phone: 202-966-7300
Fax: 202-966-2891
Website: www.aacap.org

American Art Therapy Association
225 North Fairfax Street
Alexandria, VA 22314
Toll-Free: 888-290-0878
Phone: 703-548-5860
Fax: 703-783-8468
Website: www.arttherapy.org
E-mail: info@arttherapy.org

American Association for Geriatric Psychiatry
7910 Woodmont Avenue
Suite 1050
Bethesda, MD 20814-3004
Phone: 301-654-7850
Fax: 301-654-4137
Website: www.aagponline.org
E-mail: main@aagponline.org

Information in this chapter was compiled from various sources deemed reliable. All contact information was verified and updated in June 2012. Inclusion does not imply endorsement, and there is no implication association with omission.

American Association for Marriage and Family Therapy

112 South Alfred Street
Alexandria, VA 22314-3061
Phone: 703-838-9808
Fax: 703-838-9805
Website: www.aamft.org
E-mail: central@aamft.org

American Association of Suicidology

5221 Wisconsin Avenue, NW
Washington, DC 20015
Phone: 202-237-2280
Fax: 202-237-2282
Website: www.suicidology.org

American Counseling Association

5999 Stevenson Avenue
Alexandria, VA 22304
Toll-Free: 800-347-6647
TDD: 703-823-6862
Toll-Free Fax: 800-473-2329
Fax: 703-823-0252
Website: www.counseling.org
E-mail:
webmaster@counseling.org

American Foundation for Suicide Prevention

120 Wall Street, 29th Floor
New York, NY 10005
Toll-Free: 888-333-AFSP
(888-333-2377)
Phone: 212-363-3500
Fax: 212-363-6237
Website: www.afsp.org
E-mail: inquiry@afsp.org

American Psychiatric Association

1000 Wilson Boulevard
Suite 1825
Arlington, VA 22209-3901
Toll-Free: 888-35-PSYCH
(888-357-7924)
Phone: 703-907-7300
Website: www.psych.org
E-mail: apa@psych.org

American Psychological Association

750 First Street, NE
Washington, DC 20002-4242
Toll-Free: 800-374-2721
Phone: 202-336-5500
TDD/TTY: 202-336-6123
Website: www.apa.org
E-mail: public.affairs@apa.org

American Psychotherapy Association

2750 East Sunshine Street
Springfield, MO 65804
Toll-Free: 800-205-9165
Phone: 417-823-0173
Fax: 417-823-9959
Website:
www.americanpsycho
therapy.com

Anxiety Disorders Association of America

8701 Georgia Avenue
Silver Spring, MD 20910
Phone: 240-485-1001
Fax: 240-485-1035
Website: www.adaa.org

Association for Applied Psychophysiology and Biofeedback
10200 West 44th Avenue
Suite 304
Wheat Ridge, CO 80033
Toll-Free: 800-477-8892
Phone: 303-422-8436
Website: www.aapb.org
E-mail: info@aapb.org

Association for Behavioral and Cognitive Therapies
305 7th Avenue, 16th Floor
New York, NY 10001
Phone: 212-647-1890
Fax: 212-647-1865
Website: www.abct.org

Balanced Mind Foundation
820 Davis Street, Suite 520
Evanston, IL 60201
Phone: 847-492-8510
Fax: 847-492-8520
Website:
www.thebalancedmind.org
E-mail:
info@thebalancedmind.org

Beyond Blue Ltd.
Website: www.beyondblue.org.au

Brain and Behavior Research Foundation
60 Cutter Mill Road, Suite 404
Great Neck, NY 11021
Toll-Free: 800-829-8289
Phone: 516-829-0091
Fax: 516-487-6930
Website: www.bbrfoundation.org
E-mail: info@bbrfoundation.org

Brain Injury Association of America
1608 Spring Hill Road
Suite 110
Vienna, VA 22182
Toll-Free: 800-444-6443
Phone: 703-761-0750
Fax: 703-761-0755
Website: www.biausa.org
E-mail:
braininjuryinfo@biausa.org

Canadian Mental Health Association
Phenix Professional Building
595 Montreal Road
Suite 303
Ottawa ON K1K 4L2
Fax: 613-745-5522
Website: www.cmha.ca

Canadian Psychological Association
141 Laurier Avenue West
Suite 702
Ottawa, ON K1P 5J3
Toll-Free: 888-472-0657
Phone: 613-237-2144
Fax: 613-237-1674
Website: www.cpa.ca
E-mail: cpa@cpa.ca

Caring.com
2600 South El Camino Real
Suite 300
San Mateo, CA 94403
Website: www.caring.com

Center for Mental Health Services

Emergency Services and
Disaster Relief Branch
5600 Fishers Lane, Room 17C-20
Rockville, MD 20857
Phone: 240-276-1310
Fax: 240-276-1320
Website:
mentalhealth.samhsa.gov
E-mail: info@mentalhealth.org

Center for Substance Abuse Treatment

Toll-Free: 800-662-4357
Toll-Free TDD: 800-487-4889
Phone: 240-276-2750
Website: csat.samhsa.gov

Center on Addiction and the Family

Website: www.coaf.org
E-mail: coaf@phoenixhouse.org

Depressed Anonymous

P.O. Box 17414
Louisville, KY 40217
Phone: 502-569-1989
Website:
www.depressedanon.com
E-mail: info@depressedanon.com

Depression and Bipolar Support Alliance

730 North Franklin Street
Suite 501
Chicago, IL 60654-7225
Toll-Free: 800-826-3632
Fax: 312-642-7243
Website: www.dbsalliance.org
E-mail: info@dbsalliance.org

Eating Disorder Referral and Information Center

Website: www.edreferral.com

Families for Depression Awareness

395 Totten Pond Road, Suite 404
Waltham, MA 02451
Phone: 781-890-0220
Fax: 781-890-2411
Website: www.familyaware.org

Family Caregiver Alliance

785 Market Street, Suite 750
San Francisco, CA 94103
Toll-Free: 800-445-8106
Phone: 415-434-3388
Website: www.caregiver.org
E-mail: info@caregiver.org

Geriatric Mental Health Foundation

7910 Woodmont Avenue
Suite 1050
Bethesda, MD 20814
Phone: 301-654-7850
Fax: 301-654-4137
Website: www.gmhfonline.org
E-mail: web@GMHFonline.org

Helpguide

Website: www.helpguide.org

International Foundation for Research and Education on Depression

P.O. Box 17598
Baltimore, MD 21297-1598
Fax: 443-782-0739
Website: www.ifred.org
E-mail: info@ifred.org

International OCD Foundation
P.O. Box 961029
Boston, MA 02196
Phone: 617-973-5801
Fax: 617-973-5803
Website: www.ocfoundation.org
E-mail: info@ocfoundation.org

International Society for the Study of Trauma and Dissociation
8400 Westpark Drive
Second Floor
McLean, VA 22102
Phone: 703-610-9037
Fax: 703-610-0234
Website: www.issd.org
E-mail: info@isst-d.org

International Society for Traumatic Stress Studies
111 Deer Lake Road, Suite 100
Deerfield, IL 60015
Phone: 847-480-9028
Fax: 847-480-9282
Website: www.istss.org
E-mail: istss@istss.org

Kristin Brooks Hope Center
1250 24th Street, NW, Suite 300
Washington, DC 20037
Toll-Free: 800-442-HOPE
(800-442-4673)
Toll-Free Helpline:
800-SUICIDE (800-784-2433)
Toll-Free for Veterans:
877-VET-2-VET (877-838-2838)
Phone: 202-536-3200
Fax: 202-536-3206
Website: www.hopeline.com

Mautner Project
1300 19th Street NW, Suite 700
Washington, DC 20036
Toll-Free: 866-MAUTNER
(866-628-8637)
Phone: 202-332-5536
Fax: 202-332-0662
Website:
www.mautnerproject.org
E-mail: info@mautnerproject.org

Mental Health America
(formerly National Mental
Health Association)
2000 North Beauregard Street
6th Floor
Alexandria, VA 22311
Toll-Free: 800-969-6642
Toll-Free Crisis Line:
800-273-TALK
(800-273-8255)
Phone: 703-684-7722
Fax: 703-684-5968
Website: www.nmha.org
E-mail: webmaster@
mentalhealthamerica.net

Mental Health Association of Westchester
580 White Plains Road
Tarrytown, NY 10591
Website:
www.mhawestchester.org

Mental Health Minute
Website:
www.mentalhealthminute.info

Mind
15-19 Broadway
Stratford, London
UK E15 4BQ
Phone: +44 208-519-2122
Fax: +44 208-522-1725
Website: www.mind.org.uk
E-mail: contact@mind.org.uk

**National Alliance on
Mental Illness (NAMI)**
3803 North Fairfax Drive
Suite 100
Arlington, VA 22203
Toll-Free: 888-999-NAMI
(888-999-6264)
Toll-Free: 800-950-NAMI
(800-950-6264 Helpline)
Phone: 703-524-7600
Fax: 703-524-9094
Website: www.nami.org
E-mail: info@nami.org

**National Association of
Anorexia Nervosa and
Associated Disorders
(ANAD)**
800 East Diehl Road
#160
Naperville, IL 60563
Phone: 630-577-1333
Phone: 630-577-1330 (Helpline)
Fax: 630-577-1323
Website: www.anad.org
E-mail: anadhelp@anad.org

**National Association of
School Psychologists**
4340 East West Highway
Suite 402
Bethesda, MD 20814
Toll-Free: 866-331-NASP
(866-331-6277)
Phone: 301-657-0270
TTY: 301-657-4155
Fax: 301-657-0275
Website: www.nasponline.org
E-mail: center@naspweb.org

**National Center for Child
Traumatic Stress**
Duke University
411 West Chapel Hill Street
Suite 200
Durham, NC 27701
Phone: 919-682-1552
Fax: 919-613-9898
Web site: www.nctsn.org
E-mail: info@nctsn.org

**National Center for
Posttraumatic Stress
Disorder (NCPTSD)**
U.S. Department of
Veterans Affairs (VA)
810 Vermont Avenue, NW
Washington, DC 20420
Toll-Free: 800-827-1000
Website: www.va.gov

**National Center for Victims
of Crime**
2000 M Street NW, Suite 480
Washington, DC 20036
Phone: 202-467-8700
Fax: 202-467-8701
Website: www.ncvc.org
E-mail: webmaster@ncvc.org

National Council on Problem Gambling
730 11th Street NW
Suite 601
Washington, DC 20001
Toll-Free: 800-522-4700 (Hotline)
Phone 202-547-9204
Fax 202-547-9206
Website: www.ncpgambling.org
E-mail: ncpg@ncpgambling.org

National Eating Disorders Association
165 West 46th Street
New York, NY 10036
Toll-Free: 800-931-2237
Phone: 212-575-6200
Fax: 212-575-1650
Website:
www.nationaleatingdisorders.org
E-mail: info@NationalEating
Disorders.org

National Federation of Families for Children's Mental Health
9605 Medical Center Drive
Suite 280
Rockville, MD 20850
Phone: 240-403-1901
Fax: 240-403-1909
Website: www.ffcmh.org
E-mail: ffcmh@ffcmh.org

National Institute of Mental Health
Science Writing, Press, and
Dissemination Branch
6001 Executive Boulevard
Room 8184, MSC 9663
Bethesda, MD 20892-9663
Toll-Free: 866-615-6464
Toll-Free TTY: 866-415-8051
Phone: 301-443-4513
TTY: 301-443-8431
Fax: 301-443-4279
Website: www.nimh.nih.gov
E-mail: nimhinfo@nih.gov

National Institute of Neurological Disorders and Stroke
NIH Neurological Institute
P.O. Box 5801
Bethesda, MD 20824
Toll-Free: 800-352-9424
Phone: 301-496-5751
TTY: 301-468-5981
Website: www.ninds.nih.gov

National Institute on Aging
Building 31, Room 5C27
31 Center Drive, MSC 2292
Bethesda, MD 20892
Toll-Free: 800-222-2225
Phone: 301-496-1752
Toll-Free TTY: 800-222-4225
Fax: 301-496-1072
Website: www.nia.nih.gov
E-mail: niac@nia.nih.gov

National Institute on Alcohol Abuse and Alcoholism

5635 Fishers Ln., MSC 9304
Bethesda, MD 20892
Phone: 301-443-3860
Website: www.niaaa.nih.gov
E-mail:
niaaaweb-r@exchange.nih.gov

National Institute on Drug Abuse

6001 Executive Boulevard
Room 5213, MSC 9561
Bethesda, MD 20892-9561
Phone: 301-443-1124
Fax: 301-443-7397
Websites: www.nida.nih.gov
and www.drugabuse.gov
E-mail:
information@nida.nih.gov

National Mental Health Information Center

Substance Abuse and Mental
Health Services Administration
P.O. Box 2345
Rockville, MD 20847
Toll-Free: 800-789-2647
Toll-Free TDD: 866-889-2647
Phone: 240-221-4021
TDD Phone: 240-221-4022
Fax: 240-221-4295
Website:
mentalhealth.samhsa.gov
E-mail:
nmhic-info@samhsa.hss.gov

National Women's Health Information Center (NWHIC)

Office on Women's Health
200 Independence Avenue SW
Room 712E
Washington DC 20201
Toll-Free: 800-994-9662
Toll-Free TDD: 888-220-5446
Phone: 202-690-7650
Fax: 202-205-2631
Website: www.womenshealth.gov

Office of Minority Health (OMH)

Resource Center
P.O. Box 37337
Washington, DC 20013-7337
Toll-Free: 800-444-6472
Phone: 240-453-2882
TDD: 301-251-1432
Fax: 301-251-2160
Fax: 240-453-2883
Website: minorityhealth.hhs.gov
E-mail:
info@minorityhealth.hhs.gov

Postpartum Support International

6706 SW 54th Avenue
Portland, OR 97219
Toll-Free: 800-944-4PPD
(800-944-4773)
Phone: 503-894-9453
Fax: 503-894-9452
Website: www.postpartum.net
E-mail: support@postpartum.net

Psych Central
55 Pleasant Street, Suite 207
Newburyport, MA 01950
Phone: 978-992-0008
Website: www.psychcentral.com
E-mail:
talkback@psychcentral.com

Psychology Today
115 East 23rd Street, 9th Floor
New York, NY 10010
Toll-Free: 888-875-3570
Phone: 212-260-7210
Website:
www.psychologytoday.com

Royal College of Psychiatrists
17 Belgrave Square
London SW1X 8PG
Phone: 020 7235 2351
Fax: 020 7245 1231
Website: mentalhealthuk.org

Schizophrenic.com
Website: www.schizophrenic.com
E-mail: info@schizophrenic.com

Social Phobia/Social Anxiety Association
Website: www.socialphobia.org

Substance Abuse and Mental Health Services Administration (SAMHSA)
1 Choke Cherry Road
Rockville, MD 20857
Toll-Free: 877-SAMHSA-7
(877-726-4727)
Fax: 240-221-4295
Website:
mentalhealth.samhsa.gov
Mental Health Services Locator:
mentalhealth.samhsa.gov/
databases

Suicide Awareness Voices of Education (SAVE)
8120 Penn Avenue South
Suite 470
Bloomington, MN 55431
Phone: 952-946-7998
Website: www.save.org

Suicide Prevention Resource Center (SPRC)
Education Development
Center, Inc.
43 Foundry Avenue
Waltham, MA 02453-8313
Toll-Free: 877-GET-SPRC
(877-438-7772)
TTY: 617-964-5448
Fax: 617-969-9186
Website: www.sprc.org
E-mail: info@sprc.org

Index

Index

Page numbers followed by 'n' indicate a footnote. Page numbers in *italics* indicate a table or illustration.

agoraphobia, described 189
agranulocytosis, clozapine 213, 309
Ahmed, Mansoor 41n
AIDS Alliance for Children,
  Youth and Families, hotline 656
Alaska Natives
  mental health 531
  suicide-related behaviors 113
alcohol abuse
  depression 116
  men 444–45
  trauma 520
Alcohol and Drug Helpline 656
alcoholism
  bipolar disorder 420
  described 250–51
"Alcoholism, Substance Abuse,
  and Addictive Behavior"
  (Office on Women's Health) 250n
alprazolam
  age approval 328, 331
  anxiety disorders 318
alternative therapies see
  complementary and alternative
  medicine
Alzheimer disease
  described 492–93
  overview 494–500
Alzheimer's Association, contact
  information 659
"Alzheimer's Disease Fact Sheet"
  (NIA) 494n
American Academy of Child and
  Adolescent Psychiatry, contact
  information 659
American Academy of Family
  Physicians (AAFP),
  emotional health publication 24n
American Academy of Pediatrics
  (AAP), contact information 512–13
American Art Therapy Association,
  contact information 659
American Association for Geriatric
  Psychiatry, contact information 659
American Association for Marriage
  and Family Therapy, contact
  information 660
American Association of Suicidology,
  contact information 660

American Counseling Association,
  contact information 660
American Diabetes Association,
  depression publication 585n
American Foundation for Suicide
  Prevention
  contact information 515, 660
  hotline 656
American Indians
  mental health 531
  suicide-related behaviors 113
American Psychiatric Association,
  contact information 660
American Psychological
  Association (APA)
  contact information 512, 660
  publications
    anger management 73n
    immigrants, mental health
      needs 532n
    pet ownership 90n
    sexual orientation 502n
American Psychotherapy Association,
  contact information 660
amino acids, described 358–59
amitriptyline, age approval 326, 330
amoxapine, age approval 326, 330
amphetamine,
  age approval 328, 332, *405*
amygdala
  defined 647
  described 7–8
Anafranil (clomipramine)
  age approval 326, 330
  anxiety disorders 318
anger, trauma 520
anger management,
  overview 73–80
animal-assisted therapy,
  described 303
anorexia nervosa, overview 236–39
anterior cingulate cortex (ACC)
  defined 647
  described 8
anti-anxiety medications
  anxiety disorders 318, 487
  listed 327–28, 331–32
antibiotic medications,
  streptococcal infections 439–40

Individualized Education Program
(IEP), learning disabilities 433
Individuals with Disabilities
Education Act (IDEA)
autism spectrum disorders 415
learning disabilities 433
individual therapy, children 386
infections
clozapine 213, 309
PANDAS 435–40
see also HIV infection
information processing
disorders, described 432
insomnia
acupuncture 368
depression 632–36
described 637
mood disorders 44–45
International Foundation
for Research and Education
on Depression, contact
information 662
International OCD Foundation,
contact information 663
International Society
for the Study of Trauma
and Dissociation, contact
information 663
International Society
for Traumatic Stress Studies,
contact information 663
interpersonal support,
chronic back pain 624–25
interpersonal synchrony, autism
spectrum disorders 414
interpersonal therapy (IPT)
bipolar disorder 162
described 120
epilepsy 594
overview 299–300
Intuniv (guanfacine),
age approval 328, 332
Invega (paliperidone)
age approval 325, 329
schizophrenia 214, 309
IPT *see* interpersonal therapy
isocarboxazid
age approval 326, 330
anxiety disorders 318

K

kava, described 352
Kemp, Gina 81n
ketogenic diet, described 38
Klietman, Nathaniel 42
Klonopin (clonazepam)
age approval 327, 331
anxiety disorders 318
Kristin Brooks Hope Center
contact information 663
hotline 656
kudzu, described 364–65

L

Lamictal (lamotrigine)
age approval 327, 331
bipolar disorder 158, 315
cyclothymic disorder 168
lamotrigine
age approval 327, 331
bipolar disorder 158, 315
cyclothymic disorder 168
side effects 316
Lane, Cheryl 220n
L-Arginine, described 358–59
Latinos, children of
immigrants 538–40
lavender, described 357
"Learning Disabilities"
(NICHD) 431n
learning disabilities,
overview 431–33
lemon balm, described 356–57
lesbian orientation,
described 502–3
Lexapro (escitalopram)
age approval 326, 330
anxiety disorders 317
depression 134, 311
dysthymia 141
"LGBT Depression Factsheet"
(Mautner Project:
The National Lesbian
Health Organization) 513n
LGBT persons
depression 513–15
discrimination
overview 502–13

prefrontal cortex (PFC)
  defined 652
  described 8
pregnancy
  antidepressant
    medications 459–60, 463–65
  bipolar disorder medications 162
  depression 461–65
  psychiatric medications 322–24
prejudice, LGBT persons 504–5
premenstrual dysphoric
  disorder (PMDD)
  depression 457
  described 455
premenstrual syndrome
  (PMS), overview 452–54
"Premenstrual Syndrome
  (PMS) Fact Sheet" (Office
  on Women's Health) 452n
presynaptic neurons
  brain function 10–11
  defined 652
Pristiq (desvenlafaxine),
  age approval 326, 330
problem gambling,
  overview 269–72
problem solving,
  anger management 77
Prolixin (fluphenazine),
  schizophrenia 213
propranolol,
  anxiety disorders 318
proteins, described 35
protriptyline, age approval 327, 331
Prozac (fluoxetine)
  anxiety disorders 317
  autism spectrum disorders 416
  bipolar disorder 159, 315
  bulimia nervosa 240
  depression 134, 311
  dysthymia 141
Psych Central
  contact information 667
  impulse control disorders
    publication 256n
psychiatric medications,
  described 307
psychiatric/mental health nurse,
  described 295

psychiatrists
  children 385
  defined 653
  described 294
psychiatry, defined 653
psychoanalytic therapy, children 386
psychodynamic psychotherapy,
  dysthymia 141
psychodynamic therapy,
  described 302
psychoeducation,
  bipolar disorder 162
"Psychological Factors
  of Chronic Back Pain"
  (Cleveland Clinic) 621n
psychological first aid,
  disaster survivors 523–24
Psychological First Aid Field
  Operations Guide (PFA) 525
psychological stress, cancer 568–69
"Psychological Stress
  and Cancer: Questions
  and Answers" (NCI) 568n
psychologists
  children 385
  defined 653
  described 294
"Psychology of Immigration 101"
  (APA) 532n
Psychology Today,
  contact information 667
psychosis
  defined 653
  herbal remedies 363–64
  overview 206–8
"Psychosis" (A.D.A.M., Inc.) 206n
psychosocial therapies
  children 390
  schizophrenia 215–16
psychotherapeutic medications,
  described 307
"Psychotherapies" (NIMH) 296n
psychotherapy
  anxiety disorders 488
  attention deficit hyperactivity
    disorder 407
  bipolar disorder 162–63
  borderline personality
    disorder 226–27